ADVANCES IN LIPID RESEARCH

Volume 10

Advances in Lipid Research

Volume 10

Edited by

Rodolfo Paoletti

Institute of Pharmacology
Milan, Italy

David Kritchevsky

The Wistar Institute
Philadelphia, Pennsylvania

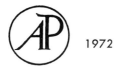 1972

ACADEMIC PRESS • New York and London

ACADEMIC PRESS, INC.
111 Fifth Avenue, New York, New York 10003

United Kingdom Edition published by
ACADEMIC PRESS, INC. (LONDON) LTD.
24/28 Oval Road, London NW1

LIBRARY OF CONGRESS CATALOG CARD NUMBER: 63-22330

PRINTED IN THE UNITED STATES OF AMERICA

CONTENTS

Application of Electron Microscopy to the Study of Plasma Lipoprotein Structure

Trudy Forte and Alex V. Nichols

Employment of Lipids in the Measurement and Modification of Cellular, Humoral, and Immune Responses

Nicholas R. Di Luzio

Microsomal Enzymes of Sterol Biosynthesis

James L. Gaylor

Brain Lipids

Robert B. Ramsey and Harold J. Nicholas

Enzymatic Systems That Synthesize and Degrade Glycerolipids Possessing Ether Bonds

Fred Snyder

Lipids in the Nervous System of Different Species as a Function of Age: Brain, Spinal Cord, Peripheral Nerve, Purified Whole Cell Preparations, and Subcellular Particulates: Regulatory Mechanisms and Membrane Structure

George Rouser, Gene Kritchevsky, Akira Yamamoto, and Claude F. Baxter

LIST OF CONTRIBUTORS

Numbers in parentheses indicate the pages on which the authors' contributions begin.

CLAUDE F. BAXTER, *Neurochemistry Laboratories, Veterans Administration Hospital, Sepulveda, California* (261)

NICHOLAS R. DI LUZIO, *Department of Physiology, Tulane University School of Medicine, New Orleans, Louisiana* (43)

TRUDY FORTE, *Donner Laboratory, Lawrence Berkeley Laboratory, University of California, Berkeley, California* (1)

JAMES L. GAYLOR, *Section of Biochemistry and Molecular Biology and the Graduate School of Nutrition, Cornell University, Ithaca, New York* (89)

GENE KRITCHEVSKY, *Division of Neurosciences, City of Hope National Medical Center, Duarte, California* (261)

HAROLD J. NICHOLAS, *Institute of Medical Education and Research and Department of Biochemistry, St. Louis University School of Medicine, St. Louis, Missouri* (143)

ALEX V. NICHOLS, *Donner Laboratory, Lawrence Berkeley Laboratory, University of California, Berkeley, California* (1)

ROBERT B. RAMSEY, *Institute of Medical Education and Research and Department of Biochemistry, St. Louis University School of Medicine, St. Louis, Missouri* (143)

GEORGE ROUSER, *Division of Neurosciences, City of Hope National Medical Center, Duarte, California* (261)

FRED SNYDER, *Medical Division, Oak Ridge Associated Universities, Oak Ridge, Tennessee* (233)

AKIRA YAMAMOTO, *Second Department of Internal Medicine, Osaka University Medical School, Osaka, Japan* (261)

PREFACE

This volume of *Advances in Lipid Research* is devoted to several special areas of lipid research which are becoming important; new frontiers of established areas of interest are also treated.

The first chapter discusses the application of electron microscopic techniques to the analysis of plasma lipoproteins, an entirely novel way of studying lipoprotein structure. The second article provides a new look at a topic that has piqued scientific interest for a long time—possible modification of reticuloendothelial function by lipids. Present awareness of the role played by lipids in membrane structure and function introduces new aspects to this field. The role of lipids in cellular, humoral, and immune responses is discussed in the second chapter. The third contribution summarizes current knowledge of the microsomal enzymes of sterol biosynthesis. With the extension of studies of lipid synthesis to tissue culture and with new methods of separation and identification of sterols, this paper should be useful to workers in a number of areas. The fifth chapter provides the latest information on one aspect (enzymatic synthesis and degradation) of glycerol lipids which contain ether bonds. This type of lipid has been found in an increasing number of tissues and cells, and its metabolic role is only now being delineated. Brain and nervous tissue research continues to expand with work covering normal development as well as genetic defects. Two chapters explore lipid neurochemistry in depth: the fourth chapter covers brain lipids (fatty acids, phospholipids, sphingolipids, galactosyl lipids, and sterols), whereas the sixth chapter is somewhat broader in scope and discusses lipids of the entire nervous system and their variation with age. Both articles contribute greatly to the knowledge of lipid neurochemistry.

RODOLFO PAOLETTI
DAVID KRITCHEVSKY

CONTENTS OF PREVIOUS VOLUMES

Application of Electron Microscopy to the Study of Plasma Lipoprotein Structure[1]

TRUDY FORTE AND ALEX V. NICHOLS

*Donner Laboratory, Lawrence Berkeley Laboratory,
University of California, Berkeley, California*

I. Introduction

A. DEFINITION OF LIPOPROTEINS

Plasma lipoproteins are macromolecules composed of proteins and lipids. They perform the important function of transporting complex lipids (triglycerides, phospholipids, unesterified cholesterol, and cholesteryl esters) in the plasma. The transported lipids are biologically important in the energy metabolism of tissues and in the structure of cell membranes.

The physical, chemical, and immunological properties of the various lipoprotein classes and their proteins (apolipoproteins) have received much attention in the past few years and several reviews have recently been published (Fredrickson *et al.*, 1967; Schumaker and Adams, 1969;

[1] This work was supported by Research Grants HE 12710-02 and HE 10878-05 from the National Heart and Lung Institute, U. S. Public Health Service, Bethesda, Maryland, and by the U. S. Atomic Energy Commission.

1

Zilversmit, 1969; Margolis, 1969; Scanu, 1965, 1969; Nichols, 1969). At this time, however, there is no comprehensive survey of available data on the microscopical visualization of plasma lipoproteins. Investigation of the various classes of plasma lipoproteins with the electron microscope has proceeded rapidly in the past few years, and in the present review we will examine the contribution of diverse electron microscopical approaches to our understanding of their morphology.

B. Scope of This Review

The present review will focus on the morphological properties of lipoproteins as shown by various electron microscopic techniques including fixation and shadowing, fixation and sectioning, freeze-etching, and negative staining. The main emphasis will be on the isolated lipoprotein fractions since such fractions are physically and chemically well defined. The lipoprotein fractions discussed are mainly those from human plasma; however, where it pertains, the review will consider plasma lipoproteins from other mammalian species. Since lipoproteins isolated from plasma and serum appear to be identical in their chemical and physical properties, the terms "plasma" and "serum" will be used interchangeably.

The aim of this review is twofold: (1) to point out the capabilities as well as the limitations of the various electron microscopic techniques in the analysis of lipoprotein structure, and (2) to stimulate further studies on morphological aspects of lipid-protein interactions in plasma lipoproteins as well as in model systems containing specific lipids and proteins.

II. Physical and Chemical Characterization of Plasma Lipoproteins

Based on many studies, four major classes of human plasma lipoproteins have been characterized by preparative and analytical ultracentrifugation and by electrophoresis. These classes are chylomicrons, very low density lipoproteins (VLDL), low density lipoproteins (LDL), and high density lipoproteins (HDL). Each of these classes can, furthermore, be ultracentrifugally fractionated into subclasses on the basis of their density. According to their electrophoretic migration on paper, the HDL are designated α-lipoproteins, LDL are designated β-lipoproteins, and VLDL are designated pre-β-lipoproteins. The chylomicrons do not migrate in the electrical field and remain at the origin.

The operational classification and compositional properties of the major classes of plasma lipoproteins are summarized in Table I.

Table I: Classification and Properties of the Major Classes of Plasma Lipoproteins

	Chylomicrons	Very low density lipoproteins (VLDL)	Low density lipoproteins (LDL)	High density lipoproteins (HDL)
Preparative ultracentrifugal density classification[a]	d < 0.95 gm/ml	d 0.95–1.006 gm/ml	d 1.006–1.063 gm/ml	d 1.063–1.21 gm/ml
Analytic ultracentrifugal flotation rate classification[b]	$S_f > 400$	S_f 20–400	S_f 0–20	$F_{1.20}$ 0–9
Paper electrophoretic migration classification	Chylomicrons	pre-β	β	α
Average composition[c]				
Phospholipid	7	19	22	24
Unesterified cholesterol	2	7	8	2
Cholesteryl esters	5	13	37	20
Triglyceride	84	51	11	4
Protein	2	8	21	50
Major protein (apolipoprotein) constituents[d]	Probably include: apoLP-ser apoLP-glu apoLP-ala₁ apoLP-ala₂	apoLDL apoLP-ser apoLP-glu apoLP-ala₁ apoLP-ala₂	apoLDL	apoLP-glnI[e] apoLP-glnII[f]

[a] d. values designate density ranges of the lipoprotein classes as isolated from plasma by sequential preparative ultracentrifugation.

[b] S_f values are ultracentrifugal flotation rates expressed as Svedbergs (10^{-13} cm/sec/dyne/gm) in a solution of density 1.063 gm/ml at 26°C (1.748 molal NaCl). $F_{1.20}$ values are flotation rates expressed in Svedbergs in a solution of density 1.20 gm/ml (Ewing *et al.*, 1965).

[c] Major compositional constituents are listed; where available, content of nonesterified fatty acids was included in compositional computation but not listed in table (Hatch and Lees, 1968; Oncley and Harvie, 1969).

[d] Protein constituents termed apolipoproteins (apoLP) are designated by their carboxyl terminal amino acids, abbreviated as follows: ala (alanine), gln (glutamine), glu (glutamic), ser (serine) (Fredrickson, 1969; Gotto *et al.*, 1971; Nichols *et al.*, 1972; Levy *et al.*, 1971; Eisenberg *et al.*, 1972).

[e] Corresponds to ApoA-I of Kostner and Alaupovic (1971); R-thr of Shore and Shore (1969); Fraction III of Scanu *et al.* (1969); and Band C of Rudman *et al.* (1970).

[f] Corresponds to ApoA-II of Kostner and Alaupovic (1971); R-gln of Shore and Shore (1969); Fraction IV of Scanu *et al.* (1969); and Band D of Rudman *et al.* (1970).

III. Various Techniques of Electron Microscopy Applied to Investigation of Liproprotein Structure

Before the initial visualization of plasma lipoproteins by electron microscopy, the sizes and possible shapes of these macromolecules were usually derived by indirect methods. The large chylomicrons, however, were detected in the conventional light microscope using dark field optics and by this method were described and named by Gage and Fish (1924). The sizes and shapes of the smaller lipoproteins (LDL and HDL) were estimated by other physical techniques. Using light-scattering measurements Bjorklund and Katz (1956) described human LDL as prolate ellipsoids, 342 by 152 Å. The size and shape of human HDL were estimated by Oncley *et al.* (1947) and these authors suggested a prolate ellipsoidal shape (300 by 50 Å) for the HDL. Lindgren and Nichols (1960) from ultracentrifugal data, assuming spherical structures for both LDL and HDL, calculated diameters of 200 Å and 78–100 Å, respectively, for these lipoproteins. Visualization of lipoproteins by electron microscopy made possible direct appraisal of their apparent sizes and shapes. The various preparative techniques used in the electron microscopy of lipoproteins together with an evaluation of their general usefulness and limitations will be discussed in the next several sections.

A. FIXATION AND SHADOW-CASTING TECHNIQUE

Application of fixation and shadow-casting for visualization of all classes of human plasma lipoproteins by electron microscopy was first carried out by Hayes and Hewitt (1957). By fixing isolated lipoproteins in buffered osmium tetroxide and then spreading and shadowing them prior to electron microscopy, they were able to determine the size and shape of the larger particles, especially those of density < 1.006 gm/ml. These larger particles appeared spherical with diameters ranging from 320 to 800 Å. The LDL after similar treatment also appeared spherical with an average diameter of 350 Å. Hayes *et al.* (1959) later used fixed and carbon-coated LDL particles for the determination of the molecular weight of these macromolecules. The calculated molecular weight value (6.0×10^6) was approximately twice the expected value from ultracentrifugal data. The authors proposed that, under the conditions of fixation, predominantly dimers of LDL had probably been formed.

According to the results of Hayes and Hewitt (1957), HDL molecules seen after fixation and shadowing were spherical with an average diameter of 150 Å. The calculated molecular weight of HDL based on this diameter was too large to be consistent with ultracentrifugal data.

The pioneering work of Hayes and Hewitt (1957) clearly pointed out the possibility of viewing plasma lipoproteins with the electron microscope. Their results also demonstrated that the use of a single electron microscopic technique (fixation with shadowing) was not adequate for definitive visualization of all classes of lipoproteins. Fixation with osmium tetroxide and shadowing worked extremely well with particles of densities < 1.006 gm/ml, i.e., the chylomicrons and VLDL, but apparently yielded data at variance with those from other physical approaches for both LDL and HDL.

1. Usefulness of Fixation and Shadow-Casting Technique

The technique of fixing and shadowing lipoproteins has been extremely useful for investigating the size distribution of chylomicrons and VLDL in conjunction with ultracentrifugal, electrophoretic, and chemical studies. Accordingly, Hayes *et al.* (1966) and Bierman *et al.* (1966) were able to demonstrate that human $S_f > 400$ subfractions containing species designated as "primary" and "secondary" particles, which have different migration rates under starch block electrophoresis, had essentially the same size distribution when visualized in the electron microscope. Similar procedures were also used by Fraser *et al.* (1968) and Lossow *et al.* (1969) to identify the size ranges of ultracentrifugally isolated VLDL and chylomicron subfractions. Fraser *et al.* (1968) were able to show the influence of time of sampling and type of diet on the size distribution of rat lymph chylomicrons from micrographs such as those in Fig. 1. The chemical compositions of the various chyle lipoprotein species were also quantified, and together with information on their volume and surface area obtained by electron microscopy, Fraser and his co-workers proposed that the chylomicron surface consists of a mixed monolayer of phospholipids, protein, and free cholesterol. A similar approach was used by Lossow *et al.* (1969) to determine the particle size and to estimate the protein coverage of several human plasma lipoprotein fractions of $S_f > 20$. Using an estimated value of 20 Å for the thickness of the VLDL protein and phospholipid surface layer, these authors calculated that the proportion of the surface covered by protein is fairly constant for lipoproteins of $S_f > 50$ (approximately 20% coverage); between S_f 20–50 the estimated protein coverage approaches 30%.

Fraser (1970) has reported that various chylomicron fractions, isolated by preparative ultracentrifugation from thoracic lymph of rabbits show an overlap in size distribution. In particular, the $S_f > 10,000$ fraction appeared to have many small particles present which may reflect incomplete fractionation or adsorption of small particles to larger ones during isolation. Electron microscopic examination of shadowed preparations

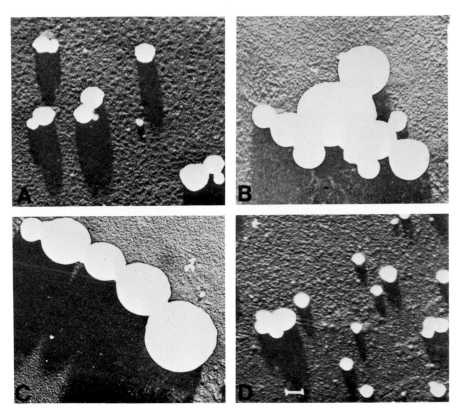

FIG. 1. Electron micrograph of fixed and shadowed rat lymph chylomicrons ($S_f > 400$). Chyle samples were taken at various time intervals after corn oil ingestion and show a significant change in size with time: (A) 0–½ hour; (B) 2–4 hours; (C) 4–6 hours; (D) 9–10 hours. Bar marker denotes 1,000 Å. Magnifications of all micrographs are approximately 30,000 ×. (Micrographs courtesy of Dr. Robin Fraser.)

can, therefore, be valuable in assessing purity of fractions isolated by ultracentrifugal, as well as other biophysical techniques.

Jones and Price (1968) demonstrated that fixation and shadow-casting are useful in the study of particle size distributions in human hyperlipemic plasma. They have shown that samples of whole plasma, after appropriate dilution, can be fixed with osmium tetroxide, shadowed, and examined within 30 minutes. The resulting micrographs give ready information on the size distribution of the lipoproteins. An example of their technique is seen in Fig. 2 which shows particles ranging in size from 500 to 5,000 Å; the pebbly background probably reflects the presence of plasma proteins and higher density plasma lipoproteins. These authors

Fig. 2. Electron micrograph of a fixed and shadowed preparation of whole plasma from a hyperlipemic patient. A wide range of particle size is evident. Bar marker represents 1,000 Å. Magnification: approximately 40,000 ×. (Micrograph courtesy of Dr. Albert Jones.)

propose that because of its rapidity and reliability this method may serve as a valuable tool in diagnosing various hyperlipidemias.

2. Limitations of Fixation and Shadow-Casting Technique

A major disadvantage of this technique is the inability to visualize the smaller lipoproteins (i.e., LDL and HDL). Although large lipoproteins are easily visualized, accumulation of the shadowing metal on small species makes size determinations inaccurate as was demonstrated in the work of Hayes and Hewitt (1957). In a critique of shadowing, Misra and Das Gupta (1965) have also shown that the size and shape of particles, such as monodisperse polystyrene latex, are distorted by the deposition of metal vapor and that this distortion is greatest with smaller particles.

Added to this, there is also a small error which can result from the uptake of osmium tetroxide by the lipids. Hayes *et al.* (1963) have shown that lipoprotein lipids take up 1 to 2 atoms of osmium per double bond. On this basis, Bierman *et al.* (1966) calculated an increase of approximately 5% in the apparent size of human lipoproteins of the S_f 20–400 class after osmication.

The technique of osmication and shadow-casting also has limitations in visualizing particles rich in saturated lipids. Several research groups have reported their lack of success in visualization of particles of density < 1.006 gm/ml which were obtained during studies employing saturated fat diets (Hayes et al., 1966; Bierman et al., 1966; Fraser, 1970; Ockner and Jones, 1970).

B. Fixation and Embedding Technique

Embedding and sectioning techniques have been extensively used to localize lipoprotein structures within cell organelles of intestinal and liver cells. To a lesser extent these techniques have also been applied to purified lipoproteins.

Kay and Robinson (1962) showed the presence of a discontinuous electron dense surface layer in fixed and embedded chylomicrons obtained from the thoracic duct of the rat. They suggested that this layer was composed of phospholipids and protein. More recent studies of Jones and Price (1968), Salpeter and Zilversmit (1968), and Schoefl (1968) indicate that the morphology observed by the above workers is apparently a general characteristic of sectioned chylomicrons. The micrograph in Fig. 3 of fixed and sectioned chylomicrons from rat lymph shows the essential features of these large particulate lipoproteins. The particles are spherical and when sectioned in the equatorial plane often appear to be bounded by a dense surface layer 50 to 100 Å wide. The general morphology and thickness of this outer layer have been shown by Schoefl (1968) to depend on such factors as lipid composition, buffer used in fixation, and the presence of additional protein. According to Schoefl, chylomicrons containing more saturated lipids appear to have a thinner surface layer. When plasma or albumin was introduced into the chylomicron sample before fixation, Schoefl found that the outer surface often contained dense thickened regions. These osmiophilic foci may represent protein adsorbed onto the surface. Investigation of the morphology of chylomicrons was noted by Schoefl to be further complicated by the nature of the buffer used during fixation. Chylomicrons fixed in veronal acetate buffer showed a smooth surface whereas those fixed in phosphate buffer had a granular surface structure.

Our own studies with fixed and sectioned human chylomicrons indicate that pH and buffer, as well as temperature during fixation, significantly influence the apparent morphological features of fixed chylomicrons. The series of micrographs in Fig. 4 present data from a study of

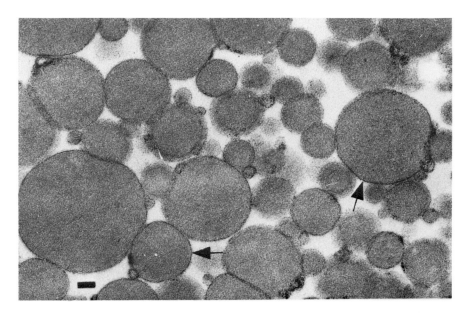

Fig. 3. Electron micrograph of fixed and sectioned rat chylomicrons. The interiors of the particles are electron dense and homogeneous. Sectioned in the equatorial plane, some of the particles appear to be bounded by a thin dense surface layer (arrows). Bar marker indicates 1,000 Å. Magnification: approximately 45,000 ×. (Micrograph courtesy of Dr. Albert Jones.)

a chylomicron sample fixed under various conditions. When fixed at 37°C in unbuffered osmium tetroxide the particles have no obvious surface layer; a few dense osmiophilic clumps are seen but these represent reduced masses of osmium not associated with the lipoprotein structures. When fixed in phosphate buffer at 37°C the particles show a definite surface layer and occasional eccentric osmiophilic foci; the surface layer has a granular appearance similar to that described by Schoefl (1968). A sample fixed in sodium cacodylate at 37°C was intermediate in its surface structure between the unbuffered and phosphate buffered samples; that is, dense eccentric osmiophilic foci are frequently seen but there appears to be no definite surface layer. Interestingly, at 4°C this latter buffer system gives a completely different picture; the particles at times appear angular and, occasionally, trilaminar structures (50 Å to 80 Å in width) similar to unit membranes can be seen. These results together with those of Schoefl demonstrate the significant influence of different preparative procedures and conditions on final electron microscopical data.

Zilversmit (1965) after freeze-thawing dog lymph chylomicrons was able to isolate a fraction rich in phospholipid and protein which he pro-

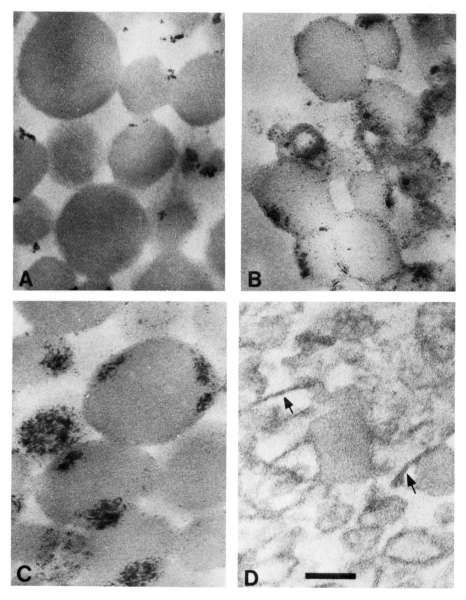

FIG. 4. Electron micrographs of a specimen of human chylomicrons fixed under varying conditions of temperature and buffer. All samples were fixed in a final concentration of 1% OsO₄ for 24 hours. (A) Unbuffered OsO₄, 37°C; (B) OsO₄ in phosphate buffer, pH 7.4, 37°C; (C) OsO₄ in sodium cacodylate buffer, pH 7.4, 37°C; (D) OsO₄ in sodium cacodylate buffer, pH 7.4, 4°C. In (D), trilaminar structures can occasionally be seen (arrows). Bar marker represents 1,000 Å. Approximate magnification of all micrographs: 130,000 ×.

posed may represent the surface layer material of chylomicrons. Electron microscopy revealed the presence of electron dense loops which were devoid of any trilaminar structure typical of biological membranes. After further studies on dog lymph chylomicrons degraded by dehydration at various temperatures, Zilversmit (1968) was able to show that the composition of the isolated surface material varies with the temperature maintained during degradation. The percentage of triglycerides in the surface material isolated after freeze-thawing was far greater than that in material isolated at 25° and 37°C. The amount of cholesterol in the surface material was greater when chylomicrons were degraded at lower temperatures. The percentage of phospholipids in the surface material obtained at 37°C was greater than that obtained at lower temperatures. It is apparent, therefore, that structures seen in fixed and sectioned material may reflect a peculiar lipid distribution which can result from the method of handling of the preparation.

1. Usefulness of the Fixation and Embedding Technique

At this stage of our knowledge, electron microscopy of fixed and embedded material can be very useful for general comparative purposes. Schoefl (1968) has noted that storage of chylomicrons produces definite structural changes. Coalescence of lipoproteins and the inclusion of small dense particles within the larger ones can be seen.

Micrographs of fixed and embedded fractions of chylomicrons and VLDL can be employed to give a gross indication of their relative content of unsaturated lipid. Schoefl (1968) has shown that chylomicrons occasionally display differential osmiophilia; smaller particles especially are more electron dense than larger ones. Although the underlying bases for the difference in osmiophilia are still obscure, it could result from a differential distribution of unsaturated and saturated triglycerides among subfractions of the chylomicrons and VLDL. Recent work of Ockner *et al.* (1969) indicates that there is indeed a differential distribution of unsaturated and saturated triglyceride fatty acids among rat chylomicrons and VLDL.

2. Limitations of Fixation and Embedding Technique

In reviewing the work on sectioned preparations it becomes quite clear that thus far there has been no comprehensive study on the effects of temperature, time, and buffer systems in procedures used during fixing and sectioning of chylomicrons or VLDL. Such a study is certainly needed for appropriate interpretation and comparison of the fine structure of these lipoproteins. In addition to difficulties encountered in interpreting the structures observed in the electron microscope, there is incomplete understanding of the precise staining properties of osmium

tetroxide in lipid-protein systems. The topic of osmium tetroxide staining, especially of lipids, has recently been reviewed by Adams (1969).

Besides the occurrence of fixation and dehydration artifacts, visualization of the smaller lipoproteins in embedded preparations is extremely
difficult if not impossible. In our laboratory we have attempted to section pelleted human LDL but because of the thickness of the plastic
section (approximately 600 Å) together with the granularity of the reduced osmium the results were uninterpretable. As would be expected,
the difficulties which beset the investigator in applying fixation and
shadowing to the study of chylomicrons and VLDL rich in saturated
lipids also are present when fixation and embedding are applied to the
same materials.

3. *Histological Localization of Lipoproteins*

Fixation and embedding techniques, often in conjunction with radio-
autography, have been useful in demonstrating sites of synthesis and
secretion of lipoproteins in cells and tissues. The literature in this field
is extensive and not within the scope of the present review. For more
information on electron microscopical studies on the formation of lipoproteins in intestinal cells the readers are directed to the works of Ashworth and Johnston (1963), Strauss (1966), McKay *et al.* (1967a,b,c).
Synthesis, storage, and transport of lipoproteins in the animal liver are
well documented in the works of Jones *et al.* (1967), Hamilton *et al.*
(1967), and Stein and Stein (1967). Chylomicrons in the vascular system of liver, mammary gland, and lung of various animals have been
described by French (1963), and Schoefl and French (1968).

Electron microscopy of lipoproteins in cells and tissues suffers from the
same disadvantages as those encountered during microscopy of isolated
lipoprotein fractions; the most pronounced being inability to visualize
the smaller lipoprotein structures and poor fixation of lipoproteins with
high content of saturated lipids. Notwithstanding these difficulties, this
technique offers valuable information on the localization of sites of
cellular production and metabolism of chylomicrons and VLDL.

C. Freeze-Fracturing and Etching Technique

The freeze-fracturing technique developed by Moor *et al.* (1961) has
been successfully applied to various types of biological specimens, and
its applicability has been reviewed by Moor (1966) and Koehler (1968).
The technique is of special value since it does not involve chemical fixation and dehydration. It is considered by Moor and Mühlethaler (1963)
to have an ultimate resolving power of 20–30 Å. The technique involves

several steps (Fig. 5) including rapid freezing, fracturing of the specimen in a vacuum, etching of the fractured surface, replication of the specimen surface, and cleaning of the replica. The fracture plane in the case of lipid bilayers (Deamer and Branton, 1967) and biological membranes (Branton, 1969) appears to be through the hydrophobic regions of these structures. This has been clearly demonstrated for cell membranes by Pinto da Silva and Branton (1970) and Tillack and Marchesi (1970). Both groups of investigators found that membranes were split along their central hydrophobic regions and thus the inner aspects of the membrane faces were displayed.

Freeze-etching can be successfully applied to the study of serum lipoproteins as shown in Fig. 6. This micrograph was taken of human lipoproteins of densities < 1.006 gm/ml and was printed so that the replica shadows appear as light regions. The smaller particles are globular while larger ones are sometimes less regular in shape with some appearing rather elongated. The surfaces of the particles are very slightly granular.

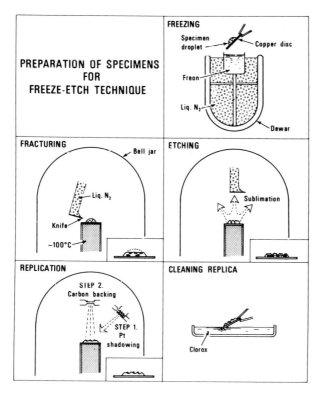

FIG. 5. Principal steps in freeze-etching technique.

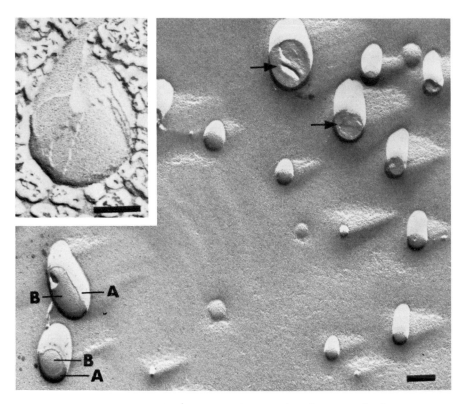

Fig. 6.   Freeze-etched chylomicrons. The particles shown in the larger micrograph are round-to-oblong in shape and their outer surfaces are fairly smooth. Fractured particles appear to have two distinct fracture faces, labeled A and B. Face A presumably corresponds to an outer surface layer while face B corresponds to the hydrophobic core material. Transversely fractured particles (arrows) show a homogeneous core. Specimen was prepared in distilled water. Bar marker represents 1,000 Å; magnification, 73,000 ×. Inset shows an unusual chylomicron particle with several onion-skin-like layers near the surface (specimen prepared in 25% glycerol). Magnification: 120,000 ×.

Occasionally two faces, labeled A and B in the figure, are seen; face A is probably the outer surface layer while face B may represent the inner lipid core. This interpretation assumes that, as in membranes, the cleavage plane follows along a hydrophobic region in proximity to the surface layer. Since there is no available evidence for the presence of a bilayer structure at the surface of these lipoproteins, the above cleavage plane might represent a region between surface phospholipids and interior triglycerides. The fractured and etched lipoprotein particles typically appear bounded by a single layer; infrequently they show several onion-skin-like layers (inset Fig. 6). The significance of the latter observation is still unclear. More typically, the core regions of the chylomicrons and VLDL, as viewed after cross fracturing, are very homogeneous and thus are comparable in appearance to fixed and sectioned material. Although it is tempting to suggest that the surface layer seen in some fractured particles may consist of a protein-phospholipid-cholesterol layer, direct evidence for such an assumption is still unavailable. Our freeze-fracture studies on stabilized commercial emulsions of unsaturated (Lipomul, The Upjohn Co., Kalamazoo, Mich.) or saturated (Lipostrate-CB, Calbiochem, Los Angeles, Calif.) triglycerides also show the appearance of two fracture faces similar to those of chylomicrons and VLDL. The triglyceride interior in both emulsions is homogeneous, indicating that the core lipids apparently have no discernible organization.

The combination of freeze-fracturing and etching provides a possible preparative method for electron microscopy of lipoproteins rich in saturated fats, thus avoiding the difficulties described in Sections III,A,2 and III,B,1. By deep-etching a specimen, it is possible to obtain size distributions of such lipoproteins. Fraser (personal communication) used this technique in an effort to characterize chylomicrons from rabbits fed butter fat and found large areas of clumped particles which did not show fracture faces and tended to be flattened, probably as a result of crowding. It is our experience that the best results are obtained by using lipoprotein concentrations calculated to allow a spacing between particles equivalent to one or two times their estimated diameter.

D. NEGATIVE STAINING TECHNIQUE

The technique of negative staining has been applied to the study of a wide variety of biological materials including bacteria, viruses, subcellular particles, proteins, and lipid dispersions (Glauert, 1965; Horne, 1965). The technique is especially useful in examining details of macromolecular structures and thus lends itself to the study of lipoproteins. Visualization of structures by this method is achieved by mixing a solution of particles with an equal volume of negative stain reagent and either applying the solution to a Formvar/carbon coated grid in droplet form or spraying it onto the grid with an atomizer. Use of fenestrated carbon films often improves contrast and resolution since particles are viewed in the stain matrix over the holes. However, these films are very fragile and subject to stretching. The stretching may distort structures trapped within the fenestrated film. The best method for applying the specimen is usually ascertained by trial and error. The use of a volatile buffer such as ammonium acetate–ammonium carbonate (Forte *et al.*,

1968), is advisable in order to avoid formation of additional salt crystals on the grid. A study of the effects of negative staining on lipoproteins by Gong *et al.* (1970) showed that upon dehydration of serum lipoproteins in sodium phosphotungstate and subsequent rehydration there was some loss of material but a considerable fraction of the lipoprotein was recovered which had normal ultracentrifugal properties. Dehydration and rehydration of the lipoproteins in the absence of phosphotungstate resulted in extensive and in certain cases almost complete degradation of the initial structures. These results supported the concept of Van Bruggen *et al.* (1962) that negatively stained molecules are trapped in a virtually frozen state.

Adequate visualization of macromolecular structures using negative staining depends on several preparative factors including stain, particle concentration, and pH. Stain concentration relative to particle concentration is critical since low concentrations show incomplete penetration by the stain while high concentrations conceal particle structure. For visualization of lipoprotein structures we have found that a final concentration of 100–250 μg lipoproteins/ml in 1% phosphotungstate gives satisfactory results.

The choice of stain and its pH also influences the visualization of macromolecular structures. The anionic phosphotungstate salts are generally used for visualizing molecules carrying a negative charge thus minimizing the problem of positive staining effects. Uranyl salts which have a low pH value and positive charge cause precipitation of both HDL and LDL.

1. *Usefulness and Limitations of Negative Staining When Applied to Lipoproteins*

Visualization of lipoproteins by negative staining has proved to be valuable since this technique fulfills several essential requirements. The method, as described earlier in this section, is very simple and specimens can be examined within minutes after preparation. Under the same conditions of preparation the method gives good reproducibility and is therefore a useful tool for comparative studies. Most important, negative staining allows visualization of the smaller, more dense lipoproteins, LDL and HDL, where other techniques such as fixation with shadowing or sectioning are inadequate.

Since extremely small samples of lipoproteins may be analyzed by negative staining, this technique lends itself to the characterization of lipoprotein samples which cannot be examined by more conventional physical and chemical means. This is especially true in some cases of lipoprotein deficiencies where it is often difficult if not impossible to obtain sufficient sample for analysis by other procedures.

The applicability of negative staining to visualizing lipoproteins is limited primarily to particles of smaller dimension than VLDL. LDL and HDL lend themselves readily to this technique while larger lipoproteins such as chylomicrons and VLDL with diameters greater than 400 Å are not adequately preserved (Forte *et al.*, 1967, 1968). These latter lipo-proteins appear to flatten and become distorted upon drying in the stain.

Perhaps the major limitation in the negative staining procedure is the inability to control the dispersion of sample material during drying. Surface tension effects may cause undesirable aggregation and may also on occasion cause distortion of particle shapes.

2. *Visualization of Lipoproteins in Whole Plasma*

The various classes of lipoproteins in unfractionated plasma can be visualized using negative staining. Normal plasma is diluted 15- to 20-fold before examination in order to dilute the plasma proteins which would otherwise tend to obscure the lipoprotein particles. A negatively stained preparation of diluted normal plasma is seen in Fig. 7. The three major classes of lipoproteins (VLDL, LDL, and HDL) can be readily distinguished; the granular background is attributed to the plasma proteins. Under the same conditions, plasma from a patient deficient in

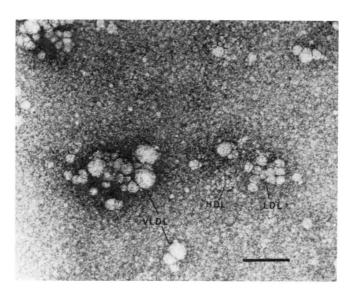

Fig. 7. Electron micrograph of negatively stained plasma. The three classes of lipoproteins can be seen: very low density (VLDL), low density (LDL), and high density (HDL) lipoproteins. Bar marker indicates 1,000 Å. Magnification: appproximately 120,000 ×.

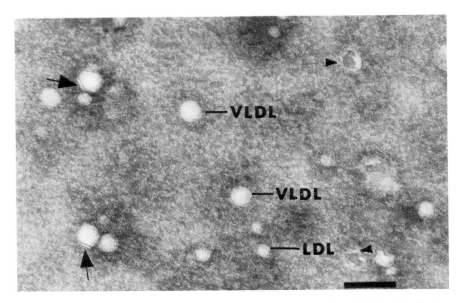

Fig. 8. Negatively stained plasma from a patient with familial lecithin:choles-terol:acyltransferase deficiency. VLDL and LDL are present but there are no recognizable HDL. Rod- or disclike structures (large arrows) primarily associated with the VLDL are found; other undefined structures are occasionally observed (small arrows). Bar marker indicates 1,000 Å. Magnification: 136,000 ×.

lecithin:cholesterol acyltransferase (LCAT) apparently lacks normal-appearing HDL particles although LDL and VLDL are recognizable (Fig. 8). The latter plasma, however, contains rod- or disclike particles not seen in normal plasma. The electron microscopical information is consistent with physical and chemical data (Norum and Gjone, 1967; Glomset *et al.*, 1970) on the plasma lipoprotein distributions observed in this disease.

Electron microscopy of whole plasma using negative staining could be a useful tool to the researcher requiring a rapid means for determining gross abnormalities in lipoprotein distribution in certain metabolic diseases. It has limitations, however, because of the presence of a relatively large amount of other protein material in the sample.

3. Structure of Isolated Lipoproteins

The various classes of lipoproteins isolated from normal plasma by preparative ultracentrifugation show a characteristic size and shape upon electron microscopy with negative staining. Furthermore, the packing of the particles upon drying in the stain matrix is very distinct for each class of lipoproteins. The size and shape as well as the packing configuration of lipoproteins from subjects in certain disease states is often completely abnormal.

    a. Normal Human HDL Structure. Free-standing, negatively stained HDL appear as particles with somewhat circular profiles which occasionally contain a dense central region (Forte *et al.*, 1967, 1968; Hamilton, 1969). On closer inspection it appears that particles in this class of lipoproteins are composed of several subunits. Figure 9 exhibits various particle structures observed during microscopy of the major subfractions of the HDL: HDL$_2$ (density 1.07–1.12 gm/ml) and HDL$_3$ (density 1.12–1.21 gm/ml). HDL$_2$ are, on the average, 95–100 Å in diameter while HDL$_3$ are 70–75 Å in diameter. The estimated diameter of the subunits is 40–50 Å for HDL$_2$ and 35–40 Å for HDL$_3$. Occasionally, structures consisting of a pair of elongated subunits can also be seen; in the HDL$_2$ fraction each elongated subunit is approximately 40–50 Å in width and 80–100 Å in length. Similar subunits in HDL$_3$ fractions are somewhat smaller; 35–40 Å in their short axis and 70–75 Å in their long axis. A diagrammatic representation of apparent HDL structure is summarized in Fig. 10. The projected side view gives two possible representations of substructure based on the various types of images seen in the micrographs. While at present it is difficult to choose unequivocally between the two representations, it should be noted that globular substructures are more frequently evident than the elongated ones.

    HDL particles, when concentrated on a grid during drying, typically form arrays displaying hexagonal packing as seen in Fig. 11. The hexagonal packing arrangement is attributable to the very uniform diameters of the particles; the center-to-center distance between particles in an HDL$_3$ preparation is 75 Å while that of HDL$_2$ is 100 Å. Determination of particle spacing and geometry of packing may be a useful means of identifying the various HDL subfractions.

    b. HDL Isolated from Other Animals. Thus far there is very little information on the morphology of HDL from other animals. As one might expect, the rat, which is a commonly used laboratory animal, has been studied in more detail than other animals. Hamilton (1969) found that the HDL fraction (density 1.06–1.21 gm/ml) of the rat consisted of particles ranging from 90 to 150 Å in diameter and appeared to be composed of several subunits. Camejo (1969) also found a very broad range of particle size for rat HDL. The observation that the HDL particles of the rat are somewhat larger than those of humans is supported by the analytical ultracentrifuge studies of Puppione (1969) and Koga *et al.* (1969).

    Other mammals which have been studied include seal, cow (Puppione *et al.*, 1970), and killer whale (Puppione *et al.*, 1971). Figure 12 shows

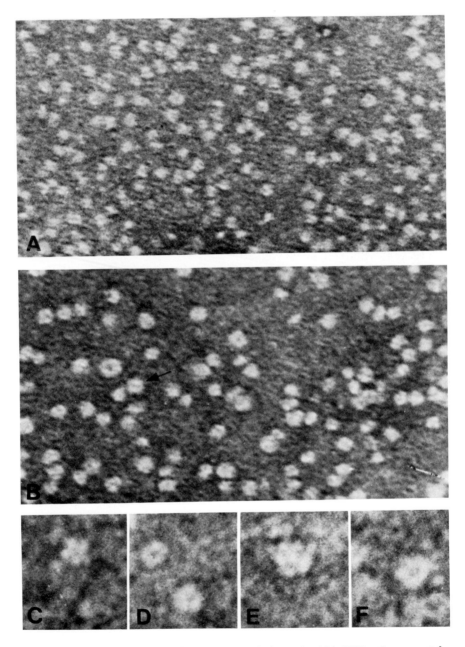

Fig. 9.   Negatively stained human HDL; (A) HDL₃, (B) HDL₂. Some particles appear to be made up of several subunits and in a few instances have a dense central region. An occasional particle (arrow) appears to have elongated subunits.

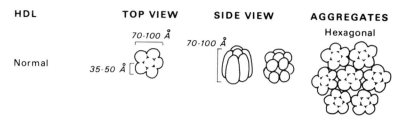

FIG. 10. Schematic representation of possible structure of HDL.

the overall structure of particles from these animals. Like human HDL, the particles pack in a hexagonal array upon drying; they also appear to be composed of several subunits. One of the particles in Fig. 12C appears to be tilted and shows subunits which may be elongated. The HDL macromolecules from all three of these mammals are somewhat larger than those of humans. Seal and cow HDL are 140 and 150 Å respectively in diameter, while whale HDL range from 70 to 130 Å. These size distributions are consistent with the higher flotation rates of these lipoproteins (Puppione *et al.*, 1970, 1971).

In a recent communication, Sardet *et al.* (1972) have described the morphology of guinea pig HDL. HDL from normal guinea pigs, although extremely low in concentration, contain both large spherical

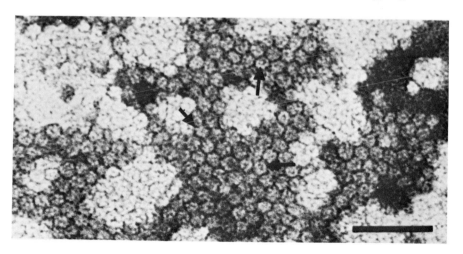

FIG. 11. Normal human HDL aggregated in a hexagonal array upon drying in sodium phosphotungstate. Arrows indicate particles which have apparent subunit structure. Bar marker represents 500 Å. Approximate magnification: 420,000 ×.

FIG. 9 (*continued*). Magnification: approximately 400,000 ×. (C) through (F) show highly enlarged HDL particles which appear to be composed of several globular subunits. Magnification: approximately 1,000,000 ×.

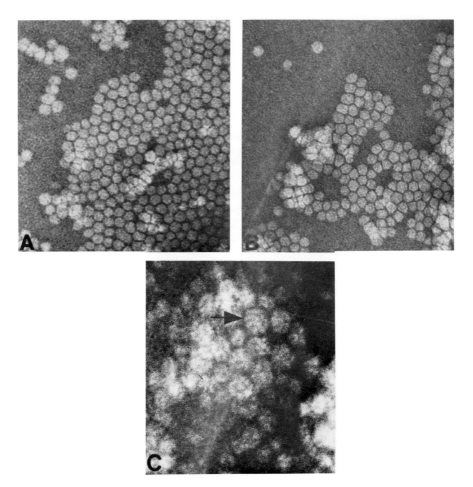

Fig. 12. Negatively stained HDL from other animals; (A) cow, (B) seal, (C) killer whale. Like human HDL these particles also aggregate in a hexagonal array and appear to have a subunit structure. One of the killer whale HDL particles is tilted and shows apparently elongated substructures (arrow). (A) and (B) magnification: 211,000 ×. (C) Approximate magnification: 494,000 ×.

particles 215 Å in diameter and small spherical particles approximately 97 Å in diameter. A striking change in HDL concentration, composition, and morphology occurs in response to dietary cholesterol. Cholesterol feeding produces a marked increase in the unesterified cholesterol to protein ratio. Negatively stained HDL preparations revealed the presence of disclike particles 250 Å in diameter which formed rouleaux with a very regular periodicity of approximately 68 Å. These disclike particles are reminiscent of the structures seen in the HDL fraction from lecithin:

cholesterol acyltransferase (LCAT) deficient patients [see Section f(1)]. Since the HDL from LCAT deficient human plasma and the cholesterol-fed guinea pigs are both extremely rich in unesterified cholesterol and both possess morphologically similar structures, the guinea pig could serve as a useful model to study aspects of the molecular basis of LCAT deficiency.

Preliminary work in this laboratory with amphibia (frog) serum indicates that, although present in extremely small quantities, the HDL particles of these animals are similar to human HDL$_2$. The HDL fraction from sardine plasma has also been examined and was found to be composed of particles which were generally equivalent to human HDL$_3$.

c. Normal Human LDL. Lipoproteins of density 1.006–1.063 gm/ml when viewed after negative staining are almost spherical (Forte *et al.,* 1967, 1968; Gotto *et al.,* 1968) and quite uniform in size; 80% of the particles are between 210 and 250 Å in diameter (Forte *et al.,* 1971a). Figure 13 is a representative micrograph showing both free-standing and packed particles. The particles are apparently highly deformable since they become flattened at their edges when apposed to each other. As a result of such deformation, the LDL particles do not show the regular packing noted in the HDL fraction. Apposed LDL structures occasionally appear to be linked together by minute strands, and in some instances (arrows in Fig. 13A) several particles are linked together in the form of a chain.

Figures 13B through E show the morphology of the LDL at high magnification; in all cases the macromolecules show fine structural detail at their surfaces. Some particles (B and E) viewed from the top clearly show edges with fine serrations, while others (C and D), which represent tilted particles, appear to show a fine structure consisting of a strandlike network on the surface of the particle. One of the images (13D) shows a girdling structure around its equator. Pollard *et al.* (1969) obtained very different micrographs after using essentially the same negative staining technique. Electron microscopy of LDL by these authors resulted in the images shown in Fig. 13F. The LDL in this micrograph are very irregular in shape and variable in size. The broad range in apparent size suggests that some of the particles may be partially buried in and obscured by the stain.

Figure 14 is a diagrammatic sketch of the top and side views of the LDL image as observed in our micrographs. The morphology suggested in Fig. 14 would account for the somewhat angular outlines of some of the free-standing particles. On the basis of their electron microscopical studies, Pollard *et al.* (1969) proposed that LDL images do show substructural detail which may consist of globular protein units, approximately 50 Å in diameter, arranged in a dodecahedral pattern with an

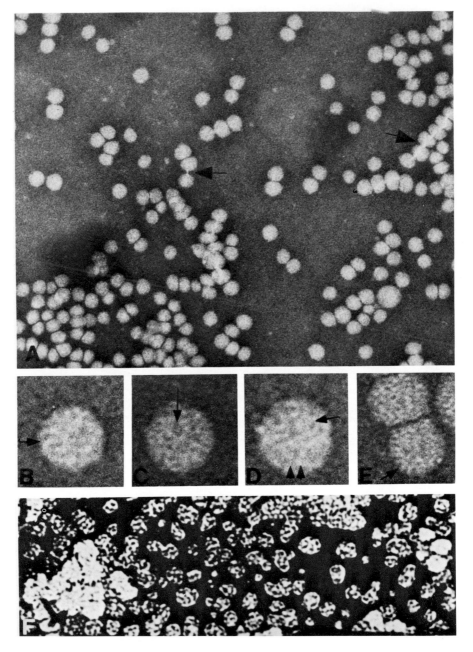

FIG. 13. Negatively stained normal human LDL. (A) Low magnification field showing both single and contiguous particles. Apposed particles often become flattened on the adjacent surfaces and occasionally appear to be fused or bridged

TOP VIEW   SIDE VIEW

Fig. 14.   Diagrammatic representation of top and side view of human LDL.

overall icosohedral symmetry for the particles (Fig. 13F). In their LDL model the pentagonal faces circumscribed by the protein would be occupied primarily by phospholipid.

Our unpublished observations (Fig. 15A through D) on degradation products formed during ether extraction of LDL (a procedure which removes most apolar and some polar lipids) suggest that the organization of protein and phospholipid moieties of the LDL may include strandlike substructures, possibly forming a surface network. In Fig. 15E some low density particles in a negatively stained preparation appear to be undergoing marked organizational changes. These changes occurred in a single isolated case and probably reflect degradation of the LDL particle due to local drying forces. It is interesting, however, that in this instance strandlike structures again appear in association with disruption of LDL surface. The ultimate resolution of the structure of LDL, in particular the possible organization of subunits or surface substructure, requires further work including investigation of products formed during reassembly of LDL apoprotein with various lipid components.

d. LDL from Other Animals. Hamilton (1969) has characterized the size and shape of rat LDL and has found them to be very similar to those of humans. LDL from whale serum have also been examined (Puppione *et al.*, 1971) and in all respects appear identical in structure to human LDL. Recently Sardet *et al.* (1972) have described LDL from normal guinea pigs; these lipoproteins, as well, closely resemble those from human plasma. Following dietary cholesterol the LDL fraction

by strandlike structures (arrows). Magnification: 212,000 ×. Micrographs (B) through (E) are highly enlarged LDL showing surface details; (B) and (E) probably represent particles seen in top view. The edges of these particles are serrated (arrows); (C) and (D) represent tilted particles which show fine structural surface detail (top centers of particles are indicated by single arrows). The image in (D) suggests that there may be a girdling substructure in the equatorial region (double arrows). Micrographs (B) through (E) are all magnified 705,000 ×. (F) A micrograph, kindly supplied by Dr. Harvey Pollard, shows the structure of negatively stained human LDL particles as prepared by the procedure of Pollard *et al.* (1969). Lipoproteins were suspended in potassium phosphotungstate and were spread on fenestrated films. Magnification: approximately 260,000 ×.

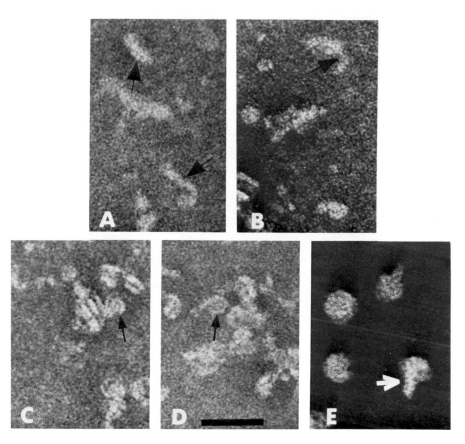

FIG. 15. (A) through (D) represent images of negatively stained structures appearing after ether extraction of human LDL. Strandlike structures are frequently seen (large arrows) and occasionally structures are present which suggest a complex network (small arrows). (E) Represents LDL which have undergone surface alterations presumably as a result of local drying conditions in the sodium phosphotungstate. On one of the particles (arrow) a strandlike structure appears to be protruding from the surface. This protruding structure is somewhat similar to the strands seen in (A) through (D). Bar marker representing 500 Å is applicable to all the micrographs. Approximate magnification: 323,000 ×.

became morphologically very heterogeneous. Besides normal appearing LDL particles, large vesicular structures 800–1100 Å in diameter were also in evidence. These latter particles resemble the large particles seen in LDL fractions from LCAT deficient plasma [Section f(1)] and those found in cases of biliary obstruction [Section f(4)].

   e. *Structure of Normal Human VLDL.* This class of lipoproteins, when visualized by negative staining, has a very broad range of particle size (300–900 Å). Like the LDL, the particles are greatly distorted when packed together during drying (Fig. 16). Smaller free-standing particles appear to be spherical; however, the larger particles often are irregular in shape due to distortion during drying. The VLDL show no obvious fine structural detail as may be seen in the higher magnification inset in Fig. 16. These particles (inset) often appear to have electron-transparent centers with a grayish halo around their periphery; the latter phenomenon is presumably due to flattening or spreading of the edges of these particles in the negative stain. Measurement of particle size from micrographs of this class of lipoproteins would probably tend to yield artifactually large values because of flattening. An alternative method for investigating VLDL structure is positive staining with osmium tetroxide

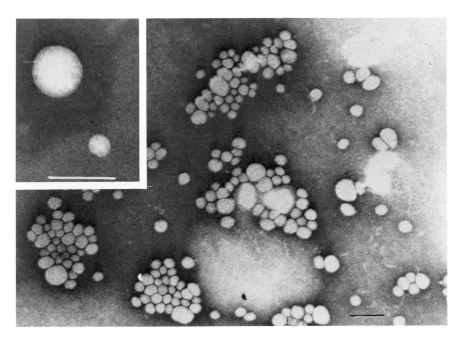

FIG. 16. Negatively stained human VLDL. Free-standing particles appear spherical; however, particles are greatly distorted in shape when aggregated. The inset shows particles at higher magnification; the edges of the large particles often appear grayish while the centers are electron transparent. These images may be the result of a flattening of the particles and a spreading of their edges in the negative stain. Bar markers represent 1,000 Å. Magnification of large micrograph is 93,000 ×. Inset magnification: 189,000 ×.

and direct examination in the microscope. This technique (Jones and Price, 1968) reduces flattening of the large particles, provided they are adequately fixed.

f. Structure of Lipoproteins in Pathological Conditions. (1) Familial lecithin:cholesterol acyltransferase deficiency. The plasma lipoproteins from patients with lecithin:cholesterol acyltransferase (LCAT) deficiency show gross abnormalities in their chemical and physical properties (Norum and Gjone, 1967; Hamnstrom *et al.*, 1969; Glomset *et al.*, 1970). Both the HDL and LDL fractions have elevated contents of unesterified cholesterol and phosphatidylcholine, while the cholesteryl ester content is abnormally low. Moreover, the total HDL concentration in the plasma of most of these patients is low.

Electron microscopic studies have shown that the morphology of certain classes of plasma lipoproteins in this disease is also abnormal (Forte *et al.*, 1971a). The HDL fraction isolated from LCAT-deficient plasma contains particles which, during drying in PTA, form stacks as shown in Fig. 17. Individual particles appear to be disclike structures; the majority show diameters between 150 and 200 Å. The discs are of uniform thickness and have a regular periodicity of 50–55 Å when stacked.

Recent studies in our laboratory on sonified mixtures of specific lipids plus HDL apoproteins indicate that the anomalous discoidal shape of

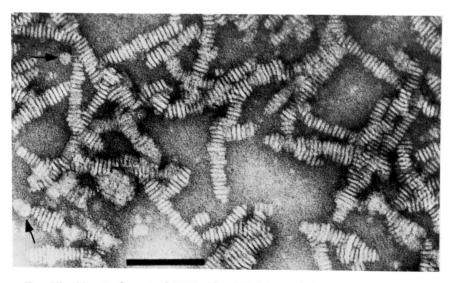

Fig. 17. Negatively stained HDL (d 1.063–1.21 gm/ml fraction) from a patient with lecithin:cholesterol acyltransferase deficiency. Particles aggregate in stacks with a 50–55 Å periodicity. The particles are disclike and profiles of free-standing particles are indicated by arrows. Bar represents 1,000 Å. Magnification: 212,000 ×.

the HDL particles from LCAT-deficient subjects may be due to their abnormal lipid composition (Forte and Nichols, 1971; Forte *et al.*, 1971b). Following sonification of mixtures of HDL apoLP-glnI (see Table I) and lecithin, the predominant structures observed were discoidal particles 100–200 Å in diameter which aggregated in stacks with a 50–55 Å periodicity (Fig. 18A). Similar structures were obtained when HDL apoLP-glnII replaced apoLP-glnI or when unesterified cholesterol was added to the mixtures (Fig. 18B). The very regular 50–55 Å repeat distance of the discoidal particles may be attributed to some bimolecular arrangement of the phospholipids stabilized by protein. Unesterified cholesterol

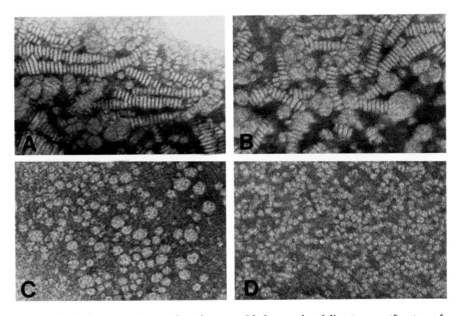

FIG. 18. Electron micrographs of reassembled particles following sonification of HDL apoproteins with various lipids. (A) ApoLP-glnI-lecithin mixture. Predominant structures are disclike particles which stack in aggregates with a 50–55 Å periodicity. (B) ApoLP-glnI-lecithin-unesterified cholesterol mixture (lecithin to cholesterol molar ratio of 1:1) again shows predominantly disclike particles. (C) ApoLP-glnI-apoLP-glnII-lecithin-unesterified cholesterol-cholesteryl ester mixture (apoLP-glnI: apoLP-glnII weight ratio was 3:1). Particles do not form stacked aggregates and appear more nearly spherical; some particles appear similar to native HDL. Particle size distribution is heterogeneous but many particles are in the range of normal HDL. (D) ApoLP-glnI-lecithin-unesterified cholesterol mixture incubated with normal d > 1.21 gm/ml ultracentrifugal protein fraction, containing lecithin:cholesterol acyltransferase. Disclike structures in d 1.063–1.21 gm/ml fraction of the sonified mixture have been transformed to small, approximately spherical, particles 50–100 Å in diameter. Magnification: (A), (B), and (D), 212,000 ×; (C), 189,000 ×.

probably inserts between the acyl chains of the phospholipids. The discoidal structures seen in these sonified preparations closely resembled those observed in the HDL fraction from LCAT-deficient plasma. The structural conformation of the sonification products was completely altered when cholesteryl esters were sonified with the apolipoprotein-lecithin-unesterified cholesterol mixtures. With the inclusion of cholesteryl ester, the reassembled particles assumed more spherical shapes (Fig. 18C) with the majority of particle diameters between 80 and 100 Å; thus they approximated normal HDL in overall structure. We also found that the discoidal particles formed by sonification of apolipoprotein-lecithin-unesterified cholesterol mixtures could be transformed into small (50–100 Å) spherical particles (Fig. 18D) upon incubation with a density > 1.21 gm/ml ultracentrifugal serum protein fraction which contains LCAT activity. When LCAT-deficient plasma was incubated with the density > 1.21 gm/ml ultracentrifugal protein fraction, the HDL underwent transformation from discs to apparently normal structures. From these studies it would appear that cholesteryl esters may play an essential role in determining the final conformation of the normal HDL macromolecule.

Although disc-shaped particles predominate in the total HDL fraction from LCAT-deficient plasma, other smaller structures are also present in this density class. Norum et al. (1971) have isolated by gel filtration a small molecular weight species which corresponds to these smaller particles. Electron microscopy (Forte et al., 1971a) of the isolated small molecular weight subfraction showed the presence of particles 45–100 Å in diameter. Some of these particles (70–100 Å) were very similar to normal HDL while those smaller than 70 Å have not been previously seen in normal serum by electron microscopy. The small molecular weight fraction serves as an effective substrate for LCAT and Glomset et al. (1970) suggest that this fraction may be a "precursor" in the formation of HDL. Previous studies of Glomset et al. (1966) showed that a small molecular weight component can be isolated from normal human and baboon HDL by gel filtration. This component appears to be present in plasma in extremely low concentrations. Since this component may play a role in HDL metabolism it warrants further investigation into its chemical, physical, and structural properties.

The LDL from plasma of patients with LCAT deficiency are abnormal in their phospholipid and unesterified cholesterol content; the content of cholesteryl esters is extremely low (Glomset et al., 1970). The density 1.019–1.063 gm/ml fraction when examined with the electron microscope consisted of at least two populations of particles as is evident in Fig. 19. The smaller particles are similar in size (210–250 Å) and shape to normal LDL. This observation is of particular interest in light of the fact

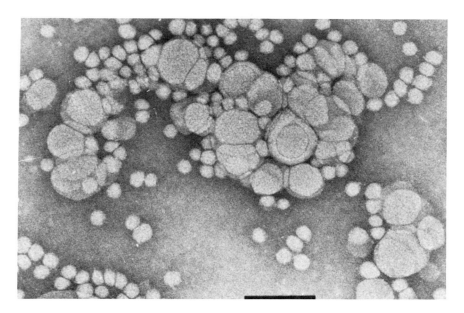

FIG. 19. Negatively stained LDL fraction (d 1.019–1.063 gm/ml fraction) isolated from plasma of a patient with lecithin:cholesterol acyltransferase deficiency. This lipoprotein fraction is characterized by the presence of small normal-appearing LDL particles as well as numerous large particles. Bar represents 1,000 Å. Magnification: 187,000 ×.

that the relative contents of phosphatidylcholine, unesterified cholesterol, and triglyceride in the fraction are disproportionately high compared to normal LDL. Unlike the HDL, however, there appears to be no drastic structural abnormality in these particles as a consequence of their lipid composition.

The larger particles in the LDL fraction from LCAT-deficient plasma are mostly between 500 and 1200 Å in size. In the electron microscope these particles appear to be rather transparent flat structures. Additional definition of these large LDL particles will require further studies utilizing such techniques as fixation and sectioning or freeze-fracturing. The large LDL components can be isolated by gel filtration, and data on their composition suggest that they are composed almost exclusively of phospholipid and unesterified cholesterol, with approximately 5% of their mass being attributable to protein (Norum *et al.*, 1971). The significance of this subfraction is yet to be established. Since similar large particles have been noted in the LDL fraction from patients with obstructive jaundice (Hamilton *et al.*, 1971), further investigation of their origin and fate would be extremely valuable.

(2) *Tangier disease.* This is a rare disease characterized by the near absence of high density lipoproteins. Plasma from patients is further characterized by reduced unesterified cholesterol and phospholipid concentrations together with elevated triglyceride concentrations (Fredrickson, 1966). Routine analytic ultracentrifugation of plasma from homozygous subjects does not detect lipoproteins of density > 1.063 gm/ml; the same is true of paper electrophoresis (Fredrickson *et al.*, 1968). However, after appropriate concentration of plasma from homozygous individuals, α-lipoproteins can be detected immunochemically (Fredrickson, 1966; Levy and Fredrickson, 1966). Tangier α-lipoproteins are immunochemically similar but not identical to normal α-lipoproteins. This lack of complete identity extends to the delipidated HDL products as well. It is possible that an abnormal apolipoprotein is present in this disease (Levy and Fredrickson, 1966).

The morphology of the ultracentrifugal HDL fraction from the plasma of homozygous Tangier patients is quite unique under electron microscopy. The structures encountered in this fraction are presented in Fig. 20. Two distinct populations of particles are immediately apparent; one consisting of relatively large, round structures 150–210 Å in diameter

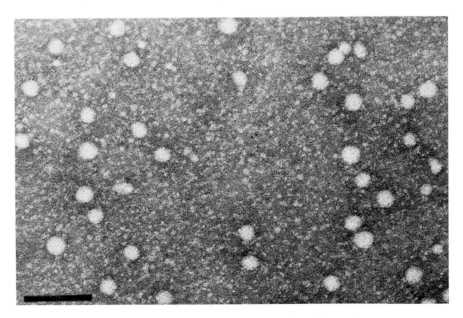

FIG. 20. Negatively stained HDL fraction from the plasma of a patient homozygous for Tangier disease. Two populations of particles are evident: large particles which may represent the Lp antigen, and small ones which are considerably smaller than normal HDL. Bar represents 850 Å. Magnification: 211,000 ×.

and the other consisting of extremely small particles less than 50 Å in size. The shape of the latter particles is difficult to define since their size approaches the limits of resolution for the negative staining technique. The larger particles may represent the Lp antigen or "sinking" pre-β subfraction (electrophoretic) described by Rider *et al.* (1970). The density (d 1.05–1.08 gm/ml), of this "sinking" pre-β component suggests that one might well expect to find it in the ultracentrifugally isolated HDL fraction.

(3) *Abetalipoproteinemia.* Individuals with the rare syndrome abetalipoproteinemia are remarkable in that they exhibit the lowest concentration of plasma lipids yet detected (Levy *et al.*, 1966; Jones and Ways, 1967). This disease is characterized by a complete absence of the β-lipoprotein band on paper electrophoresis. After appropriate concentration of the plasma, Levy *et al.* (1966) were able to demonstrate some material of d < 1.063 gm/ml which reacted immunochemically as α-lipoproteins. The amino acid composition of this lipoprotein was also found to be indistinguishable from that of HDL. Routine analytic ultracentrifugation of abetalipoproteinemia plasma (Fredrickson *et al.*, 1968) shows the presence of HDL consisting in major part of species within the $F_{1.20}$ 3.5–9.0 flotation interval.

By preparative ultracentrifugation of plasma from two subjects with abetalipoproteinemia we have been able to isolate two lipoprotein fractions containing particles demonstrable by electron microscopy. These were the d 1.006–1.063 gm/ml and d 1.063–1.21 gm/ml fractions; no material was observed in the d < 1.006 gm/ml fraction. Lipoproteins in the d 1.006–1.063 gm/ml fraction are unique in their shape and packing arrangement as shown in Fig. 21. The particles tend to aggregate in stacks not unlike those seen in the HDL fraction of LCAT-deficient patients. However, the particles are distinct in that they have an 80–90 Å periodicity (50–55 Å for LCAT deficiency) and the length of the individual rectangular-shaped units in the stack is 100–200 Å (150–200 Å for LCAT deficiency). Occasionally the particles pack in a cubelike arrangement (Fig. 21A), a feature thus far only observed in this fraction from subjects with abetalipoproteinemia. Many of the free-standing particles in Fig. 21A and B appear to have circular profiles suggesting that these particles may also be discoidal.

The d 1.063–1.21 gm/ml fraction from abetalipoproteinemia plasma contains normal-appearing HDL particles consistent with the ultracentrifugal data of others (Levy *et al.*, 1966; Fredrickson *et al.*, 1968). The majority of particles in this fraction, which includes both HDL_2 and HDL_3 subfractions, range between 65 and 100 Å.

The structural appearance of particles in the d 1.006–1.063 gm/ml

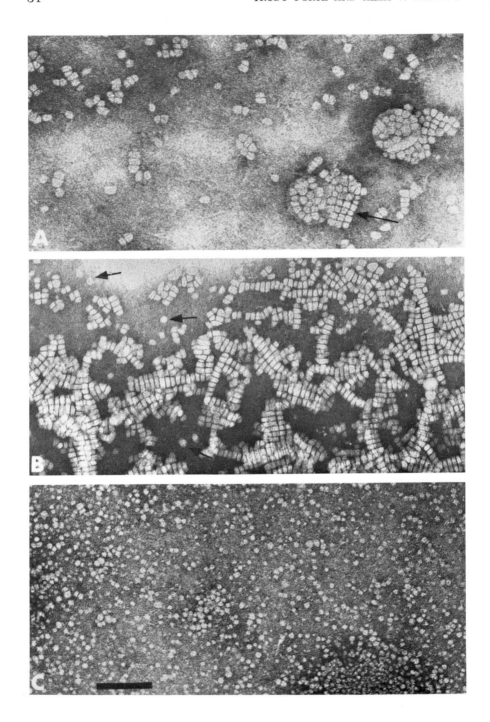

fraction in abetalipoproteinemia is abnormal. The true significance of the morphology of these particles is as yet obscure. Further characterization of the protein defect in abetalipoproteinemia has been recently reported by Gotto *et al.* (1971). Their analysis of the apolipoproteins from lipoproteins of d < 1.21 gm/ml demonstrated the presence of the major and minor apoproteins associated with normal HDL, and the absence of the major apoprotein of LDL. Since electron microscopy showed the presence of particles of d 1.006–1.063 gm/ml whose morphology is distinctly different from normal HDL or LDL, it would be valuable to characterize this fraction further.

(*4*) *Biliary obstruction.* It is well known that liver diseases of the obstructive type are accompanied by changes in the serum lipoprotein ultracentrifugal pattern (McGinley *et al.*, 1952; Eder *et al.*, 1955; Phillips, 1960). These disease states are characterized by elevated serum concentrations of cholesterol (principally unesterified cholesterol) and phospholipid. The flotation pattern of the high density lipoproteins may be highly unusual, displaying large amounts of more rapidly floating material. An LDL subfraction, which is extremely rich in phospholipid and unesterified cholesterol, has also been recently described (Seidel *et al.*, 1969, 1970). This fraction does not react with β-lipoprotein antiserum and has been designated LP-X.

The lipoprotein distribution in liver disease depends on the type of disease as well as on its severity as demonstrated by Papadopoulos and Charles (1970). Electron microscopy of lipoprotein structures in such states should be correlated with other types of chemical and clinical data. We have studied the morphology of serum lipoproteins in two cases of biliary obstruction. The HDL structures in the two subjects were considerably different as noted in Fig. 22. In the first case (Fig. 22A) the HDL appear quite normal and aggregate in a hexagonal arrangement. In the other case (Fig. 22B) hexagonal packing was not seen and particle size was less uniform; in fact, many particles were as large as 150 Å in diameter. Such large particles could account for the observation of HDL species with abnormally fast ultracentrifugal flotation rates noted in some cases of liver disease (unpublished observation).

Fig. 21. Negatively stained lipoproteins from plasma of patients with abetalipoproteinemia. (A) Density 1.006–1.063 gm/ml fraction from patient A.V. shows unusual cubelike packing (arrow) of these low density particles. (B) Density 1.006–1.063 gm/ml fraction from patient R.B. Particles often stack in aggregates having a periodicity of 80–90 Å; free-standing structures have circular profiles (arrows). (C) Density 1.063–1.21 gm/ml fraction from patient R.B. Particles in this fraction are the size and shape of normal HDL. Bar represents 1,000 Å. Magnification: 142,000 ×.

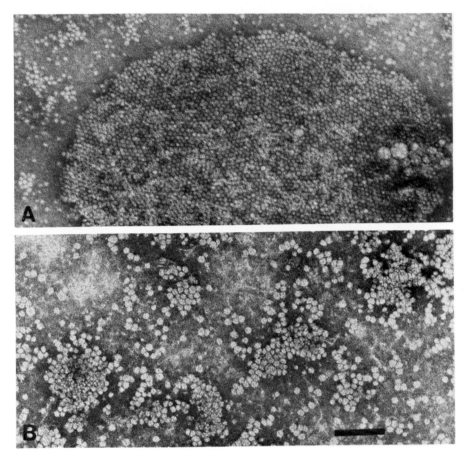

FIG. 22. Negatively stained HDL (d 1.063–1.21 gm/ml fraction) from plasma
of patients with biliary obstruction. (A) and (B) are at the same magnification.
There is a noticeable difference in size distribution of HDL particles in the two
patients. Particles in (A) appear normal and form hexagonal arrays while those in
(B) have a wide range of particle size and do not aggregate in an organized
pattern. Bar represents 1,000 Å. Magnification: 138,000 ×.

The electron microscopic studies of Hamilton *et al.* (1971) on the
structure of LDL from jaundiced patients demonstrated the presence of
two types of particles in this lipoprotein class (Fig. 23). The size and
shape of the small particles correspond closely to those of normal LDL
while the large ones had diameters in the range of 400–600 Å. These
large particles appear to be flat vesicular structures which, upon drying
in the negative stain, form stacks with a periodicity of approximately
100 Å.

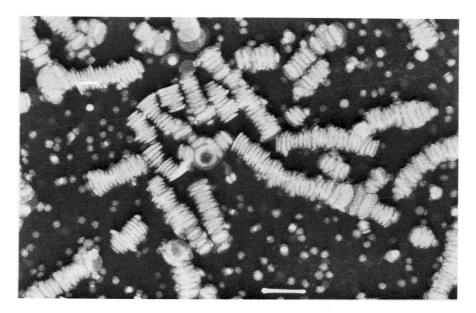

Fig. 23. Negatively stained LDL (d 1.006–1.04 gm/ml fraction) from plasma of a patient with cholestasis. Numerous, large flattened disclike structures which form stacks are characteristic. Small, normal-appearing LDL particles are also evident. Bar represents 1,000 Å. Magnification: approximately 100,000 ×. (Micrograph courtesy of Dr. Robert Hamilton.)

IV. Concluding Remarks

The various techniques of electron microscopy can be exceedingly useful for studying the fine structure of the various serum lipoprotein classes. In this review we have outlined the capabilities of techniques such as fixation and shadow-casting, freeze-etching, and negative staining. The advantages and limitations of the methods in their applicability to studies on lipoproteins have been discussed.

Electron microscopy has proved particularly useful for investigating the structure of lipoproteins in certain disease states. The unusual morphology of lipoprotein particles especially in the case of HDL from LCAT-deficient plasma has led to some basic understanding of the possible fundamental requirements for maintenance of the structure of normal HDL particles. Further, electron microscopical data on such abnormal structures have stimulated research on model systems. Electron microscopy has practical worth in this area since pertinent data can be obtained very rapidly and with extremely small samples of material. One would expect that electron microscopy will continue to provide essential information in the study of abnormal lipoprotein metabolism as well as in the evaluation of modes of interaction between protein and lipid moieties through the use of model systems.

ACKNOWLEDGMENTS

The authors gratefully acknowledge the stimulating collaboration of Dr. J. A. Glomset and Dr. K. R. Norum in the investigation of the lipoprotein abnormalities in lecithin:cholesterol acyltransferase deficiency. We wish to express our gratitude to Dr. Herbert Kayden and Dr. Robert Lees for providing samples of abetalipoproteinemia plasma and to Dr. Robert Levy and Dr. Sam Lux for samples of HDL apolipoproteins and of Tangier disease plasma. We also wish to acknowledge the excellent technical assistance of Cheryl Haden and Elaine Gong.

References

Adams, C. W. M. (1969). *Advan. Lipid Res.* **7**, 1.
Ashworth, C. T., and Johnston, J. M. (1963). *J. Lipid Res.* **4**, 454.
Bierman, E. L., Hayes, T. L., Hawkins, J. N., Ewing, A. M., and Lindgren, F. T. (1966). *J. Lipid Res.* **7**, 65.
Bjorklund, R., and Katz, S. (1956). *J. Amer. Chem. Soc.* **78**, 2122.
Branton, D. (1969). *Annu. Rev. Plant Physiol.* **20**, 209.
Camejo, G. (1969). *Biochim. Biophys. Acta* **175**, 290.
Deamer, D. W., and Branton, D. (1967). *Science* **158**, 655.
Eder, H. A., Russ, E. M., Pritchett, R. A., Wilber, M. M., and Barr, D. P. (1955). *J. Clin. Invest.* **34**, 1147.
Eisenberg, S., Bilheimer, D., Lindgren, F., and Levy, R. I. (1972). *Biochim. Biophys. Acta* **260**, 329.
Ewing, A. M., Freeman, N. K., and Lindgren, F. T. (1965). *Advan. Lipid Res.* **3**, 25.
Forte, G. M., Nichols, A. V., and Glaeser, R. M. (1967). *UCRL Semiannu. Rep.* No. 18066, p. 74, Univ. of California, Berkeley, California.
Forte, G. M., Nichols, A. V., and Glaeser, R. M. (1968). *Chem. Phys. Lipids* **2**, 396.
Forte, T., and Nichols, A. V. (1971). *Abstr. Biophys. Soc. Annu. Meet. 15th New Orleans.*
Forte, T., Norum, K. R., Glomset, J. A., and Nichols, A. V. (1971a). *J. Clin. Invest.* **50**, 1141.
Forte, T., Nichols, A. V., Gong, E. L., Lux, S., and Levy, R. I. (1971b). *Biochim. Biophys. Acta* **248**, 381.
Fraser, R. (1970). *J. Lipid Res.* **11**, 60.
Fraser, R., Cliff, W. J., and Courtice, F. C. (1968). *Quart. J. Exp. Physiol. Cog. Med.* **53**, 390.
Fredrickson, D. S. (1966). *In* "The Metabolic Basis of Inherited Diseases" (J. B.

Stanbury, J. B. Wyngaarden, and D. S. Fredrickson, eds.), pp. 486–508. McGraw-Hill, New York.

Fredrickson, D. S. (1969). *Proc. Nat. Acad. Sci. U. S.* **64**, 1138.

Fredrickson, D. S., Levy, R. I., and Lees, R. S. (1967). *New Engl. J. Med.* **276**, 32.

Fredrickson, D. S., Levy, R. I., and Lindgren, F. T. (1968). *J. Clin. Invest.* **47**, 2446.

French, J. E. (1963). *In* "Biochemical Problems of Lipids" (A. C. Frazer, ed.), pp. 296–303. Elsevier, Amsterdam.

Gage, S. H., and Fish, P. A. (1924). *Amer. J. Anat.* **34**, 1.

Glauert, A. M. (1965). *Lab. Invest.* **14**, Part 2, 331.

Glomset, J. A., Janssen, E. T., Kennedy, R., and Dobbins, J. (1966). *J. Lipid Res.* **7**, 638.

Glomset, J. A., Norum, K. R., and King, W. (1970). *J. Clin. Invest.* **49**, 1827.

Gong, E. C., Forte, G. M., and Nichols, A. V. (1970). *Physiol. Chem. Phys.* **2**, 180.

Gotto, A. M., Levy, R. I., and Fredrickson, D. S. (1968). *Lipids* **3**, 463.

Gotto, A. M., Levy, R. I., John, K., and Fredrickson, D. S. (1971). *New Engl. J. Med.* **284**, 813.

Hamilton, R. L. (1969). *In* "Proceedings of the 1968 Deuel Conference on Lipids" (G. Cowgill, D. L. Estrich, and P. D. Wood, eds.), pp. 3–28. U. S. Govt. Printing Office, Washington, D. C.

Hamilton, R. L., Regen, D. M., Gray, M. E., and LeQuire, V. S. (1967). *Lab. Invest.* **16**, 305.

Hamilton, R. L., Havel, R. J., Kane, J. P., Blaurock, A. E., and Sata, T. (1971). *Science* **172**, 475.

Hamnstrom, B., Gjone, E., and Norum, K. R. (1969). *Brit. Med. J.* **ii**, 283.

Hatch, F. K., and Lees, R. S. (1968). *Advan. Lipid Res.* **6**, 1.

Hayes, T. L., and Hewitt, J. E. (1957). *J. Appl. Physiol.* **11**, 425.

Hayes, T. L., Murchio, J. C., Lindgren, F. T., and Nichols, A. V. (1959). *J. Mol. Biol.* **1**, 297.

Hayes, T. L., Lindgren, F. T., and Gofman, J. W. (1963). *J. Cell Biol.* **19**, 251.

Hayes, T. L., Freeman, N. K., Lindgren, F. T., Nichols, A. V., and Bierman, E. L. (1966). *Protides Biol. Fluids, Proc. Colloq.* **14**, 273.

Horne, R. W. (1965). *Lab. Invest.* **14**, Part 2, 316.

Jones, A. L., and Price, J. M. (1968). *J. Histochem. Cytochem.* **16**, 366.

Jones, A. L., Ruderman, N. B., and Herrera, M. G. (1967). *J. Lipid Res.* **8**, 429.

Jones, J. W., and Ways, P. (1967). *J. Clin. Invest.* **46**, 1151.

Kay, D., and Robinson, D. S. (1962). *Quart. J. Exp. Physiol. Cog. Med.* **47**, 258.

Koehler, J. K. (1968). *Advan. Biol. Med. Phys.* **12**, 1.

Koga, S., Horwitz, D. L., and Scanu, A. M. (1969). *J. Lipid Res.* **10**, 577.

Kostner, G., and Alaupovic, P. (1971). *FEBS Lett.* **15**, 320.

Levy, R. I., and Fredrickson, D. S. (1966). *Circulation* **34**, Suppl. 3, 156. (Abstr.)

Levy, R. I., Fredrickson, D. S., and Laster, L. (1966). *J. Clin. Invest.* **45**, 531.

Levy, R. I., Bilheimer, D. W., and Eisenberg, S. (1971). *In* "Plasma Lipoproteins" (R. M. S. Smellie, ed.), pp. 3–17. Academic Press, New York.

Lindgren, F. T., and Nichols, A. V. (1960). *In* "The Plasma Proteins" (F. W. Putnam, ed.), Vol. 2, pp. 1–58. Academic Press, New York.

Lossow, W. J., Lindgren, F. T., Murchio, J. C., Stevens, G. R., and Jensen, L. C. (1969). *J. Lipid Res.* **10**, 68.

McGinley, J., Jones, H., and Gofman, J. (1952). *J. Invest. Dermatol.* **19**, 71.

McKay, D. G., Kaunitz, H., Csavossy, I., and Johnson, R. E. (1967a). *Metab. Clin. Exp.* **16**, 111.

McKay, D. G., Kaunitz, H., Csavossy, I., and Johnson, R. E. (1967b). *Metab. Clin. Exp.* **16**, 127.

McKay, D. G., Kaunitz, H., Csavossy, I., and Johnson, R. E. (1967c). *Metab. Clin. Exp.* **16**, 137.

Margolis, S. (1969). In "Structural and Functional Aspects of Lipoproteins in Living Systems" (E. Tria and A. M. Scanu, eds.), pp. 369–424. Academic Press, New York.

Misra, D. N., and Das Gupta, N. N. (1965). *J. Roy. Microsc. Soc.* **84**, 373.

Moor, H. (1966). *Int. Rev. Exp. Pathol.* **5**, 179.

Moor, H., and Mühlethaler, K. (1963). *J. Cell Biol.* **17**, 609.

Moor, H., Mühlethaler, K., Waldner, H., and Frey-Wyssling, A. (1961). *J. Biophys. Biochem. Cytol.* **10**, 1.

Nichols, A. V. (1969). *Proc. Nat. Acad. Sci. U. S.* **64**, 1128.

Nichols, A. V., Lux, S., Forte, T., Gong, E., and Levy, R. I. (1972). *Biochim. Biophys. Acta* **270**, 132.

Norum, K. R., and Gjone, E. (1967). *Scand. J. Clin. Lab. Invest.* **20**, 231.

Norum, K. R., Glomset, J. A., Nichols, A. V., and Forte, T. (1971). *J. Clin. Invest.* **50**, 1131.

Ockner, R. K., and Jones, A. L. (1970). *J. Lipid Res.* **11**, 284.

Ockner, R. K., Hughes, F. B., and Isselbacker, K. J. (1969). *J. Clin. Invest.* **48**, 2367.

Oncley, J. L., and Harvie, N. R. (1969). *Proc. Nat. Acad. Sci. U. S.* **64**, 1107.

Oncley, J. L., Scatchard, G., and Brown, A. (1947). *J. Phys. Chem.* **51**, 184.

Papadopoulos, N. M., and Charles, M. A. (1970). *Proc. Soc. Exp. Biol. Med.* **134**, 797.

Phillips, G. B. (1960). *J. Clin. Invest.* **39**, 1639. (Abstr.)

Pinto da Silva, P., and Branton, D. (1970). *J. Cell Biol.* **45**, 598.

Pollard, H., Scanu, A. M., and Taylor, E. W. (1969). *Proc. Nat. Acad. Sci. U. S.* **64**, 304.

Puppione, D. L. (1969). Ph.D. Thesis, UCRL Rep. No. 18821. Univ. of California, Berkeley, California.

Puppione, D. L., Forte, G. M., Nichols, A. V., and Strisower, E. H. (1970). *Biochim. Biophys. Acta* **202**, 392.

Puppione, D. L., Forte, G. M., and Nichols, A. V. (1971). *Comp. Biochem. Physiol.* **39B**, 673.

Rider, A. K., Levy, R. I., and Fredrickson, D. S. (1970). *Circulation* **42**, Suppl. 3, 10.

Rudman, D., Garcia, L. A., and Howard, C. H. (1970). *J. Clin. Invest.* **49**, 365.

Salpeter, M. M., and Zilversmit, D. B. (1968). *J. Lipid Res.* **9**, 187.

Sardet, C., Hansma, H., and Ostwald, R. (1972). *J. Lipid Res.* (in press).

Scanu, A. (1965). *Advan. Lipid Res.* **3**, 63.

Scanu, A. (1969). In "Structural and Functional Aspects of Lipoproteins in Living Systems" (E. Tria and A. M. Scanu, eds.), pp. 425–445. Academic Press, New York.

Scanu, A., Toth, J., Edelstein, C., Koga, S., and Stiller, E. (1969). *Biochemistry* **8**, 3309.

Schoefl, G. I. (1968). *Proc. Roy. Soc. Ser. B* **169**, 147.

Schoefl, G. I., and French, J. E. (1968). *Proc. Roy. Soc. Ser. B* **169**, 153.

Schumaker, V. N., and Adams, G. H. (1969). *Annu. Rev. Biochem.* **38**, 113.

Seidel, D., Alaupovic, P., and Furman, R. H. (1969). *J. Clin. Invest.* **48**, 1211.

Seidel, D., Alaupovic, P., Furman, R. H., and McConathy, W. J. (1970). *J. Clin. Invest.* **49**, 2396.

Shore, B., and Shore, V. (1969). *Biochemistry* **8**, 4510.

Stein, A., and Stein, Y. (1967). *J. Cell Biol.* **33**, 319.

Strauss, E. W. (1966). *J. Lipid Res.* **7**, 307.

Tillack, T. W., and Marchesi, V. T. (1970). *J. Cell Biol.* **45**, 649.

Van Bruggen, E. F. J., Wiebenga, E. H., and Gruber, M. (1962). *J. Mol. Biol.* **4**, 1.

Zilversmit, D. B. (1965). *J. Clin. Invest.* **44**, 1610.

Zilversmit, D. B. (1968). *J. Lipid Res.* **9**, 180.

Zilversmit, D. B. (1969). *In* "Structural and Functional Aspects of Lipoproteins in Living Systems" (E. Tria and A. M. Scanu, eds.), pp. 329–368. Academic Press, New York.

Employment of Lipids in the Measurement and Modification of Cellular, Humoral, and Immune Responses

NICHOLAS R. Di LUZIO

*Department of Physiology, Tulane University School of Medicine,
New Orleans, Louisiana*

I. Introduction

The main purpose of this review is to accent the use of lipids to modify reticuloendothelial (RE) function and to indicate the consequences, either beneficial or detrimental, on the host when particulate lipid preparations are administered intravenously. The uniqueness of lipids in their ability to modify RE function suggests that circulating plasma lipids may be an integral part of the as yet undefined control mechanism which regulates the activity of the reticuloendothelial system (RES).

Since certain phases of the involvement of the macrophage cell in health and disease processes cannot be considered in this review, the reader's attention is called to previous reviews (Jaffe, 1931; Halpern, 1959; Hirsch, 1959) and to the very recent books of Stuart (1970), Pearsall and Weiser (1970), and Nelson (1969) for further information on the multifacet reticuloendothelial system.

The discovery by Elias Metchnikoff, that mobile cells of the starfish larvae serve in the defense of the organism against foreign agents, initiated the concept of phagocytosis (Metchnikoff, 1905). That phagocytic cells play an essential role in host-defense against a variety of invading foreign agents has clearly remained undisputed. The concept advanced by Aschoff (1924), that phagocytic cells constitute a system, was based upon the functional properties of these cells of ingesting various vital dyes or other particulate agents. This was the unifying feature which led to the introduction of the term "Reticuloendothelial System" in 1924 by Aschoff. In the approximately 50 years which have elapsed since the functional designation was given to the RES, it has become obvious that the phagocytic act is but one small facet of the functional contribution of the RES to the well-being of the host. In view of the multipotential nature of the RES, it would appear to be advisable now to consider the RES as a "host-defense system."

At the present time, studies have amply demonstrated that the RES is involved in what might be considered three major areas: (A) metabolic, (B) immunologic, and (C) phagocytic. In considering phagocytosis, the processes of the phagocytic event are generally now considered to require the following steps which are briefly listed.

1. Recognition or discrimination, i.e., the ability of the RES to identify "self" from "altered-self" and "non-self."

2. Opsonization, i.e., preparation of the particulate entity for macrophage ingestion through the expression of either natural or acquired antibodies.

3. Attachment phase.

4. Ingestion.

5. Killing.

6. Digestion.

7. Excretion and/or storage.

The metabolic phase of RE cell involvement includes two major areas: the first is detoxification, as in the modification of endotoxins, certain steroidal hormones, as well as other macromolecular pharmacological agents; and the second is the participation of RE cells in such overt metabolic processes as carbohydrate, lipid, and protein metabolism, as well as production of bile pigments and its involvement in iron metabolism.

Currently attracting greater interest than the metabolic participation of the RES is the involvement of the RES in the physiology of the immune response which includes: (a) antigen clearance, (b) antigen-antibody removal, (c) formation of a "processed" or super-antigen, (d) antigen persistence, and (e) the possible production of so-called natural antibodies. It is the reviewer's opinion that the use of lipids to modify functional expression of the RES and to test its behavioral patterns under varying conditions will do much to enhance our knowledge of this system.

II. Problems Relative to the Evaluation of Reticuloendothelial Function

From an anatomical viewpoint, while admirably arranged for the optimal expression of its functional activity, the RES is uniquely characterized by its diffuse nature as noted by the following outline of the anatomical localization of the RES.

Anatomy of the Reticuloendothelial System
A. Fixed Sinusoidal Cell Populations
   1. Kupffer cells (most important quantitatively)
   2. Splenic macrophage
   3. Bone marrow macrophages (possible stem cell macrophages)
   4. Adrenal macrophages
   5. Lymph node macrophages
   6. Pulmonary macrophages (may also be "wandering" variety)
B. Wandering Macrophages
   1. Peritoneal macrophages
   2. Other serous cavity macrophages
   3. Blood monocytes
   4. Polymorphonuclear leukocytes
   5. Lymph macrophages
C. Histiocytes of connective tissue
D. Microglia of central nervous system
E. Endothelial cells with ultimate phagocytic potential

The classical technique of inducing a deficiency syndrome by surgical removal of the system under study is, in the case of the RES, obviously incompatible with continued existence of the organism due to the diffuse anatomical nature of the system. Studies to elucidate the physiology of the RES have, therefore, concentrated on inducing functional disturbances. Initial considerations involved attempts to saturate the system with dyes or colloidal agents to possibly induce a physical type of impairment in function (Jaffe, 1931; Smith, 1930a,b). More recent studies indicated that because of the proliferative ability of the RES, the administration of large amounts of colloidal materials actually can induce stimulation and hyperfunction rather than hypofunction (Blickens and Di Luzio, 1964). Thus, the present concept is that while the RES may be physically saturated by large quantities of one colloid or particulate agent, the system is neither permanently impaired nor "blocked" in its ability to remove other colloids from the circulation (Saba and Di Luzio, 1969a).

III. Employment of Lipids to Measure Reticuloendothelial Function *in Vivo*

The employment of artificial lipid emulsions to measure RE phagocytic function essentially dates back to the initial observations of Saxl and Donath (1925). Saxl and Donath employed a 20% oil emulsion which was administered in doses of 5 ml to control and experimental human subjects. Fingertip blood samples were obtained every 3 minutes for 30 minutes and the relative presence of lipid particles was determined by counting the number of lipid particles by means of dark field microscopy.

Saxl and Donath reported an increased removal of lipid emulsion particles in hyperthyroidism and decreased removal in conditions of uremia, infection, jaundice, and liver cirrhosis. In this study they also made a series of observations on the pharmacological effects of certain administered agents on the RES. This study constituted the initial attempt to measure RE function in man and the influence of disease processes and pharmacological agents on RE function. The validity of employing such a lipid emulsion to measure RE function was, in this author's opinion, never ascertained although there appears to be little doubt the emulsion behaved as a foreign particulate.

The subsequent histological studies of Jaffe and Berman (1928) in experimental animals suggested that particulate lipid emulsions were rapidly transferred from hepatic Kupffer cells to hepatic parenchymal cells, and that such lipid preparations could not be employed as a phagocytic test lipid emulsion. Waddell *et al.* (1953, 1954) also demonstrated the effective removal of artificial lipid emulsions by liver, but did not delineate the relative participation of hepatic parenchymal and Kupffer cells in this process.

Studies by Di Luzio and Riggi (1964) have led to the development of an artificial lipid emulsion, designated "RE test lipid emulsion" by these authors, which was and still is effectively employed as an agent to measure phagocytic function. The validity of employing the intravascular clearance of this emulsion as an index of phagocytic function was clearly demonstrated by the observation that reticuloendothelial hyperfunction and hyperplasia, induced in rats by the administration of glucan (Riggi and Di Luzio, 1961, 1962), significantly augmented the vascular removal of this particulate lipid preparation (Table I). Lipid emulsions such as Intralipid did not possess this feature of RE removal (Di Luzio and Riggi, 1964). Similarly, chylomicrons (Di Luzio *et al.*, 1965a,b) and a lipoprotein preparation (Di Luzio and Bierman, 1964) were not removed by a phagocytic process (Fig. 1). Light and electron microscopic studies (Fig. 2), which were also conducted to evaluate the validity of employing this lipid emulsion, clearly indicated the selective removal of this emulsion by macrophages in both experimental animals (Ashworth *et al.*, 1963) and man (Di Luzio *et al.*, 1965a,b; Ladman *et al.*, 1963, 1964). The nontoxic, nonimmunogenic nature of the RE test lipid emulsion, as well as its kinetics of clearance (Di Luzio and Riggi, 1964, 1967) and its vascular removal in the absence of intravascular hydrolysis, demonstrated its applicability in evaluating RE function in man (Salky *et al.*, 1964).

In general, studies in man employing the RE test lipid emulsion denoted that patients with bacterial infections (Salky *et al.*, 1964) as well as neoplasia (Salky *et al.*, 1967) and autoimmune disorders (Salky *et al.*,

Table I

DISAPPEARANCE AND TISSUE DISTRIBUTION OF TRIPALMITIN-^{14}C-LABELED ARTIFICIAL RE TEST LIPID EMULSION IN GLUCAN-TREATED RATS[a,b]

Group	Intravascular t/2 (minutes)	Liver %ID/gm[c]	Liver %ID/TO[d]	Spleen %ID/gm	Spleen %ID/TO	Lung %ID/gm	Lung %ID/TO
Saline	30.4	3.04	30.65	5.49	4.11	1.01	1.53
Glucan	3.5	6.37	67.88	0.99	1.60	0.50	1.14

[a] From Di Luzio and Riggi (1964).

[b] Male rats weighing approximately 200 gm were injected with either saline or glucan for 5 days. On the sixth day, the rats were killed 10 minutes after administration of the RE test lipid emulsion in the amount of 61 mg of triglyceride/100 gm of body weight. Mean values are derived from 8 saline and 6 glucan-treated rats. Glucan is a profound activator of RE function.

[c] %ID/gm = percent of the injected tripalmitin-^{14}C recovered per gram of liver.

[d] %ID/TO = percent of the injected tripalmitin-^{14}C recovered per total organ.

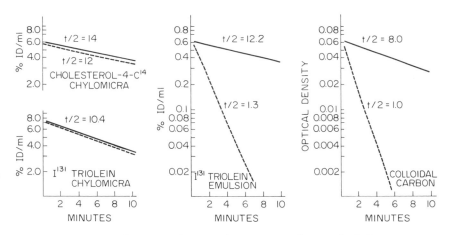

Fɪɢ. 1.   Intravascular removal rates of RE test emulsion and chylomicrons compared with colloidal carbon. Upper solid lines indicate disappearance rate of each substance in normal, sodium chloride-injected rats. Lower broken lines indicate disappearance rates of each substance in rats whose RE system was stimulated and made hyperfunctional by injection of glucan, a neutral polysaccharide. From Salky et al. (1964).

1965) have enhanced functional activity of the RES (Table II). Sex and age did not alter the rate of vascular clearance of this emulsion. Since the "RE test lipid emulsion" in its native state does not apparently require the presence of opsonins or recognition factor (Saba and Di Luzio, 1965; Saba et al., 1966) for its phagocytosis, the enhanced vascular clearance rates observed in patients with such diverse clinical conditions denotes RE cellular hyperfunction. Subsequent studies have revealed that the emulsion, when prepared in gelatin, becomes dependent upon the presence of an intact opsonic, or, as now designated by this laboratory, a humoral recognition factor system for phagocytosis to occur (Filkins and Di Luzio, 1966a,b; Saba et al., 1966; Di Luzio et al., 1971).

IV. *In Vitro* Employment of Lipids for Evaluation of Cellular and Humoral Events in Phagocytosis

Since methyl palmitate-induced RE hypofunction (see Section VI) is associated with a profound depression in hepatic phagocytosis, and since Kupffer cell phagocytosis of foreign material is highly dependent upon the presence of opsonins or recognition factors (Rowley, 1962; Saba et al., 1966; Saba and Di Luzio, 1965; Pisano and Di Luzio, 1970a; Filkins and Di Luzio, 1966a,b; Saba and Di Luzio, 1969b) studies were undertaken to develop an *in vitro* method whereby it would be possible to

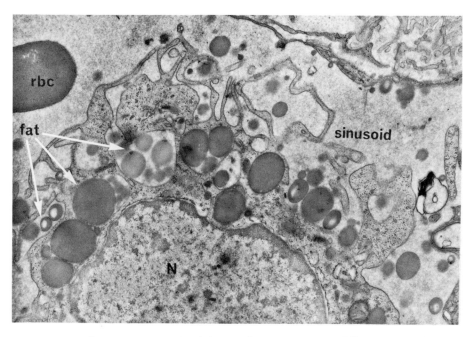

FIG. 2. Electron micrograph of human liver 10 minutes following the administration of "RE test lipid emulsion." The exclusive accumulation of the particulate lipid preparation in the Kupffer cells characterizes the behavior of this lipid preparation. rbc → red blood cell, n, nucleus. From Ladman *et al.* (1964).

evaluate the importance of cellular and humoral mechanisms in methyl palmitate-induced RE depression.

In these studies liver slices were incubated *in vitro* with various colloidal particles, and the uptake of the labeled particle by the Kupffer cells of the liver slice was determined under various conditions. Employing microaggregated heat-denatured human serum albumin, approxi-

Table II

RETICULOENDOTHELIAL FUNCTION IN NORMAL AND CLINICAL SUBJECTS[a]

Group	Number	t/2 (minutes)
Normal	24	7.42 ± 0.55
Acute bacterial infection	7	1.30 ± 0.37
Subacute bacterial infection	6	3.75 ± 0.07
Chronic bacterial infection	7	4.27 ± 0.29
Pulmonary tuberculosis-treated	12	5.40 ± 0.51
Rheumatoid arthritis	20	4.2 ± 0.2
Neoplasia	53	4.0 ± 0.4

[a] From Salky *et al.* (1964, 1965, 1967).

mately 10–20 mμ in size, the phagocytosis of this denatured protein was
not influenced by the presence of plasma factors. However, further degradation of the albumin particles to produce microaggregates of 1–3 μ in
size resulted in a particle whose phagocytic uptake was profoundly enhanced by the presence of recognition factors in plasma (Saba and
Di Luzio, 1965). Radioactive colloidal gold also required the presence
of plasma recognition factors for its phagocytosis (Table III). It was
observed that plasma which was depleted of its humoral recognition
factor activity by preincubation with a specific particulate suspension
was rendered incapable of supporting active cellular recognition and
phagocytosis of the particle that was used for depletion; however, it still
possessed recognition activity toward a different type of particle. These
findings suggested that there exists a multiple humoral recognition factor
system, that is, each particle requires a specific recognition factor for
identification and phagocytosis (Saba et al., 1966), a concept which is
supported by the observations of Vaughn (1965).

The reticuloendothelial test lipid emulsion which we have employed
extensively to evaluate phagocytosis in experimental and clinical studies
was found to be phagocytized and metabolized in the absence of plasma
factors (Saba et al., 1966). It appears that the lipophilic nature of the
lipid emulsion apparently is already identified as "non-self" by the
macrophage, suggesting the possibility that the lipophilic groupings on
the surface of the particulate are identical to that which would be
present with opsonin-dependent particles after the interaction of the
recognition factor and particle has occurred. In essence, these findings

Table III

UPTAKE OF COLLOIDAL GOLD (^{198}AU) BY RAT LIVER SLICES AS A FUNCTION
OF PLASMA CONCENTRATION IN THE INCUBATION MEDIUM[a]

% Plasma in medium[b]	Phagocytic uptake %ID/100 mg[c]
0.0	0.9 ± 0.2
6.25	3.3 ± 1.1
12.5	5.9 ± 2.0
25.0	8.6 ± 2.0
50	12.4 ± 1.9
100	22.8 ± 3.0

[a] From Saba and Di Luzio (1965).

[b] Krebs-Ringer phosphate (pH = 7.4) was used as the diluent. Incubation volume in
all experiments was 3 ml. Values are expressed as means ± standard error. Incubation
time was 30 minutes. The concentration of colloidal gold in each incubation vial was
191 μg.

[c] Liver weight on a wet weight basis.

imply that the RE test lipid emulsion is already what might be considered "self-opsonized." The behavior of the lipid emulsion parallels that of polystyrene latex particles whose phagocytic uptake by macrophages occurs independent of plasma factor activity (Sbarra and Karnovsky, 1959).

The *in vitro* liver slice technique clearly appears to be a sensitive, efficient quantitative model system for evaluating a variety of factors which might influence the phagocytic and metabolic function of the macrophage as well as for serving as a basis for humoral recognition factor assay in man and experimental animals (Saba and Di Luzio, 1968; Pisano and Di Luzio, 1970b; Pisano *et al.*, 1970a,b; Di Luzio *et al.*, 1971).

In an effort to evaluate the general significance of humoral recognition factors in various animal species that are extensively employed in studies of phagocytosis, a comparative study of *in vitro* phagocytosis was conducted employing mice, dogs, rats, and rabbits. It was observed that the plasma from the mouse, rat, and dog supported enhanced phagocytosis of colloidal radiogold by their respective liver slices employed *in vitro*. It was observed, however, that rabbit plasma was found to lack the specific plasma factor which was essential for the *in vitro* phagocytosis of colloidal gold (Filkins and Di Luzio, 1966a). In continuing studies to define the mechanism of phagocytosis and the manner by which recognition of foreignness is conferred upon particulate agents, it was observed that the addition of gelatin to the RE test lipid emulsion resulted in profound augmentation of the intravascular removal of the lipid emulsion *in vitro* (Filkins and Di Luzio, 1966a,b; Saba *et al.*, 1966).

It was proposed that the gelatin interacted with the lipid particle and, in essence, "coated" the surface of the lipid particle. By covering the lipophilic nature of the lipid particle with a protein coat, the particle now requires the presence of plasma humoral recognition factors for its phagocytosis. In all studies to date, the presence of heparin was essential for the expression of optimum phagocytosis (Filkins and Di Luzio, 1966b; Saba *et al.*, 1966; Pisano and Di Luzio, 1970a). In studies on the properties of the recognition factor, it was found that the recognition factor essential for colloidal gold phagocytosis was destroyed by heating serum to 60°C. The pH optimum for gold was 7.2 to 8.5 and differed significantly from that of albumin which was 6.2 to 7.0 denoting the possibility of a different recognition factor system for each of these particles. Anaerobic incubation resulted in slight impairment in phagocytosis due to its influence on the particle ingestion phase rather than the initial phase of particle attachment to the macrophage.

In attempting to isolate and identify the recognition factor, it was found that barium sulfate absorption of serum markedly depleted serum recognition factor activity (Saba *et al.*, 1966). It was possible to restore, to a significant extent, humoral recognition factor activity by addition to the incubation medium of the barium sulfate eluate. In attempting to characterize the factor, cellulose acetate electrophoretic studies demonstrated a selective depletion of the α-2-globulin fraction in barium sulfate absorbed serum.

These studies indicated that the *in vitro* phagocytosis of a variety of particulate preparations can be markedly augmented by a plasma system which we consider to be a humoral factor recognition moiety. In an effort to determine whether these recognition factors are in essence "natural antibodies," an evaluation of plasma humoral recognition factor activity in germ-free rats was conducted (Saba *et al.*, 1967).

The results indicated that the humoral recognition factor system relative to the colloidal gold phagocytosis is functionally developed in germ-free animals. Liver tissue obtained from germ-free and conventional control rats manifested similar phagocytic capabilities when incubated in either germ-free or conventional serum. These studies support the concept that the recognition factor system may be similar to "natural antibody" since it exists in germ-free animals which have minimal exposure to antigenic stimulation, and indeed, the recognition factor activity in the germ-free animals might well be equated with that which is demonstrated in invertebrates (Stuart, 1968).

In studies evaluating the role of serum recognition factors on the phagocytic activity of fixed macrophages, the influence of recognition factor activity on splenic and alveolar phagocytosis of particulate materials was also undertaken and contrasted with that of liver. It was observed that when the particulate preparations were incubated in the presence of plasma rather than artificial buffer medium, liver and spleen phagocytosis increased 30- to 40-fold. In contrast, the enhancement in particulate uptake by lung was approximately 11-fold. This difference in enhancement between liver, lung, and splenic tissue appears to reflect the variable populations of macrophage cells which are present in these two tissues. These studies support the concept that the membrane sites involved in cellular recognition and binding of the opsonized or "prepared" particulate material are fundamentally similar for liver, lung, and spleen macrophages, since all three populations responded with increased activity to the same type of opsonized particles.

In an attempt to further evaluate the assay system for the determination of humoral recognition factor activity in plasma, rat Kupffer cells were isolated by the use of collagenase and trypsin digestion of liver tissue (Pisano *et al.*, 1968a). The isolated Kupffer cells possessed the ability to phagocytize particulate materials in the presence of serum and

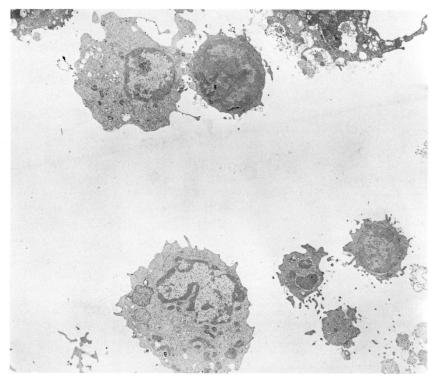

Fig. 3.   Electron microscopic section of isolated rat Kupffer cell preparations. From Hoffman, Lentz, Pisano, and Di Luzio (unpublished observations).

heparin. Metabolic studies indicated the cells possessed a significant fatty acid metabolism and the phagocytic processes of the isolated Kupffer cells were both cyanide and iodoacetate sensitive. Microelectrophoretic studies suggested that the surface integrity of the isolated Kupffer cells, as measured by its zeta potential, remain intact during the isolation procedure (Pisano *et al.*, 1968a). An electron microscopic study of the isolated Kupffer cells is presented in Fig. 3.

V. Evaluation of Plasma Humoral Recognition Factor Activity in Human Subjects

Since our previous studies indicated that the phagocytic activity of the reticuloendothelial system as measured by the intravascular removal of the RE test lipid emulsion was significantly enhanced in patients with neoplasia (Salky *et al.*, 1967), and since the RE test lipid emulsion did not require humoral recognition factor activity for its phagocytosis, studies were undertaken in which recognition factor activity was measured in plasma of normal subjects as well as those with neoplasia (Pisano and Di Luzio, 1970b; Pisano et al., 1970a,b; Di Luzio et al., 1971). A variety of other disease states were employed as control groups to determine the specificity of humoral recognition factor alterations. In agreement with previous observations, it was observed that normal human serum, in the presence of heparin, was as effective as rat serum in promoting the phagocytosis by rat liver slices, indicating that human humoral recognition factor activity can also enhance the phagocytic expression of the rat macrophage (Fig. 4). This would imply that the receptors on the macrophage, both rat and man, are essentially identical since the recognition factor in human plasma can support the uptake of foreign particles by rat macrophages. The converse is also true, i.e., rat plasma is as effective as human plasma in supporting the uptake of gelatinized RE test lipid emulsion particles by human alveolar macrophages (Di Luzio et al., 1971).

In contrast to the observation of the pronounced enhancement in phagocytosis which is observed when normal human serum is employed as the incubation medium, it was found that when serum derived from patients with untreated carcinoma, either metastatic or nonmetastatic was employed, an approximate 90% reduction in particle uptake oc-

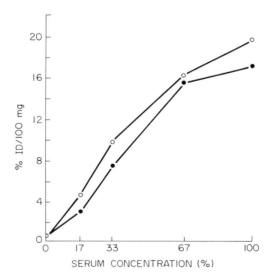

FIG. 4. Humoral recognition factor activity of serum of normal rats (○) and "normal" human subjects (●) as reflected by its ability to promote the phagocytosis of gelatinized RE test lipid emulsion. From Pisano and Di Luzio (1970b).

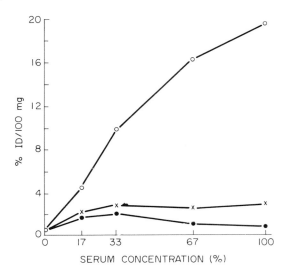

Fɪɢ. 5.   Opsonic activity of serum from normal human (○———○) and carcinoma patients, either nonmetastatic (x) or metastatic (●———●). Rat liver slices were incubated with gelatinized RE test lipid emulsion for 30 minutes at 37°C in appropriate serum concentration and heparin. Each point represents a mean of 16 determinations with 8 serum samples, i.e., subjects, per group. From Pisano and Di Luzio (1970b).

curred (Fig. 5). This finding denotes essential loss of humoral recognition factor activity in the presence of neoplasia. In five individuals who had undergone either radiation or surgical therapy, all manifested four- to six-fold elevations in humoral recognition factor as denoted by the ability of their serum to support Kupffer cell phagocytosis within 1 to 9 days following treatment.

In contrast to the observations that patients with neoplasia show profound loss of recognition factor activity, it was observed that patients with certain other clinical disorders, such as pneumonia, diabetes, and hypertension were found to have essentially normal recognition factor activity (Table IV). Since depletion of recognition factor activity was not observed when benign tumors were present, these findings denote that neoplastic disease in man is associated with considerable decrease in humoral recognition factor activity. In view of the partial restoration of humoral factor activity with treatment, it was suggested that loss of humoral recognition factors may be an important element in neoplasia (Fig. 6) (Pisano *et al.*, 1970a; Di Luzio *et al.*, 1971).

The mechanism of induction of so-called reticuloendothelial "blockade," which is the phagocytic depression developed following the administration of colloidal particulate materials, was also evaluated by our

Table IV

PLASMA HUMORAL RECOGNITION FACTOR ACTIVITY IN PATIENTS WITH UNTREATED NONMETASTATIC OR METASTATIC CARCINOMA AS COMPARED TO TREATED PATIENTS OR THOSE WITH OTHER DISEASE STATES[a]

Group	Phagocytic uptake, %ID/100 mg				
	Serum concentration:				
	0.0	16.7	33.3	66.7	100.0
Normal control	0.6	4.5	9.9	16.3	19.6
Carcinoma patients[b]	0.7	2.3	2.8	2.6	3.1
Metastatic carcinoma patients[c]	0.6	1.8	2.1	1.3	1.0
Carcinoma patients in therapy[d]	0.7	2.7	4.2	5.8	8.7
Non-neoplastic disease group[e]	0.6	4.2	9.9	11.8	13.5

[a] From Di Luzio *et al.* (1971).

[b] Carcinoma patients were four males and four females, ranging in age from 40 to 75 years. The site of lesion was liver (2), lung (4), and bronchogenic (2).

[c] Metastatic group consisted of five females and four male subjects ranging in age from 54 to 78 years. Liver and intra-abdominal involvement generally characterized this population.

[d] Group, consisting of five subjects, was assayed 1 to 9 days following treatment which consisted of cobalt irradiation and/or surgical removal of the tumor.

[e] Noncancerous group consisted of nine males, ages ranging from 42 to 61 years. Clinical disorders include such diverse entities as diabetes, hypertension, gastric and duodenal ulcers, pneumonia, emphysema, and hepatitis.

in vitro technique (Saba and Di Luzio, 1969a,b). It was observed that the intravenous administration of gelatinized RE test lipid emulsion induced a state of phagocytic depression as indicated by impairment in intravascular phagocytosis and depressed hepatic uptake of the test

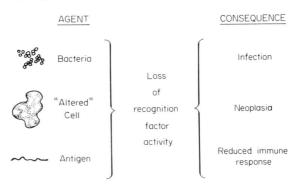

FIG. 6. Postulated importance of loss of recognition factor activity by which macrophages detect the presence of foreign particles in their environment to the development of a disease state. This working hypothesis is presently under investigation and evaluation.

emulsion. The depression, which occurred within 30 minutes after the administration of the particulate gelatinized RE test lipid emulsion, was found to be temporary and followed by a period of recovery which was completed in 2 hours. It was also observed that, in support of the concept of the existence of a multiple recognition factor system, blockade was specific for the particle employed in that a dissimilar particle was removed at normal clearance rates in animals which were blockaded with gelatinized RE test lipid emulsion. In support of the concept that RE blockade is related to the loss of recognition factor activity in plasma, the administration of a gelatinized lipid emulsion, which was preopsonized by incubation with normal serum, was found to completely eliminate the manifestations of RE depression in blockaded rats.

In further evaluation of the mechanism of RE blockade, humoral recognition factor activity which was evaluated before, during, and following blockade, revealed that a profound depression in opsonic activity occurred during RE blockade (Pisano *et al.*, 1968b; Saba and Di Luzio, 1969a). A restoration in humoral recognition factor activity occurred during the postblockade interval, and indeed, an excellent temporal relationship existed between RE blockade and recovery, with opsonin depletion in the former state and opsonic elevation in the latter state, clearly demonstrating that blockade is due to depletion of recognition factors from plasma (Saba and Di Luzio, 1969a). The rapid compensatory response of the recognition factor system suggests the presence of a physiological mechanism, yet to be elucidated, which controls the circulating plasma recognition factor levels and thus directly influences the expressed activity of the reticuloendothelial system (Saba and Di Luzio, 1969a).

In continuing studies as to the mechanism of recovery from RE blockade, it was observed that restoration of plasma humoral recognition factor activity was inhibited by the administration of puromycin (Pisano *et al.*, 1968b). The effect of puromycin appears to be mediated by an inhibition of recognition factor activity rather than by any puromycin-induced macrophage defect (Pisano *et al.*, 1968b). These studies clearly indicate that recognition factor activity in plasma relates to *de novo* synthesis of protein following the administration of an RE blocking agent which depletes plasma of its recognition factor activity. Thus, a sensitive control mechanism which regulates plasma levels of recognition factor activity appears to exist.

At the present time the phagocytosis of the gelatinized RE test lipid emulsion clearly requires the presence of serum factors or opsonins. In an attempt to isolate and characterize the recognition factor, four major protein fractions were obtained from rabbit serum (Pisano and Di Luzio, 1970a). It was observed that only that fraction which remained soluble at 50% ammonium sulfate saturation, consisting principally of α-globulins, manifested humoral recognition factor activity as measured by its ability to enhance normal intravascular clearance rates and induce recovery from RE blockade.

It is anticipated that further studies defining the mechanism of humoral recognition factor activity and its interaction with foreign particulate agents will greatly contribute to an appreciation of the mechanism by which discrimination of the macrophage population is manifested. It can also be predicated that if recognition factor activity can be modified toward a specific antigenic entity, shall we say a cardiac cell, then it would be possible, in essence, to transplant this particular cell and not have rejection occur, as the subject would be internally blinded to the presence of this particular cell population since the exclusive recognition factor is absent. It would, therefore, be possible to transplant specific cell populations in the absence of immunosuppressive therapy while maintaining intact the defense system of the body toward other invading microorganisms or foreign cell species. While at the present this concept is still in the development state, initial studies have also already been conducted in this laboratory which reveal the potentiality of such a concept.

VI. Employment of Lipids to Depress Phagocytic Activity of the Reticuloendothelial System

Stuart et al. (1960a,b) initially evaluated the role of glyceryl and ethyl esters of fatty acids upon the phagocytic function of the reticuloendothelial system as evaluated by the rate of removal of injected colloidal carbon from the vascular system. They found that the administration of ethyl stearate resulted in profound impairment in the rate of clearance of colloidal carbon. The duration of depression persisted for 3 or 4 days after a single intravenous injection, with restoration of normal phagocytic activity at that time. Ethyl oleate was also found to depress the phagocytic system.

The studies of Stuart et al. (1960a,b) were preceded by the observation of Shivas and Fraser (1959) that the interperitoneal administration of ethyl stearate produced profound necrosis of the abdominal lymphoid structures and, indeed, these authors initially suggested that administration of ethyl stearate may well be a useful technique for altering the reticuloendothelial system. Stuart (1960, 1962), in attempting to develop chemical control over reticuloendothelial activity, essentially reconfirmed the induction of necrosis of lymphoid structures by the use of ethyl palmitate. Profound depression of phagocytosis was manifested following the administration of ethyl palmitate to mice in doses of 25 mg per 20 gm of body weight. Widespread destructive changes were observed in the spleen, changes which extended to both the pulp and Malpighian bodies. The pulp was profoundly acellular. The existing cells showed pronounced nuclear changes and nuclear vacuolation and a loss of staining properties. In certain instances, a total loss of lymphoid cells was observed, leaving only a central arteriole surrounded by isolated and dead lymphocytes. These observations have been confirmed in the reviewer's laboratory where pronounced splenic necrosis was induced with massive doses of methyl palmitate as well. It is interesting to note that Stuart's observations, as well as those in the author's laboratory, showed no significant lesions or loss of nuclear material within liver cells. These findings are quite surprising and suggest a pronounced sensitivity of the splenic cells to fatty acid esters since the accumulation of injected labeled fatty acid esters in the spleen is essentially similar to that which was observed in the liver on a per gram basis (Blickens and Di Luzio, 1965).

Stuart (1960) also noted the pronounced regional differences in the ethyl palmitate-induced reticuloendothelial function and sensitivity, a fact which has been stressed by a variety of experimental studies in our laboratory. Stuart (1960) proposed a concept that chemical splenectomy induced by ethyl palmitate is probably related to high concentrations of ethyl palmitate achieved within the splenic macrophages. The intracellular accumulation of ethyl palmitate was predicated to result in cell damage and the release of cytotoxic materials from ethyl palmitate-damaged cells which alter the remaining lymphoid structures of the spleen. Clearly, the employment of fatty acid esters is a simple means of inducing chemical splenectomy for investigative studies.

Stuart (1962) also tested the ability of cholesterol oleate, which was prepared as a suspension with a particle size of 5 to 15 μ by homogenization with Tween 20, to alter phagocytic activity. The intravenous administration of cholesterol oleate to mice in the amount of 10 to 30 mg resulted in phagocytic depression for a period of approximately 4 days. The degree and duration of phagocytic impairment was similar to that noted with ethyl palmitate. Lower doses in the amount of 50 mg of cholesterol oleate produced profound structural alterations of the spleen and liver. These studies further demonstrate that a variety of fatty acid esters are capable of modifying reticuloendothelial activity.

Stuart and Davidson (1963) extended the study of the effects of purified cholesterol oleate preparations on RE function and splenic structure. Cholesterol oleate produced a significant stimulation of phagocytic activity at low dose levels, i.e., 2.5 mg, while pronounced depression occurred at doses extending from 10 mg and above. Repeated injections of cholesterol oleate for 3 days in the amount of 30 mg per day induced pronounced histological alterations characterized by splenic vacuolization. Stuart and Davidson (1963) noted that plasma cells were unaltered by cholesterol oleate administration and lymph follicles did not develop any lesions. They suggest the possibility that cholesterol oleate may be a useful technique for dissecting the relative roles of lymphoid and phagocytic cells in respect to relative functional activities.

Wooles and Di Luzio (1963) stressed the employment of methyl palmitate as the lipid of choice in inducing reticuloendothelial depression. Pronounced impairment of colloidal carbon phagocytosis was induced by the administration of methyl palmitate. The depression in phagocytic activity of the reticuloendothelial system by methyl palmitate was not correlated with the destruction of hepatic and splenic RE cellular elements as noted with ethyl stearate. Di Luzio and Wooles (1964), employing highly purified methyl palmitate, showed pronounced impairment in phagocytosis for a 10-day period after methyl palmitate administration. The depression in phagocytic activity was not associated with any alteration in Bromsulphalein (BSP) clearance (Table V), a reflection of hepatic parenchymal cell activity. These studies suggested that the employment of purified fatty acid esters could be advantageous in evaluating the relative functional role of hepatic parenchymal and Kupffer cells since a selective alteration of only Kupffer cells was induced by methyl palmitate administration. Histological studies indicated that the uptake of colloidal carbon by macrophage cells of spleen was comparable in the methyl palmitate and control group and no alteration in architecture of the spleen was observed. The degree of phagocytosis by pulmonary macrophages was also comparable. A comparison of a number of macrophage cells in the liver indicated no change in macrophage cell number following methyl palmitate administration, however,

Table V

PHAGOCYTIC ACTIVITY, ORGAN WEIGHTS, AND PLASMA BROMSULPHALEIN IN
CONTROL AND RETICULOENDOTHELIAL-DEPRESSED MICE[a]

Group	Number	Colloidal carbon half-time (minutes)	BSP (mg/ml)
Tween	8	7.85	0.175
Methyl palmitate	10	49.20	0.153

[a] From Di Luzio and Wooles (1964).

the degree of Kupffer cell phagocytosis of colloidal carbon was profoundly reduced and many Kupffer cells exhibited a complete absence of carbon particles.

Since lipids offer convenient means to chemically control RE activity, studies were undertaken in our laboratory (Di Luzio and Blickens, 1966) to evaluate the influence of a variety of lipid preparations on phagocytic activity of the RES. Highly purified saturated and unsaturated fatty acid esters, as well as different classes of phospholipids, were studied for their influence on RE activity. These studies revealed that the administration of an emulsion of methyl palmitate to mice by oral or intraperitoneal injections induced no alteration in phagocytic activity. In contrast, intravenous administration produced a profound impairment in the intravascular clearance of colloidal carbon. Dose response data indicated a most severe depression was obtained by 35-mg doses of methyl palmitate administered to mice weighing approximately 20 gm.

The depression in phagocytosis was not immediate upon administration but was induced approximately 4.5 to 5 hours after the administration of the methyl palmitate emulsion (Fig. 7). Phagocytosis remained depressed for a period of 10–17 days after methyl palmitate administration. Maximum depression was observed at the 2 to 5-day period following methyl palmitate administration.

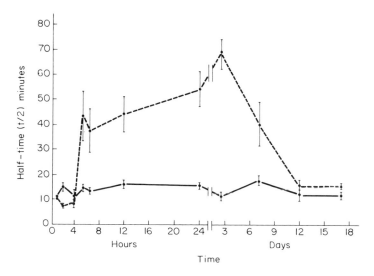

Fig. 7. Phagocytic function, as indicated by the intravascular clearance of colloidal carbon in Tween control (————) and methyl palmitate-treated mice (- - - - - -). Each point represents the mean value of 5 to 13 mice. Vertical lines represent standard error. From Di Luzio and Blickens (1966).

Table VI

INTRAVASCULAR REMOVAL AND 10-MINUTE TISSUE DISTRIBUTION OF AN "RE
TEST LIPID EMULSION" IN TWEEN- AND METHYL PALMITATE-TREATED
MICE[a,b]

Activity	Tween (6)	Methyl palmitate (6)
Liver ($\%ID$/TO)	77.0 ± 7.8	12.7 ± 0.8
Lung ($\%ID$/TO)	2.2 ± 0.2	7.6 ± 0.6
Spleen ($\%ID$/TO)	4.9 ± 0.9	2.0 ± 0.4
Adipose ($\%ID$/gm)	2.2 ± 0.7	1.5 ± 0.1
Blood ($\%ID$/ml)	6.6 ± 1.2	44.2 ± 2.8
Half-time (minutes)	6.9 ± 1.33	23.9 ± 7.8

[a] From Di Luzio and Blickens (1966).

[b] Mice were injected with 35 mg of methyl palmitate. Intravascular removal of 37 mg
triglyceride/100 gm as ^{14}C-tripalmitin-labeled RE test lipid emulsion was evaluated
24 hours after methyl palmitate or Tween injection. Values expressed as percentage of
injected dose (ID) per gram of tissue, per milliliter of blood, or per total organ (TO), are
means $\pm$ standard error. Number in parentheses denotes number of mice.

In evaluating the mechanism of the reduced intravascular clearance
of colloids in animals treated with fatty acid ester derivatives, studies
were undertaken to determine the tissue distribution of the "RE test
lipid emulsion" in methyl palmitate-treated animals (Table VI). It was
observed that the decreased phagocytic activity was related to impairment of hepatic and splenic macrophage activity with minimal alterations in lung phagocytosis. The administration of methyl palmitate to
splenectomized mice produced a greater degree of phagocytic depression
than that which was observed in intact mice (Di Luzio and Blickens,
1966) (Table VII).

In agreement with the observations of Stuart *et al.* (1960a,b; Stuart
and Cooper, 1963), the glyceryl ester of oleic acid induced a mild, but

Table VII

INFLUENCE OF SPLENECTOMY ON THE PHAGOCYTIC RESPONSE OF MICE TO
METHYL PALMITATE ADMINISTRATION AS DETERMINED BY THE
INTRAVASCULAR CLEARANCE OF COLLOIDAL CARBON[a,b]

Group	Number	Colloidal carbon $t/2$ (minutes)
Sham-Tween	5	17.9 ± 4.5
Sham-methyl palmitate	11	29.9 ± 3.8
Splenectomized-Tween	5	19.0 ± 3.7
Splenectomized-methyl palmitate	10	57.0 ± 8.0

[a] From Di Luzio and Blickens (1966).

[b] Values are expressed as means $\pm$ standard error.

Table VIII

PHAGOCYTIC ACTIVITY 24 HOURS AFTER INTRAVENOUS ADMINISTRATION OF
VARIOUS UNSATURATED FATTY ACID ESTERS[a,b]

Group	Number	Colloidal carbon t/2 (minutes)
Tween 20 control	48	14.8 ± 0.5
Methyl palmitoleate	15	24.5 ± 1.3
Methyl oleate	12	31.7 ± 4.2
Methyl elaidate	13	27.9 ± 0.4
Methyl linoleate	8	27.6 ± 4.5
Methyl linolenate	9	19.7 ± 2.0
Methyl arachidonate	4	26.9 ± 3.0
Triolein	13	9.4 ± 1.3

[a] From Di Luzio and Blickens (1966).

[b] Male C57BL/6J mice were injected intravenously with 0.7 ml of an emulsion of 0.1% Tween 20 in 5% dextrose and water containing 35 mg of the ester or 0.7 ml of the suspending agent. The intravascular removal of colloidal carbon (16 mg/100 gm body weight) was measured 24 hours after injection of the fatty acid esters. Values are expressed as means ± standard error.

measurable stimulation of RE function (Table VIII). In contrast, certain methyl, ethyl, and butyl esters of fatty acids containing 14 to 20 carbon atoms and varying degrees of saturation all induced a depression of phagocytic activity of the reticuloendothelial system (Tables VIII and IX). Fatty acid esters containing 6 to 13 carbon atoms induced immedi-

Table IX

PHAGOCYTIC ACTIVITY OF MICE 24 HOURS AFTER INTRAVENOUS ADMINISTRATION
OF VARIOUS SATURATED FATTY ACID ESTERS[a,b]

Group	Number	Colloidal carbon t/2 (minutes)
Tween 20 controls	48	14.8 ± 0.5
Methyl myristate	11	32.3 ± 8.2
Methyl pentadecanoate	14	29.7 ± 2.8
Methyl palmitate	29	32.3 ± 2.7
Ethyl palmitate	8	21.2 ± 1.9
n-Butyl palmitate	9	26.3 ± 3.4
Methyl stearate	7	39.8 ± 4.1

[a] From Di Luzio and Blickens (1966).

[b] Male C57BL/6J mice were injected intravenously with 0.7 ml of an emulsion of 0.1% Tween 20 in 5% dextrose and water containing 35 mg of the ester or 0.7 ml of the suspending agent. Colloidal carbon removal of 16 mg/100 gm body weight was measured 24 hours after injection of the fatty acid esters. Methyl myristate was employed in doses of 17.5 mg because of toxicity at the higher dose. Values are expressed as means ± standard error.

ate death upon intravenous administration and could not be employed.

Studies were also undertaken in the author's laboratory of cholesterol derivatives, such as cholesterol palmitate, cholesterol oleate, and cholesterol acetate. However, in contrast to the reports of Stuart's group (Stuart, 1962; Stuart and Davidson, 1964), suitable emulsions could not be prepared either by sonification or microhomogenization; therefore, an evaluation of ester derivatives of cholesterol could not be undertaken.

Relative to the influence of the phospholipids on phagocytic activity, lecithin was found to induce a significant impairment in phagocytosis while cephalin and sphingomyelin emulsions did not alter phagocytic activity (Table X). These studies demonstrate that a wide variety of saturated and unsaturated fatty acid esters, when administered intravenously, exerted profound effects on the phagocytic activity. Studies on the influence of lipids on RE function of dogs could not be carried out because of the extreme sensitivity of dogs to the suspending medium, resulting in a severe allergic response.

Cooper (1964) attempted to relate the physical or chemical properties of a series of saturated triglycerides on RE activity both *in vitro* and *in vivo*. The triglycerides employed were tricaproin, tricaprylin, tricaprin, trilaurin, trimyristin, tripalmitin, tristearin, and triolein. Variations in particle size were induced by the use of a variety of emulsifying agents. Employing labeled triolein preparations, 80% of the administered activity was removed from the blood within 2 minutes of injection. However, at 1 hour the localization of the intravenous preparation showed 80% uptake by lung, suggesting the mechanical trapping of the large lipid particles by the lung due to particle instability. Liver activity approximated 18% during the 4-hour period. At 24 hours, approximately 99% of the activity

Table X

PHAGOCYTIC ACTIVITY OF MICE 24 HOURS AFTER INTRAVENOUS ADMINISTRATION OF EGG LECITHIN, CEPHALIN, AND SPHINGOMYELIN[a]

Group	Number	Colloidal carbon t/2 (minutes)
Tween 20	12	14.4 ± 0.8
Egg lecithin[b]	8	23.8 ± 4.3
Cephalin	8	13.8 ± 1.6
Sphingomyelin	9	15.2 ± 2.3

[a] From Di Luzio and Blickens (1966).

[b] Male C57BL/6J mice were injected intravenously with either an emulsion of 0.7 ml of 0.1% Tween 20 in 5% dextrose and water containing 35 mg of egg lecithin, cephalin, or sphingomyelin. Values are means ± standard error.

was not present in the tissues studied, suggesting a relatively rapid metabolism of the iodinated lipid which was associated with the release of ^{131}I in the urine. Cooper (1964) found that tricaprin was the most potent substance in the series of triglyceride preparations studied. Deviations from a carbon chain length of 10 resulted in a decrease in stimulatory activity of the preparation. Tripalmitin and tristearin produced an early depression of phagocytic activity which was followed 3 days later by mild stimulation.

The influence of saturated triglyceride on the phagocytic activity of peritoneal macrophages was also investigated (Cooper, 1964). Tricaproin and trimyristin produced moderate increases in phagocytic activity of peritoneal macrophages but did not enhance the ability of the macrophage to destroy the ingested organism. Tripalmitin and tristearin did not improve the phagocytic activity of isolated macrophages at all. Large doses of tricaprylin, tricaprin, and trilaurin appeared to inhibit phagocytosis. These data suggest that the chemical nature of the triglyceride is important in determining if alterations in phagocytic activity would occur or whether a change in intracellular digestive ability is induced. These findings, that varying preparations of lipids consisting of fatty acids of different carbon chain lengths and structures are able to modify the cellular activity of macrophages, again stressed the possibility that the macrophage cell itself may be regulated, in part, through the carbon chain length of the fatty acid radical, the nature of the fatty acid itself, and the particle size of specific lipid moieties which exist in the environment of the macrophage.

In attempting to evaluate the mechanism of methyl palmitate-induced RE depression, Blickens and Di Luzio (1965) demonstrated that methyl palmitate-induced paralysis of RE activity was not related to prolonged storage of methyl palmitate in macrophages, nor was it associated with methanol formation following a very rapid hydrolysis of methyl palmitate (Tables XI and XII).

Since methyl palmitate-induced RE hypofunction is associated with a profound and almost exclusive depression in Kupffer cell phagocytosis, and since Kupffer cell uptake of particulate material is dependent to a great extent upon humoral mechanisms or plasma phagocytic-promoting factors which have been designated as opsonins (Wright and Douglas, 1903), studies were undertaken (Saba and Di Luzio, 1968) to evaluate the humoral and cellular aspects of methyl palmitate-induced RE depression. Opsonin or, as currently designated, humoral recognition factor activity was studied by *in vitro* techniques in which liver slices were incubated in the presence of serum and the uptake of a gelatinized RE

Table XI

TISSUE DISTRIBUTION OF LABELED METHYL PALMITATE AT
24 HOURS IN MICE[a]

Group[b]	Liver (%ID/ TO)[c]	Lung (%ID/ TO)	Spleen (%ID/ TO)	Adipose (%ID/ gm)[d]	Blood (%ID/ ml)[e]
Methyl-C-14-palmitate	0.91	0.03	0.02	0.62	0.05
(Methyl-labeled)	±0.04	±0.01	±0.01	±0.09	±0.01
Methyl palmitate-U-C-14	7.12	0.25	2.81	3.53	0.41
(Fatty acid-labeled)	±0.30	±0.01	±0.34	±0.44	±0.18

[a] From Blickens and Di Luzio (1965).
[b] Means and standard errors are derived from 4 mice per group.
[c] %ID/TO = percent of the injected dose per total organ.
[d] %ID/gm = percent of the injected dose per gram of adipose tissue.
[e] %ID/ml = percent of the injected dose per milliliter of whole blood.

test lipid emulsion was studied. The gelatinized state of the lipid emulsion was employed since its uptake by macrophages is dependent upon opsonins.

In agreement with previous observations (Blickens and Di Luzio, 1964; Di Luzio and Blickens, 1966), it was found that methyl palmitate administration greatly reduced intravascular clearance of the gelatinized ^{131}I-labeled RE test lipid emulsion. Spleen uptake was also significantly decreased while localization of the emulsion in lung was enhanced slightly. The gelatinized RE test lipid emulsion was also administered in its opsonized state to determine whether or not the prior opsonization of the RE test lipid would result in normalization of its clearance rate. It was found that opsonization of the emulsion with normal serum prior to its administration to methyl palmitate-RE-depressed rats resulted in an increased vascular clearance of the gelatinized RE test lipid emulsion.

Table XII

ACCUMULATIVE $^{14}CO_2$ EXCRETION OF LABELED METHYL PALMITATE[a]

Group[b]	Accumulative $^{14}CO_2$ excretion %ID recovered[c]			
	2 hours	4 hours	6 hours	24 hours
Methyl-C-14 palmitate	14.29	37.64	67.07	84.83
(Methyl-labeled)	±4.56	±10.17	±13.57	±4.83
Methyl palmitate-U-C-14	19.80	27.56	34.20	53.67
(Fatty acid-labeled)	±1.04	±1.37	±1.48	±1.00

[a] From Blickens and Di Luzio (1965).
[b] Mean and standard errors are derived from 4 mice per group.
[c] %ID = percent of the injected dose recovered.

The splenic and hepatic defect in phagocytosis was still altered, suggesting that the increased vascular clearance noted was related to removal of the opsonized particles by other macrophage populations such as bone marrow. It was also observed that when methyl palmitate serum was evaluated for its opsonic activity by *in vivo* analysis, it appeared to have slightly less opsonin levels than that of normal serum. These studies indicate that opsonic activity is slightly depressed after methyl palmitate administration, but the major defect in phagocytosis induced by methyl palmitate is related to an impaired hepatic and splenic phagocytic event. The importance of this impaired phagocytic event to altered immunologic responses observed in methyl palmitate-treated animals is as yet to be determined.

VII. Employment of Lipids to Stimulate Phagocytic Activity of the Reticuloendothelial System

Stuart *et al.* (1960a) studied the influence of the intravenous administration of various lipid emulsions on the phagocytic function of the reticuloendothelial system as evaluated by the rate of vascular clearance of intravenously administered colloidal carbon. The emulsions employed were olive oil and glyceryl trioleate. The emulsions were prepared in Tween although other emulsifying agents such as soya lecithin and Pluronic F^{68} were also used. Twenty-four hours after the administration of glyceryl trioleate a considerable increase in the rate of clearance of colloidal carbon was observed. The injected dose was 25 mg of lipid to a 20- to 25-gm mouse. The RE stimulatory effect of glyceryl trioleate was also maximal at 24 hours and the RES remained hyperactive for a period of 5 to 6 days after which normal phagocytic function was manifested. Emulsified olive oil also resulted in stimulation of the RES while glyceryl mono-oleate exerted no alteration in phagocytic function. The ethyl ester of oleic acid also produced a severe depression of phagocytic activity.

Stuart *et al.* (1960a) proposed that the functional changes induced by the intravenous injection of various lipid moieties were related to the intracellular accumulation of lipid and that the chemical nature of the lipid determines the effect produced. A notation is made that the stimulatory activity of olive oil and glyceryl trioleate only occurred in about 80% of the animals. Reason for failure of stimulation in the remaining 20% of the population was unknown. Stuart *et al.* (1960a) also noted that the fatty acid ethyl esters could, if administered repeatedly at 4-day intervals, maintain prolonged depression in phagocytosis. However, studies in our laboratory employing methyl palmitate indicated that when methyl palmitate is repeated at 5-day intervals the animals become refractory to subsequent injections of methyl palmitate so that it is impossible to maintain a prolonged and sustained depression of phagocytosis by methyl palmitate administration.

It is clear that the regulation of RE function by rather simple lipid moieties makes these lipids extremely valuable agents in exploring the effects of the RE system on a variety of immunological, metabolic, and other functional activities of the RES. Stuart *et al.* (1960a) also note the possibility that circulating blood lipids may exert a measure of control on RE activity; this point is as yet to be established.

Cooper and West (1962), in an attempt to evaluate the mechanisms of macrophage alteration by various lipids, developed an *in vitro* system to study the mechanism by which glyceryl trioleate stimulates macrophage activity. Peritoneal macrophages were found to be stimulated by the addition of glyceryl trioleate to the medium. The stimulation was found to be both time and dose dependent relative to the ability of peritoneal macrophages to ingest a variety of bacterial preparations. An enhanced capacity of peritoneal macrophages obtained from treated animals toward the phagocytosis of poorly opsonized bacterial organisms which normally are virtually resistant to phagocytosis by normal macrophages was also observed. These studies indicate that the extent of phagocytosis is not entirely dependent on the existence of circulating humoral recognition factors but may also be determined by certain unknown physiological or metabolic charactristics of the macrophage cells.

Cooper and West (1962) postulated that the stimulation of phagocytosis by triolein is undoubtedly related to the effect of triolein on macrophage cells, as exposure of the organisms to triolein either before or after opsonization did not increase the phagocytosis of bacteria by normal cells. These studies clearly indicate that the activity of triolein is related to the effects of the lipid on the macrophage population of cells rather than the particle or preparation which is undergoing phagocytosis. Cooper and West (1962) also noted that the triolein particles were phagocytized by peritoneal macrophages without prior serum treatment, that is, the triolein particles do not require opsonization per se; however, as noted by these investigators, one cannot establish whether or not cyto-opsonin or cell-bound opsonin was present on the macrophage cell itself which could opsonize the triolein particles directly or whether this particle, much like polystyrene latex and RE test lipid particles, does not require the presence of opsonins for phagocytosis.

The above-noted studies further substantiate the possibility that various lipids may well exert a modifying effect on macrophage cell activity. Stuart and Cooper (1963) also prepared suspensions employing Tween

20, glyceryl tricaprate, or 2-oleodistearin with an average particle size of 4 to 12 μ and 4 to 18 μ respectively. Stuart and Cooper (1963) observed that glyceryl tricaprate resulted in RE stimulation which persisted for approximately 3 days. In contrast, the 2-oleodistearin produced a biphasic response in which 5- to 20-mg injected doses in mice produced stimulation, while larger doses resulted in unaltered activity. The evaluation of the time response indicated that the depression of activity observed shortly after the administration of 2-oleodistearin was followed at 1 day by normal activity and in a subsequent increase in activity for a 4- or 5-day period. These studies stress the importance of dose responses in the analysis of lipid agents which modify RE function. The authors postulated that the biphasic response was probably related to initial saturation of the macrophage cell with lipid and the associated recovery was due to the metabolism of lipid moiety. Studies in the author's laboratory do not support the concept of lipid-induced cell saturation as a factor in lipid-induced RE alteration (Blickens and Di Luzio, 1965).

Stuart and Cooper (1963) note that glyceryl tricaprate is less toxic than triolein and was well tolerated in experimental animals, despite heterogeneity of the particle size. Histological studies indicate that the hyperphagocytic state induced by tricapratin occurs in the absence of any granulatomous or plasma cell reactions. Biozzi *et al.* (1963) reported that the stimulatory effect of glyceryl trioleate could be maintained for 20 days or more as long as the injections are continued, while ethyl stearate significantly decreased the phagocytic activity of the RES for periods of 25 days if injections are repeated at 4-day intervals. Surprisingly, our studies indicate an inability to maintain the methyl palmitate-induced impairment in phagocytic function when methyl palmitate is administered at 5-day intervals.

Biozzi *et al.* (1963) demonstrated that the distribution of ^{131}I-labeled glyceryl trioleate was principally in liver, with lung and spleen showing very moderate localization of the emulsion. Histological observations of liver of rats treated with triolein showed an enhanced localization of colloidal carbon in Kupffer cells. Thus, the stimulation of the RES induced by triolein is accompanied by a great increase in the number of Kupffer cells in the liver. Cooper and Houston (1964) showed that triolein-treated peritoneal macrophage cell populations contain significantly greater numbers of phagocytizing macrophage cells than normal populations of cells. They observed that a certain percentage of peritoneal macrophage cells are immediately capable of phagocytosis. This percentage has been estimated to be approximately 40% of the peritoneal macrophage populations. Functional changes occur in the remaining macrophage cell populations which are associated with the development of their phagocytic activity. It was impossible to distinguish whether the triolein stimulatory effect is related to the enhancement in the numbers of peritoneal macrophage cells which phagocytize, or to an enhanced ingestion of bacteria by those macrophage cells which already were involved in previous phagocytic events. Microscopic examinations tend to indicate that the enhancement in phagocytosis in triolein-treated cell populations is related to an increase in the number of phagocytically active cells. Thus, triolein may function as an activating agent to induce the transition of a resting macrophage cell to an active macrophage cell in the presence of ingested particulate materials. In essence, triolein confers, as Cooper and Houston (1964) express it, "a possibility of phagocytic maturity that conceivably is related to changes in morphological, biochemical and/or physical-chemical characteristics of the individual cell." The mechanism by which a simple lipid like triolein can produce phagocytic maturity is currently unanswered.

In an attempt to extend these studies regarding the mechanism of action of triolein, the electrophoretic mobility of mouse peritoneal macrophages was studied (Cooper and Houston, 1964). It was found that the electrophoretic mobility of peritoneal macrophage cells declined rapidly during *in vitro* incubation. The cells derived from triolein-treated animals, in agreement with previous observations, possess significantly greater phagocytic activity than normal macrophage cell populations and also possess a greater electrophoretic mobility. The incubation of normal peritoneal macrophages, in Hank's solution in the presence of triolein, was associated with increased mobility of peritoneal macrophages. Maximal mobility was obtained with 20 μg of triolein per 10^6 cells which is similar in concentration to the amount of triolein which enhances phagocytic activity. Another observation made by these investigators (Cooper and Houston, 1964) was that the pronounced decrease in macrophage mobility which occurred when untreated macrophage cell populations were incubated for a 30-minute period was not observed when triolein was added to the incubation medium. The effect of triolein in altering the electrophoretic mobility of macrophages appeared to be specific to the macrophage cell, as human red cells which were exposed to triolein *in vitro* showed no alteration in electrophoretic mobility. These findings are suggestive of a lipid-induced alteration in the cellular membrane of the macrophage cell.

Lee and Cooper (1964) also conducted a series of biochemical studies which indicated that acid phosphatase activity of triolein-treated macrophages was not significantly different from that of control groups. These studies are in profound contrast to other types of RE stimulating agents which markedly increase acid phosphatase activity of macrophages. In addition, the respiratory activity of triolein-treated macrophage cells or macrophage cells derived from triolein-treated animals was not significantly different from normal cells. The addition of opsonized bacteria produced an early and rapid increase in respiratory activity of control macrophages which was comparable to that observed in the triolein-treated macrophage populations.

Carr and Williams (1967), attempting to determine the cellular basis of RE stimulation with glyceryl trioleate, undertook autoradiographic and electron microscopic studies. In agreement with the previous observations of Lee and Cooper (1964), no increase in acid phosphatase activity was observed when peritoneal macrophages were incubated in the presence of triolein; however, it was observed that there was an increase in the length of macrophage cell processes induced by triolein. The extended processes of the macrophages persisted for several days and could be induced by repeated contact with triolein particles. The *in vitro* incubation of macrophage cells with tritiated trioleate indicated the localization of the tritiated label on the surface of the cell in the area of the prominent cell membrane processes as well as in the nuclei and other cell organelles (Williams and Carr, 1968).

In agreement with the observations of Cooper and Stuart (1962), the studies of Carr (1968; Williams and Carr, 1968) indicate a direct stimulation of macrophages with triolein which relates to a change in the surface configuration of the cell. The high concentration of labeled lipids in the extended cell processes of the macrophage cell suggests the direct action of the lipid on the macrophage cell surface. Since glyceryl trioleate also enters the macrophage in considerable amounts and is actively metabolized by the macrophage, the possibility of an intracellular event to induce cell stimulation cannot be excluded. Since the composition of certain intracellular radioactive lipids was closely related to that of the administered lipid, and since surface lipases were not demonstrated in macrophage cells, it is possible that the ingested lipid enters in intact form. Indeed, relatively large particles of lipid were found existing within the cytoplasm (Williams and Carr, 1968).

Since lipids offer a convenient means for chemically controlling reticuloendothelial activity, studies were undertaken by Di Luzio and Blickens (1966) to evaluate the relationship of a variety of lipids on reticuloendothelial activity. Relative to the reticuloendothelial stimulatory lipids, triolein was the only lipid which induced a stimulatory influence on reticuloendothelial function as reflected by colloidal carbon.

Whether circulating or tissue lipids can exert a pronounced effect on reticuloendothelial activity remains to be established. However, it is suggested by the above observations of particulate lipids exerting a regulatory role on reticuloendothelial functions, that plasma lipids may conceivably influence the activity of the RE system. Indeed, the present difficulty in defining the mechanism of control relative to RE function may well reside in the possibility that the RES is controlled by circulating lipids, possibly due to their particulate nature. While further efforts are essential to define this possibility, there is little question that various intravenous artificial lipid preparations do offer unique means to chemically regulate and modulate certain functional activities of the reticuloendothelial system.

VIII. Modification of Endotoxin Responses by Lipids

The observations that endotoxins, which were administered intravenously, are rapidly removed from the circulation and accumulate in liver and spleen (Braude et al., 1958; Di Luzio and Crafton, 1969) suggest the importance of the reticuloendothelial system (RES) in endotoxemia. There is little question today that endotoxin preparations are indeed phagocytized by macrophage cells. The endotoxin preparations themselves have a very pronounced stimulatory activity on the RES (Biozzi et al., 1955; Benacerraf and Sebestyen, 1957; Filkins and Di Luzio, 1967, 1969) and indeed, resistance to endotoxin has been considered to develop on the basis of the stimulatory effect of endotoxin on the RES (Zweifach et al., 1957). Studies indicate that resistance of animals to the pyrogenic and lethal effects of bacterial endotoxins is largely dependent upon the state of the RES (Beeson, 1947a; Benacerraf et al., 1959; Crafton and Di Luzio, 1969; Di Luzio and Crafton, 1970; Lemperle, 1966; Suter et al., 1958). Thus, stimulation of the RES with nonlethal doses of bacterial lipopolysaccharides results in protection of the animal against the subsequent lethal dose of endotoxin. So-called "blockade" of the RES by a variety of colloidal particles such as saccharated iron oxide, thorotrast, and trypan blue were found to increase the sensitivity of animals to toxic effects of endotoxin (Beeson, 1947a,b).

More recent studies have indicated that under certain circumstances it is possible to produce an enhancement of phagocytic activity and yet induce extreme sensitivity to the lethal effects of endotoxin. Cooper and Stuart (1961) studied the influence of triolein stimulation and ethyl stearate depression of the RES on endotoxin toxicity in mice. Triolein, which induced a hyperphagocytic state of the RES, rendered mice significantly more susceptible to endotoxin effects, while ethyl stearate did not appreciably enhance susceptibility to endotoxin.

Subsequently, Stuart and Cooper (1962) reported additional details of the influence of RE stimulatory and depressive lipids on endotoxin responsiveness. Glycerol trioleate, which activated the RES as denoted by enhanced vascular clearance of colloidal carbon, also enhanced the vascular clearance of chromium-labeled endotoxin. During initial states of RE activation, the animals were found to be hypersensitive to the lethal effects of endotoxin. In ethyl stearate-treated animals, no alteration in endotoxin susceptibility was observed (Stuart and Cooper, 1962). The ethyl stearate-treated animals manifested a decreased number of Kupffer cells in contrast to the increased number of Kupffer cells which were found in triolein-treated animals. These investigators concluded that phagocytosis per se is of relatively little importance in resistance to endotoxin. More important than the modification of endotoxemia by possible changes in phagocytosis may be the possible ability of RE modifying agents to alter macrophage intracellular detoxification mechanisms. It is quite obvious that the influence of a variety of RE lipid modifying agents on intracellular metabolic, digestive, and killing abilities of the macrophage is as yet to be elucidated.

Previous studies from the author's laboratory have indicated that heparin, which can enhance phagocytic activity (Filkins and Di Luzio, 1966b), also modifies endotoxin responses (Filkins and Di Luzio, 1968). The administration of heparin, either prior to, or at early intervals after endotoxin administration reduced the endotoxin-induced lethality. These findings suggested that modification of RE activity, in a manner as yet undefined, by agents which influence macrophage function, can profoundly alter endotoxin-induced lethality.

Since methyl palmitate is an effective RES depressant, studies were undertaken by Crafton and Di Luzio (1969) to evaluate the influence of selective chemical-induced RES depression induced by methyl palmitate on endotoxin-induced lethality. Surprisingly, it was found that the administration of methyl palmitate prior to endotoxin administration induced profound resistance to lethal and indeed superlethal doses of endotoxin (Table XIII). These studies indicated that there is a disassociation between the phagocytic act per se and alterations in endotoxin lethality.

In an effort to evaluate whether or not a plasma factor was present in methyl palmitate-treated animals which conferred host resistance to endotoxin preparations, plasma from methyl palmitate-treated animals was administered to normal animals prior to administration of endotoxin. No effect was manifested when plasma was transferred from methyl palmitate-treated animals to normal animals relative to endotoxin lethality, suggesting that the protective effect of methyl palmitate is not mediated by a plasma humoral factor.

Table XIII

MODIFICATION OF LETHALITY TO INTRAVENOUSLY ADMINISTERED *Salmonella enteritidis* ENDOTOXIN IN METHYL PALMITATE-INDUCED RE-DEPRESSED RATS[a]

Group	Endotoxin[b] dose (mg/100 gm body wt)	Number of rats	Percent mortality[c]
Normal	0.5	8	38
Control (Tween)	0.5	12	0
Methyl palmitate	0.5	12	0
Normal	0.75	10	60*
Control (Tween)	0.75	11	0
Methyl palmitate	0.75	13	0
Normal	1.00	10	70*
Control (Tween)	1.00	10	30
Methyl palmitate	1.00	12	0
Normal	1.50	11	100*
Control (Tween)	1.50	11	91*
Methyl palmitate	1.50	11	9
Normal	2.00	10	100*
Control (Tween)	2.00	30	74*
Methyl palmitate	2.00	21	14
Normal	3.00	9	100*
Control (Tween)	3.00	10	80
Methyl palmitate	3.00	10	0

[a] From Crafton and Di Luzio (1969).

[b] *Salmonella enteritidis* endotoxin was suspended in pyrogen-free saline and adminis- tered via the dorsal vein of the penis. Methyl palmitate was suspended in Tween 20 and in dextrose-in-water solution and injected 48 and 24 hours prior to endotoxin.

[c] The percent mortality in the groups marked with an asterisk is significantly ($P <$ 0.025) greater than the death rate in the methyl palmitate group which received the same dose of endotoxin.

The striking protective influence of methyl palmitate administration on endotoxin lethality, which occurs in the association of a selective chemical-induced depression in reticuloendothelial phagocytosis, ap- pears to be in direct contrast to the past findings of Beeson (1947a) on the influence of so-called particle-induced depression and subsequent enhancement in endotoxin lethality. Beeson initially reported that the functional state of the reticuloendothelial system was a determining fac- tor in the extent of the endotoxin-induced injury. He speculated that in the presence of RE-induced depression, which was induced by the ad- ministration of particulates such as Thorotrast, endotoxin would continue to circulate for a greater period of time in the blood and thus exert its deleterious effect on the body before it was cleared from the vascular system by RE cells. More recently, Fisher (1967) reported that endotoxin labeled with ^{131}I was removed more rapidly in the "RE blockaded" rabbits and mice than in normal animals and proposed that the sensitivity of "RE blockaded" animals to endotoxin was a function of delay in cellular disposal of endotoxin and not delayed phagocytosis of the endotoxin preparation from the vascular compartment.

In evaluating the mechanism by which methyl palmitate-induced RE alterations alter endotoxin lethality, studies were undertaken by Di Luzio and Crafton (1969) on the influence of methyl palmitate administration on the vascular clearance and tissue distribution of ^{51}Cr-labeled *Salmonella enteritidis* endotoxin in rats which received methyl palmitate. The vascular clearance of the labeled endotoxin preparation was found to be biphasic consisting of an early, or fast, component and a slow component (Table XIV). The RES-depressing agent, methyl palmitate, exerted essentially no influence on the vascular clearance of labeled endotoxin, but did significantly decrease splenic uptake. In general, these studies, which also employed other RE modifying agents which alter endotoxin lethality in varying directions, did not reveal any association between the vascular clearance and/or tissue distribution of the labeled endotoxin and lethality. These findings suggest the possibility of a macrophage-mediated cellular response to endotoxemia which is altered in methyl palmitate-treated animals and is the major determinant of endotoxin-induced lethality. The precise cellular response in endotoxemia, be it the detoxification potential of the macrophage cell and/or the lysosomal enzyme activities of the macrophage cell, remains to be ascertained.

Table XIV

VASCULAR CLEARANCE AND TISSUE DISTRIBUTION OF ^{51}Cr-LABELED *Salmonella enteritidis* ENDOTOXIN IN TWEEN AND METHYL PALMITATE-TREATED RATS[a,b]

| | Intravascular t/2 (minutes) | | Tissue activity | | | | | |
| | Fast component | Slow component | Liver | | Lung | | Spleen | |
Treatment			%ID/ gm	%ID/ TO	%ID/ gm	%ID/ TO	%ID/ gm	%ID/ TO
Tween	18.3 ±0.7	85.3 ±8.5	3.9 ±0.57	28.7 ±4.42	2.1 ±0.14	3.7 ±0.34	5.6 ±0.73	3.5 ±0.25
Methyl palmitate	21.3 ±2.0	67.0 ±3.3	2.7 ±0.15	24.4 ±1.70	2.4 ±0.23	4.1 ±0.30	0.8 ±0.22	0.6 ±0.13

[a] From Di Luzio and Crafton (1969).

[b] Values, expressed as means ± SE, are derived from 6 Tween control and 8 methyl palmitate-treated rats. The tissue distribution data are expressed as percentage of injected dose per gram of wet weight (%ID/gm) and total organ (%ID/TO).

Table XV

MODIFICATION OF TOURNIQUET SHOCK MORTALITY IN RATS BY METHYL
PALMITATE PRETREATMENT

Group	Tourniquet duration[a]	Number of rats	Percent mortality[b]
Normal	4	25	36
Tween	4	26	27
Methyl palmitate	4	22	73
Normal	6	22	59
Tween	6	18	56
Methyl palmitate	6	19	84
Normal	8	22	73
Tween	8	12	83
Methyl palmitate	8	21	95

[a] Rubber bands were applied to both hind limbs and released 4, 6, or 8 hours after application.
[b] Mortality was calculated 24 hours after tourniquet release.

In contrast to the protective effect of methyl palmitate on endotoxin shock, a detrimental effect of methyl palmitate-induced RE suppression was observed in the tourniquet shock model (Table XV) (Trejo et al., 1971). The percent mortality was increased approximately 60% when tourniquets were applied for 4–8 hours. The mechanism of this differential sensitivity of methyl palmitate-treated animals to endotoxin and tourniquet shock is presently unknown.

IX. Role of Intravenous Lipids in Modifying Infectious Processes

In 1925, Nakahara reported that rabbits which received interperitoneal injections of olive oil survived fatal doses of staphylococci and pneumococci. Triolein-treated mice also manifested increased resistance to bacterial infection with *Diplococcus pneumoniae* (Cooper and Stuart, 1962). Cooper and Stuart (1962) studied the susceptibility of mice to pneumococcal infection following the administration of either ethyl stearate or triolein. Depression of the RE activity with ethyl stearate did not influence the course of infection following the administration of *Diplococcus pneumoniae*, while triolein administration exerted marked protective ability on the infectious processes. The duration of protection was a maximum of 3 days after triolein and the protective effect was lost the fifth day. These events essentially coincided with the changes in phagocytic activity.

Phagocytic alterations during pneumococcal infection were pronouncedly enhanced in triolein-treated mice when compared to normal mice, as well as those which received ethyl stearate (Cooper and Stuart, 1962). Phagocytic capacity decreased markedly as the animals reached terminal stages of their infection. Surprisingly, changes in total white cell counts did not reflect any alteration in susceptibility of the animals to the bacterial agent, suggesting a predominant fixed macrophage cellular response. While ethyl stearate administration did not modify the blood concentration of pneumococci during the infectious state, the triolein-treated groups showed decreased levels of pneumococci and manifested an enhanced ability to remove bacteria from the vascular system.

Cooper and Stuart (1962) observed that ethyl stearate could reduce the phagocytic activity of mice that were previously treated with triolein. Under these conditions, the protective effect of triolein, in respect to pneumococci infection, was lost. Thus, there is an apparent correlation between level of phagocytic activity at the time of the administration of bacteria and survival rates.

Lavelle and Starr (1969) studied the pathogenicity of mouse hepatitis virus (MHV-1) in mice following the intraperitoneal administration of triolein. Significant protection, as denoted by the extent of liver damage, was observed in triolein-treated mice which received intraperitoneal injections of MHV-1. Cortisone suppression of RES function and enhancement in virus-induced hepatic injury could be modified by triolein administration.

Nakahara (1925) reported that mice which received intraperitoneal injections of olive oil were significantly protected against pneumococci, and this protection was associated with pronounced phagocytosis of the bacterial organisms. Cooper (1965) subsequently investigated the influence of triolein on *Klebsiella pneumoniae* infection. Significant resistance to *K. pneumoniae* infection was observed following triolein administration. Analysis of the number of organisms found in the peritoneal cavity during the course of infection revealed significant decreases in triolein-treated animals. Likewise, the number of viable organisms in blood was markedly decreased in the triolein-treated group suggesting a very pronounced impairment in multiplication of the infectious organisms. The number of polymorphonuclear and mononuclear cells in the peritoneum of triolein-treated animals was greatly increased. However, in studies where normal macrophage cells were administered to animals which were challenged with *K. pneumoniae* organisms, cell transfer studies did not indicate a significant modification in lethality resulting from the bacterial challenge. These studies do not suggest an enhanced activity of triolein macrophages toward either phagocytosis of the bacterial organisms or to the killing process itself. In view of these observations, Cooper (1965) also evaluated the relative participation of a humoral component in lipid-induced protection against *Klebsiella* infection and found that the opsonic activity of serum collected from trioleintreated animals was notably enhanced in contrast to that of the normal group. These studies suggest that triolein may act as a potent adjuvant, causing significant antibody production or that it is able to enhance opsonin formation in some as yet undefined manner. The role of endotoxins in modifying humoral factors in blood was also emphasized in the studies of Filkins and Di Luzio (1968).

X. Influence of Intravenously Administered Lipids on the Immune Response

The theory of phagocytosis as proposed by Metchnikoff contributed greatly to the appreciation of immunology by stressing the importance of phagocytosis in the protection of the organism from a variety of disease states.

There is little question today that in the chronological order of cellular involvement in the immune reaction the macrophage is the initial cell. Since lipids can so profoundly modify phagocytosis, Di Luzio's group studied the influence of intravenously administered methyl palmitate on the primary and secondary immune response of animals to particulate antigens, that is, sheep red blood cells. It was found (Wooles and Di Luzio, 1963; Di Luzio and Wooles, 1964) that the administration of methyl palmitate, which markedly reduced reticuloendothelial cell phagocytosis, was associated with a significant depression in both the primary and secondary immune response (Table XVI). Subsequently, Stuart and Davidson (1964) studied the effect of both stimulation and depression of the RES induced by various lipid moieties on the production of antibodies to foreign red cells. They observed that the administration of glycerol trioleate, which greatly stimulated the activity of RES, did not modify the production of antibody when the antigen was given 24 or 72 hours after the administration of the lipid emulsion. That is, antibody formation was not enhanced at the time of maximal stimulation of phagocytic activity. More importantly, profound depression of the RES which was induced by cholesterol oleate administration in emulsified form was associated with a significant reduction in antibody formation if the antigen was administered during the period of RE depression. It was postu-

Table XVI

PRIMARY AND SECONDARY HEMOLYSIN RESPONSE IN
RETICULOENDOTHELIAL-DEPRESSED MICE[a]

	Primary[b]		Secondary	
Group	Log$_2$ titer	1 : Titer	Log$_2$ titer	1 : Titer
Tween	7.17 ± 0.29	$1:198 \pm 45$	7.23 ± 0.18	$1:192 \pm 18$
Methyl palmitate	3.27 ± 0.61	$1:18 \pm 4$	4.53 ± 0.75	$1:52 \pm 4$

[a] From Di Luzio and Wooles (1964).

[b] Values expressed as means $\pm$ SE. Primary response evaluated 7 days after initial injection of sheep cells. Secondary titer evaluated 7 days after second injection of sheep erythrocytes.

lated by Stuart and Davidson (1964) that the reduction of immunological responsiveness in cholesterol oleate-treated animals might be due to a diminished uptake of the antigen by immunocompetent cells because of alteration in cell receptors or cell uptake of the antigen due to the saturation of the macrophages with the lipid preparations. Indeed, histological sections showed considerable accumulation of lipid in various portions of the spleen.

In agreement with the observations with cholesterol oleate, the administration of methyl palmitate before or shortly after antigen administration also caused a reduction in antibody formation which paralleled the inhibition of phagocytic function. Large doses of the methyl palmitate preparations induced extensive splenic necrosis which may well relate to the reduction in antibody formation. Indeed, previous studies by Di Luzio *et al.* (1964) demonstrated that the removal of the spleen results in total inhibition of antibody formation following the intravenous administration of sheep red blood cells. The studies of Stuart and Davidson (1964) further confirm the importance of the macrophage in immune response and indeed the macrophage currently can be considered as the afferent limb of the immune reflex arc.

In studying the manner by which ethyl palmitate suppresses reticuloendothelial function, Buchanan and MacGregor (1964) studied the administration of ethyl palmitate on the vascular clearance of chromium-labeled foreign blood cells, as well as hemoglobin. These studies, as well as others, indicated that ethyl palmitate administration induced extensive splenic necrosis. The vascular clearance of labeled red cells was greatly diminished in ethyl palmitate-treated animals. Indeed, half-times increased approximately eightfold in the ethyl palmitate group. The impairment in phagocytosis was associated with a decrease in both spleen and liver uptake. It is interesting to note that hemoglobin, which was cleared from the vascular system at a rapid rate, was not altered by ethyl palmitate administration, suggesting either that soluble antigens are not removed by macrophage cells or that agents which profoundly altered RE function to particulate antigens need not manifest a similar behavior toward soluble antigens.

Buchanan and MacGregor (1964) pointed out that there is a need for a simple, safe method for widespread depression of phagocytic function in clinical medicine. It may well be that certain lipid substances may provide practical therapeutic measures through their ability to either stimulate or depress the RES.

That the fatty acid ester-induced destruction of the spleen need not be associated with depression of phagocytic activity or impaired immune response induced by fatty acid esters is obvious from the studies of Di Luzio and Wooles (1964). These investigators demonstrated that the intravenous administration of methyl palmitate, which resulted in depression of phagocytic activity of the reticuloendothelial system, did not destroy RE cellular elements or induce altered numbers of hepatic or splenic red cells. These studies also indicated that when BSP retention in plasma was evaluated in methyl palmitate-treated animals in an effort to evaluate hepatic parenchymal cell activity, normal parenchymal cell function was manifested, suggesting that methyl palmitate exerts an exclusive action on Kupffer cells.

A severe depression of phagocytic activity of the RES, induced by methyl palmitate at the time of injection of foreign sheep red cells, was associated with a marked decrease of primary hemolysin response (Table XVI). When compared to the control group, the degree of depression of antibody formation was approximately 95%. Similarly, a decreased antibody formation, which approximated 75% occurred in the secondary immune response. When these data were correlated with the observations of Swartzendruber et al. (1961), a single injection of methyl palmitate appeared equivalent in reducing antibody formation, following the administration of foreign red cells, to that of splenectomy combined with lymphadenectomy and thymectomy. These studies (Di Luzio and Wooles, 1964) clearly indicate that methyl palmitate can be employed on an experimental basis in not only producing phagocytic impairment, but also in inducing an immune paralysis to particulate antigens. The reduced antibody formation which was observed with methyl palmitate was not associated with an alteration in total circulating leukocytes or in the percentage of lymphocytes in peripheral blood. Obviously, the employment of such chemical agents should greatly contribute to further understanding of the kinetics of the immune process and the role of the macrophage in immune events as well as the further evaluation of the physiopathology of the reticuloendothelial system.

Table XVII
BLOOD CLEARANCE OF ^{51}Cr-LABELED SHEEP ERYTHROCYTES
IN RE-HYPOFUNCTIONAL MICE[a,b]

Group	Blood radioactivity[c]				Intravascular clearance t/2 (minutes)
	5 min	20 min	30 min	60 min	
Tween	81.9 ± 3.7	44.0 ± 3.7	28.0 ± 5.6	16.8 ± 5.3	16.5
Methyl palmitate	98.8 ± 3.3	95.8 ± 4.9	86.0 ± 2.5	81.5 ± 4.8	209

[a] From Morrow and Di Luzio (1965b).
[b] Values expressed as means ± standard error.
[c] Expressed as percent of injected dose per total blood volume.

In studying the mechanism by which methyl palmitate induced a depression of immunological phenomena, Morrow and Di Luzio (1965b) studied the fate of chromium-labeled foreign red cells in mice with altered RE function. It was demonstrated that RE depression induced by methyl palmitate administration was associated with a marked decrease in the vascular clearance of chromium-labeled sheep red blood cells (Table XVII) due to a failure of phagocytosis by both Kupffer cells and splenic macrophages (Table XVIII). These findings denote that alterations in RE function induced by methyl palmitate, as related to changes in antibody formation, are associated with at least two events: an alteration in vascular clearance of the particulate antigenic material and the organ distribution of the foreign cell. These studies also demonstrated the ability to transplant heterologous red cells by depression of the macrophage population.

Ohbuchi (1968) reported that methyl palmitate suppressed antibody formation against bovine serum albumin. As noted in our previous studies, Ohbuchi confirmed the observation that lymph nodes and hematopoietic structures were unaltered by methyl palmitate administration.

Table XVIII
DISTRIBUTION OF ^{51}Cr-LABELED SHEEP ERYTHROCYTES IN
RE-HYPOFUNCTIONAL MICE[a,b]

Group	Time: 1 hr		Time: 24 hr	
	Tween	Methyl palmitate	Tween	Methyl palmitate
Liver	37.4 ± 4.3	7.7 ± 0.5	24.1 ± 2.0	35.8 ± 2.0
Lung	3.3 ± 0.6	4.8 ± 0.2	0.3 ± 0.02	4.6 ± 1.2
Spleen	10.3 ± 1.8	0.6 ± 0.1	8.9 ± 0.9	3.2 ± 0.5

[a] From Morrow and Di Luzio (1965b).
[b] Values, as percent of injected dose per organ, are expressed as means ± standard error.

Ohbuchi (1968) suggested the possibility that saturated lipids such as methyl palmitate and ethyl stearate may be incorporated into the cell membrane, resulting in a "rigid cell membrane." Triolein, as an unsaturated lipid, would permit greater flexibility of the membrane, enhancing the process of phagocytosis by increasing the engulfing process. This concept is not supported by the metabolism which methyl palmitate undergoes when it is administered (Blickens and Di Luzio, 1965) nor is it suggested by the fact that fatty acid esters of unsaturated fatty acids are also depressant compounds (Di Luzio and Blickens, 1966). The macrophage impairing activity, however, may well reside in its ability to induce changes in the cell receptor to which the particle and its opsonin is complexed prior to the phagocytic event.

Frei *et al.* (1965) have reported that the fraction of the antigen which is susceptible to the phagocytic event induces the immune response while the nonphagocytizable fraction induces tolerance. These studies indicate that modification in the phagocytic event would change antibody formation, as indeed, it has been previously demonstrated (Wooles and Di Luzio, 1963). In essential support of this concept, Schoenberg *et al.* (1964) demonstrated the direct cytoplasmic connection between macrophages and potential antibody forming cells. By such a direct cytoplasmic connection, the transfer of cytoplasmic substance, possibly processed antigen, from macrophage to cells of the lymphocytic series could be achieved. Thus, it is possible that in RE depression a failure in phagocytosis or in an intracellular processing event also results in a depression of transfer of the processed antigen from the macrophages to antibody forming cells. The ability to alter phagocytic activity may be an important initial step in altering the immune response. Indeed, the chromium-labeled red blood cell data of Morrow and Di Luzio (1965a,b) suggest a significant inhibition of antigen processing by the macrophage cell itself by methyl palmitate administration. These findings again clearly demonstrate that methyl palmitate and other lipids have the ability to influence the fate of particulate antigens, through their modifying effect on the behavior of macrophages, thereby ultimately determining the response of the immune system.

XI. Influence of Intravenously Administered Lipids on Transplantation Reactions

The RES, which has been considered as one of the most important sources of protection which the host possesses against a variety of pathogenic invaders, plays a major function in transplantation reactions. The reactions of the macrophage against foreign tissues or cells is essentially similar to its reactions against pathogenic organisms. Indeed, one of the principal roles of antibody is to react with an antigen so that the antigen-antibody complex is removed by a phagocytic mechanism at a more rapid rate, thereby reducing the degree of antigen-induced injury. Thus, the process of discriminative phagocytosis plays a major role in systemic defenses against foreign agents.

In studying the response of an altered functional state of the RES to the acceptability of xenogenetic or allogenic bone marrow cells which were transplanted into lethally irradiated mice, Wooles and Di Luzio (1962) initially demonstrated that a relationship existed between RE status at the time of transplantation and the acceptance of foreign bone marrow transplants. Subsequently, Wooles and Di Luzio (1964) indicated a relationship between the activity of the RES at the time of transplantation and survival of lethally irradiated mice which received allogenic bone marrow. More recent studies by our group (Table XIX) revealed that methyl palmitate administration induced a 63% prolongation in survival time of allogenic skin grafts.

Relative to selective chemical modification of the reticuloendothelial system on transplantation reactions, studies were undertaken of the influence of RE cell depression on the classical graft-versus-host reaction (Simonsen, 1962). The graft-versus-host (GVH) reaction can be induced by the injection of F_1 hybrid mice with immunocompetent cells derived from the parent strain. Previous studies have demonstrated that during the period of graft-versus-host reaction, a pronounced hypersplenism occurs (Simonsen, 1962; Howard, 1964). An increase in phagocytic activity also characterized the GVH reaction (Howard, 1964; Di Luzio, 1967). These events have provided a convenient, effective, and reproducible assay of the graft-versus-host reaction. The depression of the functional state of the reticuloendothelial system of the host did not influence the development of the graft-versus-host reaction; however, the administration of spleen cells derived from RE-depressed donor mice resulted in normal phagocytic activity and in reduced splenomegaly

Table XIX

ENHANCED ACCEPTANCE OF SKIN HOMOGRAFTS BY METHYL
PALMITATE ADMINISTRATION

Group	Number	Average survival time (days)
Control	6	12.6
Methyl palmitate	11	20.6

(Di Luzio, 1967). These studies suggested that modification of reticulo-endothelial function of animals which serve as lymphoid cell donors is associated with corresponding alteration in the immunological capabilities of the transplanted spleen cells. Thus, methyl palmitate not only alters phagocytic function and immunological responsiveness of the animals, but also modifiies the immune competency of splenic lymphoid cells. Thus, the modification of donor lymphoid cell by agents which affect the reticuloendothelial system was proposed by Di Luzio to be effective in the control of transplantation reactions such as the graft versus-host response. Indeed, it was postulated that the technique of modification of RE donor cell activity to alter the severity and the nature of the transplantation reaction may be of value in the ultimate control of the variety of transplantation response.

In an effort to evaluate the hypothesis that transplantation should be readily effected in methyl palmitate-treated mice, the transplantation of either a lymphosarcoma or adenocarcinoma from C3H mice to control and Re-depressed C3H or incompatible C57BL mice was conducted (Di Luzio, 1965). Phagocytic activity and tumor and organ weights were determined at 0–5–10–15 days following transplantation. While phago-cytic depression did not influence the initial growth of the lymphosar-coma in C3H mice, the methyl palmitate-treated mice had significantly greater tumors at 15 days. Incompatible C57BL mice manifested com-plete rejection of both tumors. However, in the methyl palmitate-depressed mice, gross and histological evidence indicated tumor accept-ance in all instances. These studies denote that depression of phagocytic and immunological response by a simple fatty acid ester effectively pro-motes the transplantation of foreign neoplastic cells.

Subsequently, Di Luzio (1968) demonstrated that the enhanced phagocytic activity which characterized the graft-versus-host reaction is due to an increase in hepatic localization of an RE test lipid emulsion. Surprisingly, although profound splenomegaly was manifested in the graft-versus-host response, the splenic and pulmonary uptake of the test colloid was significantly reduced, denoting that neither the splenic nor the pulmonary macrophage cells contribute to the enhanced phagocytic state. These studies clearly demonstrated that in evaluating altered RE responses, tissue distribution data become an essential part in the inter-pretation of altered vascular rates.

Kauffman et al. (1967) employed methyl palmitate as an RE depres-sant and utilized second set renal transplants as an assay for homograft sensitization. These investigators demonstrated that methyl palmitate treatment considerably inhibited homograft rejection. Comparison of methyl palmitate with azathioprine and local graft radiation indicated that methyl palmitate is as effective in preventing sensitization to renal homografts as azathioprine or radiation. It is entirely possible, in view of the pronounced and rather exclusive RES-modifying activity of particulate lipids, that further use of lipids in modifying RES function will not only contribute to defining the physiopathology of the RES but be of benefit in resolving transplantation reactions.

XII. Summary

The reticuloendothelial system (RES) is a fundamental host-defense system of the body. It plays a major role in defense of the host against bacterial, viral, and parasitic infections, in part by its role as the afferent limb of the immune reflex arc as well as its expression of intracellular killing. The RES is also involved in neoplasia, transplantation, inflammation, and host response to traumatic, hemorrhagic, endotoxic, and burn shock. In view of its multifacet expression and its unique anatomical localization, the further delineation of the role of the RES to the well-being of the host requires that specific chemical agents be developed which have the ability to selectively enhance or depress the functional expression of this unique system. This review considers the very unusual property of a variety of intravenously administered lipid preparations to either enhance or impair the homeostatic expression of the RES in a variety of physiological and pathological responses. The employment of lipids has and will continue to facilitate the delineation of the role of macrophage cells in cellular and humoral immunity. The extremely diverse effects of intravenously administered lipids on RES function including its phagocytic, metabolic, and immunologic activity will continue to stimulate investigative studies into the role of RES in body economy. On the basis of current knowledge, it can be anticipated that lipids will be of potential value in enhancing host resistance to a variety of infectious agents, modulating inflammation and neoplasia, as well as altering transplantation events. The delineation of how diverse lipids modify RE function may also contribute to resolving the as yet unclarified mechanism of RES regulation.

ACKNOWLEDGMENTS

The studies of the author and colleagues have been supported, in part, by the Atomic Energy Commission, American Heart Association, American Cancer Society, National Institutes of Health, and the Edward Schleider Educational Foundation.

References

Aschoff, L. (1924). "Lecture on Pathology," pp. 1–33. Hoeber, New York.
Ashworth, C. T., Riggi, S. J., and Di Luzio, N. R. (1963). *Exp. Mol. Pathol. Suppl.* **1**, 83.
Beeson, P. B. (1947a). *J. Exp. Med.* **86**, 39.
Beeson, P. B. (1947b). *Proc. Soc. Exp. Biol. Med.* **64**, 146.
Benacerraf, B., and Sebestyen, M. M. (1957). *Fed. Amer. Soc. Exp. Biol.* **16**, 860.
Benacerraf, B., Thorbecke, G. J., and Jacoby, D. (1959). *Proc. Soc. Exp. Biol. Med.* **100**, 796.
Biozzi, G., Benacerraf, B., and Halpern, B. N. (1955). *Brit. J. Exp. Pathol.* **36**, 226.
Biozzi, G., Stiffel, C., and Mouton, D. (1963). *Rev. Fr. Etud. Clin. Biol.* **8**, 341.
Blickens, D. A., and Di Luzio, N. R. (1964). *J. Reticuloendothel. Soc.* **1**, 68.
Blickens, D. A., and Di Luzio, N. R. (1965). *J. Reticuloendothel. Soc.* **2**, 60.
Braude, A. I., Carey, F. J., Sutherland, D., and Zalesky, M. (1958). *J. Clin. Invest.* **34**, 850.
Buchanan, K. D., and MacGregor, R. F. (1964). *Brit. J. Exp. Pathol.* **45**, 248.
Carr, I. (1968). *Z. Zellforsch. Mikrosk. Anat.* **89**, 355.
Carr, I., and Williams, M. A. (1967). *Advan. Exp. Med. Biol.* **1**, 98.
Cooper, G. N. (1964). *J. Reticuloendothel. Soc.* **1**, 50.
Cooper, G. N. (1965). *J. Pathol. Bacteriol.* **89**, 665.
Cooper, G. N., and Houston, B. (1964). *Aust. J. Exp. Biol. Med. Sci.* **42**, 429.
Cooper, G. N., and Stuart, A. E. (1961). *Nature (London)* **191**, 295.
Cooper, G. N., and Stuart, A. E. (1962). *J. Pathol. Bacteriol.* **83**, 227.
Cooper, G. N., and West, D. (1962). *Aust. J. Exp. Biol. Med. Sci.* **40**, 485.
Crafton, C. G., and Di Luzio, N. R. (1969). *Amer. J. Physiol.* **217**, 736.
Di Luzio, N. R. (1965). *Fed. Proc. Fed. Amer. Soc. Exp. Biol.* **24**, 614.
Di Luzio, N. R. (1967). *J. Reticuloendothel. Soc.* **4**, 459.
Di Luzio, N. R. (1968). *J. Reticuloendothel. Soc.* **5**, 368.
Di Luzio, N. R., and Bierman, E. L. (1964). *Proc. Soc. Exp. Biol. Med.* **116**, 1045.
Di Luzio, N. R., and Blickens, D. A. (1966). *J. Reticuloendothel. Soc.* **3**, 250.
Di Luzio, N. R., and Crafton, C. G. (1969). *Proc. Soc. Exp. Biol. Med.* **132**, 686.
Di Luzio, N. R., and Crafton, C. G. (1970). *Advan. Exp. Med. Biol.* **9**, 27.
Di Luzio, N. R., and Riggi, S. J. (1964). *J. Reticuloendothel. Soc.* **1**, 136.
Di Luzio, N. R., and Riggi, S. J. (1967). *Advan. Exp. Med. Biol.* **1**, 382.
Di Luzio, N. R., and Wooles, W. R. (1964). *Amer. J. Physiol.* **206**, 939.
Di Luzio, N. R., Wooles, W. R., and Morrow, S. H. (1964). *J. Reticuloendothel. Soc.* **1**, 429.
Di Luzio, N. R., Salky, N. K., Riggi, S. J., and Ladman, A. J. (1965a). *Proc. Jap. Soc. Reticuloendothel. Syst.* **4**, 389.
Di Luzio, N. R., Salky, N. K., Riggi, S. J., and Ladman, A. J. (1965b). *In* "The Reticuloendothelial System," p. 389. Nissha Printing Co., Kyoto.
Di Luzio, N. R., Pisano, J. C., and Salky, N. K. (1971). *Advan. Exp. Med. Biol.* **15**, 373.
Filkins, J. P., and Di Luzio, N. R. (1966a). *Proc. Soc. Exp. Biol. Med.* **122**, 177.
Filkins, J. P., and Di Luzio, N. R. (1966b). *Proc. Soc. Exp. Biol. Med.* **122**, 548.
Filkins, J. P., and Di Luzio, N. R. (1967). *Proc. Soc. Exp. Biol. Med.* **125**, 908.
Filkins, J. P., and Di Luzio, N. R. (1968). *Amer. J. Physiol.* **214**, 1074.
Filkins, J. P., and Di Luzio, N. R. (1969). *J. Reticuloendothel. Soc.* **6**, 287.
Fisher, S. (1967). *Nature (London)* **213**, 511.

Frei, P. C., Benacerraf, B., and Thorbecke, G. J. (1965). *Proc. Nat. Acad. Sci. U. S.* **53**, 20.

Halpern, B. N. (1959). *J. Pharm. Pharmacol.* **11**, 321.

Hirsch, J. (1959). *Bacteriol. Rev.* **23**, 48.

Howard, J. G. (1964). *J. Reticuloendothel. Soc.* **1**, 29.

Jaffe, R. H. (1931). *Physiol. Rev.* **11**, 277.

Jaffe, R. H., and Berman, S. L. (1928). *Arch. Pathol. Lab. Med.* **5**, 1020.

Kauffman, H., Humphrey, L., Hanback, L., Davis, F., Madge, G., and Rittenbury, M. (1967). *Transplantation* **5**, 1217.

Ladman, A. J., Salky, N. K., and Di Luzio, N. R. (1963). *J. Appl. Physiol.* **34**, 2504.

Ladman, A. J., Salky, N. K., and Di Luzio, N. R. (1964). *J. Reticuloendothel. Soc.* **1**, 365.

Lavelle, G. C., and Starr, T. J. (1969). *Brit. J. Exp. Pathol.* **50**, 475.

Lee, A., and Cooper, G. N. (1964). *Aust. J. Exp. Biol. Med. Sci.* **42**, 725.

Lemperle, G. (1966). *Proc. Soc. Exp. Biol. Med.* **122**, 1012.

Mitchnikoff, E. (1905). "Immunity in Infective Diseases" (Engl. transl. by F. G. Binnie). Cambridge Univ. Press, London and New York.

Morrow, S. H., and Di Luzio, N. R. (1965a). *J. Reticuloendothel. Soc.* **2**, 355.

Morrow, S. H., and Di Luzio, N. R. (1965b). *Proc. Soc. Exp. Biol. Med.* **119**, 647.

Nakahara, W. (1925). *J. Exp. Med.* **42**, 201.

Nelson, D. S. (1969). "Macrophages and Immunity." North-Holland Publ., Amsterdam.

Ohbuchi, S. (1968). *Acta Med. Okayama* **22**, 137.

Pearsall, N. M., and Weiser, R. S. (1970). "The Macrophage." Lea & Febiger, Philadelphia, Pennsylvania.

Pisano, J. C., and Di Luzio, N. R. (1970a). *J. Reticuloendothel. Soc.* **7**, 386.

Pisano, J. C., and Di Luzio, N. R. (1970b). *Tulane Med.* **2**, 7.

Pisano, J. C., Filkins, J. P., and Di Luzio, N. R. (1968a). *Proc. Soc. Exp. Biol. Med.* **128**, 917.

Pisano, J. C., Patterson, J. T., and Di Luzio, N. R. (1968b). *Science* **162**, 565.

Pisano, J. C., Di Luzio, N. R., and Salky, N. K. (1970a). *J. Lab. Clin. Med.* **76**, 141.

Pisano, J. C., Salky, N. K., and Di Luzio, N. R. (1970b). *Nature (London)* **226**, 1049.

Riggi, S. J., and Di Luzio, N. R. (1961). *Fed. Proc. Fed. Amer. Soc. Exp. Biol.* **21**, 265.

Riggi, S. J., and Di Luzio, N. R. (1962). *Nature (London)* **193**, 1292.

Rowley, D. (1962). *Advan. Immunol.* **2**, 241.

Saba, T. M., and Di Luzio, N. R. (1965). *J. Reticuloendothel. Soc.* **2**, 437.

Saba, T. M., and Di Luzio, N. R. (1968). *Life Sci.* **7**, 337.

Saba, T. M., and Di Luzio, N. R. (1969a). *Amer. J. Physiol.* **216**, 197.

Saba, T. M., and Di Luzio, N. R. (1969b). *Amer. J. Physiol.* **216**, 910.

Saba, T. M., Filkins, J. P., and Di Luzio, N. R. (1966). *J. Reticuloendothel. Soc.* **3**, 398.

Saba, T. M., Filkins, J. P., and Di Luzio, N. R. (1967). *Proc. Soc. Exp. Biol. Med.* **125**, 630.

Salky, N. K., Di Luzio, N. R., P'Pool, B., and Sutherland, A. J. (1964). *J. Amer. Med. Ass.* **187**, 744.

Salky, N. K., Mills, D., and Di Luzio, N. R. (1965). *J. Lab. Clin. Med.* **66**, 952.

Salky, N. K., Di Luzio, N. R., Levin, A. G., and Goldsmith, H. S. (1967). *J. Lab. Clin. Med.* **70**, 393.

Saxl, P., and Donath, F. (1925). *Wien. Klin. Wochenschr.* **38,** 66.

Sbarra, A. J., and Karnovsky, M. C. (1959). *J. Biol. Chem.* **243,** 1355.

Schoenberg, M. D., Mumaw, V. R., Moore, R. D., and Weisberger, A. S. (1964). *Science* **143,** 964.

Shivas, A. A., and Fraser, G. P. (1959). *Nature* (*London*) **184,** 1813.

Simonsen, M. (1962). *Progr. Allergy* **6,** 349.

Smith, H. P. (1930a). *J. Exp. Med.* **51,** 379.

Smith, H. P. (1930b). *J. Exp. Med.* **51,** 395.

Stuart, A. E. (1960). *Lancet* ii, 896.

Stuart, A. E. (1962). *Nature* (*London*) **196,** 78.

Stuart, A. E. (1968). *J. Pathol. Bacteriol.* **96,** 401.

Stuart, A. E. (1970). "The Reticuloendothelial System." Livingstone, Edinburgh.

Stuart, A. E., and Cooper, G. N. (1962). *J. Pathol. Bacteriol.* **82,** 245.

Stuart, A. E., and Cooper, G. N. (1963). *Exp. Mol. Pathol.* **2,** 215.

Stuart, A. E., and Davidson, A. E. (1963). *Brit. J. Exp. Pathol.* **44,** 24.

Stuart, A. E., and Davidson, A. E. (1964). *J. Pathol. Bacteriol.* **87,** 305.

Stuart, A. E., Biozzi, G., Stiffel, C., Halpern, B. N., and Mouton, D. (1960a). *Brit. J. Exp. Pathol.* **41,** 599.

Stuart, A. E., Biozzi, G., Stiffel, C., Bernard, M., Halpern, B. N., and Mouton, D. (1960b). *C. R. Acad. Sci.* **250,** 2779.

Suter, E., Ullman, E. G., and Hoffman, R. G. (1958). *Proc. Soc. Exp. Biol. Med.* **99,** 167.

Swartzendruber, D. C., Bigelow, R. R., Congdon, C. C., and Makinodan, T. (1961). *Amer. J. Physiol.* **200,** 1272.

Trejo, R., Crafton, C. G., and Di Luzio, N. R. (1971). *J. Reticuloendothel. Soc.* **9,** 299.

Vaughn, R. B. (1965). *Brit. J. Exp. Pathol.* **46,** 71.

Waddell, W. R., Geyer, R. P., Clarke, E., and Stare, F. J. (1953). *Amer. J. Physiol.* **175,** 299.

Waddell, W. R., Geyer, R. P., Clarke, E., and Stare, F. J. (1954). *Amer. J. Physiol.* **177,** 90.

Williams, M. A., and Carr, I. (1968). *Exp. Cell. Res.* **51,** 196.

Wooles, W. R., and Di Luzio, N. R. (1962). *Amer. J. Physiol.* **203,** 404.

Wooles, W. R., and Di Luzio, N. R. (1963). *Science* **142,** 1078.

Wooles, W. R., and Di Luzio, N. R. (1964). *Proc. Soc. Exp. Biol. Med.* **115,** 756.

Wright, A. E., and Douglas, S. R. (1903). *Proc. Roy. Soc., London* **72,** 357.

Zweifach, B. W., Benacerraf, B., and Thomas, L. (1957). *J. Exp. Med.* **106,** 403.

Microsomal Enzymes of Sterol Biosynthesis

JAMES L. GAYLOR

*Section of Biochemistry and Molecular Biology and the Graduate
School of Nutrition, Cornell University, Ithaca, New York*

I. Introduction

This chapter is not a review of progress in sterol biosynthesis. Excellent review articles have been published. For example, see reviews by Clayton (1965), Olson (1965), Bloch (1965), Frantz and Schroepfer (1967), Sih and Whitlock (1968), Staunton (1969), and Yamamoto and Bloch (1970a). Furthermore, methods of great value to investigators of sterol biosynthesis were collected in a volume of *Methods in Enzymology* (Clayton, 1969). More specialized articles on methods may be helpful, such as the concise review by Frantz *et al.* (1969) that deals with the preparation of labeled sterols. Rather, this chapter deals specifically with only a narrow segment of methods that have been used to study sterol biosynthesis—the solubilization and purification of microsomal enzymes that catalyze the conversion of lanosterol to cholesterol (Fig. 1). As a result, the three very specific purposes of the chapter are: to place in sequence the position of enzymatic studies as part of the investigation of sterol biosynthesis; to provide experimental methods for solubilization and some of the reasons for choosing various methods in a study of a

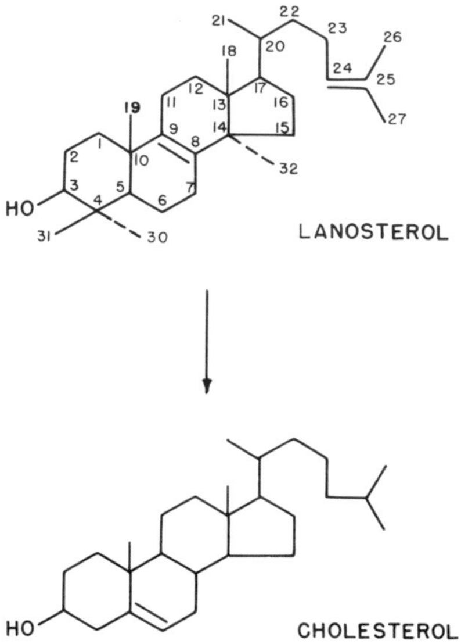

FIG. 1. Enzymatic conversion of lanosterol to cholesterol.

microsomal enzyme; and, most importantly, to convince the reader that investigation of microsomal enzymes has progressed satisfactorily in order to encourage others to carry out similar studies, even though they may have had little previous experience in this area.

This chapter is not a general, comprehensive compilation of methods used to solubilize particle-bound enzymes; this article deals with enzymes of sterol biosynthesis and closely related enzymatic processes. Many enzymes that are bound to other particles have been studied in detail. For example, some of the techniques described herein were taken primarily from analogous investigations of mitochondrial enzymes. More specifically, most of the methods described in this chapter have been used in the author's laboratory, and details about each method appropriately come from experience rather than from literature citations. Even at that, we were aware that a rather useless, sterile chapter might result because simply presenting methods without discussion would not be particularly useful, even to investigators in a closely related area. On the other hand, we have attempted to illustrate the progress of the solubilization of microsomal enzymes of sterol biosynthesis by including the mistakes (and, when possible, reasons for making them), negative results, and some of the extensive trials and errors that generally are omitted from published results. Thus, in a subsection below, in addition to a description of procedures, a narrative on the sequence of events in the investigation of methods used to solubilize one specific enzyme is included as an illustrative example (see Section II,B,4).[1]

Finally, this author agrees completely with the comment of Yamamoto, Lin, and Bloch (1969), that there are as yet no "standard procedures" of isolation[2] of microsomal enzymes. Accordingly, for any specific enzymatic study envisioned by the reader, at best this chapter may offer suggestions, but it certainly should not be considered a laboratory manual.

A. MICROSOMES AS ENZYMES

Microsomes are prepared by differential centrifugation of broken-cell preparations (for discussion, see Siekevitz, 1965). The microsomes result from cellular endoplasmic reticulum that has been shown to be the site of cholesterol biosynthesis in mammalian liver cells (Chesterton, 1968). The reticulum develops at early stages of fetal life but not all enzymatic, electron carrier, and lipid components are present in microsomes isolated from neonatal livers (Ernster and Orrenius, 1965). However, Chevallier (1964) presented convincing evidence that at the time of birth, 80 to 85% of the cholesterol is of fetal and not maternal origin. Thus, the full complement of microsomal enzymes of sterol biosynthesis is present in neonatal liver.

Various marker enzymes and pigments have been used to distinguish microsomes from preparations of other particles; in addition, similar investigations have shown that microsomal membranes may be distinguished from membranes of other cellular organelles (Brunner and

---

[1] Most of the experimental work reported herein has been supported by Research Grants AM-10767 and AM-04505 from the National Institute of Arthritis and Metabolic Diseases, G-19556 from the National Science Foundation, and by funds made available through the State University of New York. The author is very grateful for this decade af generous support. A preliminary report of this material was given in a symposium held in April, 1970, in connection with the Annual Meeting of the American Oil Chemists Society (Gaylor *et al.*, 1970b).

[2] The term "solubilization" will be used rather freely in this chapter as an operational definition *in lieu* of a single word that says, "freed from the main bulk of residual particulate material that is collected as a particle after highspeed centrifugation." Toward the end of the chapter, some criteria used to claim solubility will be enumerated but not discussed. There are several reasons for not simply pursuing purification of a solubilized enzyme to homogeneity: the sought-for enzyme may be inactive in a lipid-free, solubilized form; reconstitution of multienzyme systems may require fragments of retained microsomal membrane; the primary purpose in many studies is to remove a contaminating enzyme (see Section II,A,2), rather than to obtain homogeneous preparations of soluble enzymes; etc.

Bygrave, 1969; Van Tol, 1970; Fleischer *et al.*, 1971). Thus, published methods are available for the preparation and characterization of liver microsomes that contain the enzymes needed to catalyze the multistep conversion of lanosterol into cholesterol.

In 1962, our work on the microsomal enzymes of sterol biosynthesis was initiated by repeating the earlier observation of Olson *et al.* (1957) who showed that the "extra" methyl groups of lanosterol (carbon atoms 30, 31, and 32 shown in Fig. 1) were oxidized to carbon dioxide by a fortified preparation of liver microsomes. We prepared biosynthetically labeled lanosterol[3] (Moller and Tchen, 1961), suspended the steroid in an excess of the detergent, Tween 80, and incubated the suspension far too long with an overwhelming excess of microsomes. [14C]Carbon dioxide was collected, and the "rate" of lanosterol demethylation[4] was calculated from the known specific activity of the substrate. The use of inappropriate conditions was particularly revealing, though, because this preliminary observation led to extensive investigation of optimal conditions for studying the properties of the microsomal enzymes of lanosterol demethylation.

Briefly, the selection of optimal conditions for study of the composite enzymes of microsomes was possible because the collection of enzymes (i.e., microsomes) had properties that were quite analogous to properties observed for any soluble enzyme. That is, initial velocity of oxidative methyl sterol demethylation that is catalyzed by microsomes remained constant for a measurable period of time (Gaylor, 1964), and, under appropriate conditions of saturation by oxygen and needed cofactors, initial velocity measurements were adequately proportional to variations of the concentration of substrate to allow calculation of apparent values of K_m and V_{max} from reciprocal plots.[5] Furthermore, the measured rates of "microsomal" demethylation have been shown to re-

---

[3] Common names of some sterols are used for simplicity: lanosterol is 4,4,14α-trimethyl-5α-cholesta-8,24-dien-3β-ol; the "4α-methyl sterol" (Fig. 3, IV) is 4α-methyl-5α-cholest-7-en-3β-ol; the "4α-carboxylic acid" (V of Fig. 3) is 3β-hydroxy-5α-cholest-7-ene-4α-carboxylic acid; zymosterol is 5α-cholesta-8,24-dien-3β-ol.

[4] Demethylation refers to the process of conversion of each methyl group into carbon dioxide (Fig. 3, I → III or IV → VI).

[5] Throughout the course of these studies, apparent calculated values, designated K'_m and V'_{max}, have been reported because it seems inappropriate to extend the analogy to soluble enzymes to the extent of a claim for real kinetic values. Furthermore, the reader must realize that these measurements were carried out with suspensions of insoluble enzymes that were incubated with suspensions of insoluble substrate (see Section II,A,3) that were brought into contact with the enzyme by dissolution in a detergent solution and dilution with warm buffer to the desired substrate concentration.

spond to changes in the amounts of microsomal protein, pH, cofactor concentrations, and temperature regardless of the source of microsomes: rat liver (Gaylor, 1964); rat skin (Gaylor *et al.*, 1966a); yeast (Moore and Gaylor, 1968); or testicular tissue (Gaylor and Tsai, 1964). In addition, the observed rates of demethylation responded to addition of competitive and noncompetitive inhibitors (Gaylor, 1964; Lee and Gaylor, 1968; Gaylor *et al.*, 1965). The main point of these studies should be obvious. Because the collection of enzymes in microsomes has been shown to respond in a predictable way to variations of these conditions, it is appropriate to carry out investigations of rates of microsomal enzyme-catalyzed processes to solve some of the interesting problems of pathway, control, stereochemistry, etc., of sterol biosynthesis. In these experiments, microsomes were used as one would normally study the properties of a soluble enzyme. Thus, for multienzymatic transformation or for a single enzyme in a multistep enzymatic conversion (see Voigt *et al.*, 1970), once appropriate conditions are established investigations of relative rates of transformation may be undertaken.

B. Enzymatic versus Organic Approach

A brief analysis of the approaches used to investigate complex, multienzymatic processes should help to fix the position of enzyme characterization into the time-frame of other aspects of study of sterol biosynthesis. About 2 years ago, Professor A. R. Battersby was a visiting lecturer on our campus. During his lecture series on alkaloid biosynthesis, he analyzed the sequence of events in the investigation of a complex biosynthetic process such as alkaloid formation. An unworthy[6] parallel to the events of alkaloid biosynthesis is given in Table I for sterol biosynthesis. Initially, precursor-product relationships were established by inspection of structural analogy. Accordingly, simplification such as the impact of the isoprene rule developed into relationships that were tested experimentally with the *organic approach*. In the organic approach, substrates were synthesized, and the compounds generally contained isotopically labeled atoms. The labeled substrate was introduced into a minimally altered enzymatic system that catalyzed either the entire biosynthetic process or a number of transformations in sequence. Frequently an intact organism was used. The analysis of the abundance and

---

[6] The author wishes to make clear that Dr. Battersby developed this concept; it is only applied to sterol biosynthesis in this report. Those wishing to study his analysis more fully are encouraged to read review articles by Professor Battersby (1963, 1967) that contain many experimental analyses in addition to the development of the concept of approach.

Table I

APPROACHES USED TO STUDY COMPLEX BIOSYNTHETIC PROCESSES

Approach	Substrate	Enzyme	Sequence in the study
Organic	Synthetic containing ^{14}C, ^{3}H, ^{15}N	Whole organism, minimally altered enzymatic system	First
Enzymatic	Isotope for assay only	Purified enzyme	Second

position of isotopic atoms in the sought-for product allowed the organic approach to be used for the study of precursor-product relationships, the origin of each atom stereochemically in the product, and, to some extent, knowledge of the actual enzymatic process. The latter was accomplished by inference from the conditions under which certain conversions were found to occur; sometimes alternatives between possible enzymatic transformations were excluded by the conditions selected (e.g., anaerobic incubation to limit mixed-function oxidative attack).[7]

In the *enzymatic approach,* the sought-after enzyme is purified free from other enzymes that act either on the substrate or on the product. Substrates may or may not be isotopically labeled; occasionally, label is introduced to afford either a sensitive or a simple assay. It should be obvious that the organic approach must be taken first. The investigation of oxidative demethylation of methyl sterols may be used to illustrate the *transition from the organic to the enzymatic approach* in our laboratory. Lindberg and co-workers (1963) reported that when 4-methyl sterols labeled with $3\alpha[^3$H] were converted enzymatically into C_{27}-steroids, the tritium label was lost. Similarly, 3α-tritium label was not quantitatively removed from C_{27}-sterols in control incubations in which oxidative 4-demethylation did not occur. Accordingly, they proposed that 3-ketosteroids may be obligatory intermediates in oxidative demethylation (Fig. 2, top line). This is an excellent application of the organic approach. Dr. Swindell, while a graduate student in this laboratory, observed that oxidative demethylation of 4,4-dimethyl sterol substrates was incomplete when the compounds were incubated with thoroughly washed microsomes and NADPH was omitted from the medium (Swindell and Gaylor, 1968). 3-Ketosteroids accumulated, and the 4α-methyl-5α-cholest-7-en-3-one was shown to be formed quantitatively from the 4,4-dimethyl-5α-cholest-7-en-3β-ol substrate (Fig. 2, line 2). Later, Dr.

---

[7] Simply referring to these approaches as organic or enzymatic does not imply that the tools of the organic chemist are not used in the latter approach. For example, substrates must be prepared (Frantz *et al.,* 1969), and products must be analyzed.

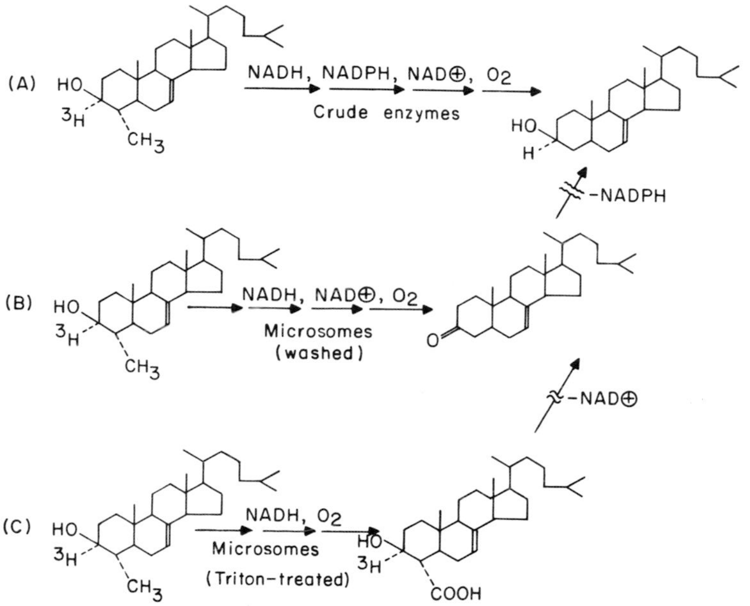

FIG. 2.   Dissection of reactions of methyl sterol demethylase. (A) Lindberg *et al.* (1963). (B) Swindell and Gaylor (1968). (C) Miller and Gaylor (1970a).

Miller, a more recent graduate student, found that effective elimination of endogenous pyridine nucleotides from these enzymatic processes of liver microsomes by Triton treatment (Miller *et al.*, 1967) and aerobic incubation of Triton-treated microsomes with 4,4-dimethyl substrate and an NADH-generating system (to keep the pyridine nucleotide in the reduced form) yielded the 4α-carboxylic acid product (Miller and Gaylor, 1970a; line 3 of Fig. 2 in this chapter). 3α[^{3}H] of the 4,4-dimethyl sterol substrate was fully retained in the carboxylic acid product. Thus, the organic approach was very useful; precursor-product relationships were predicted for oxidative demethylation. In addition, the transition between the organic and enzymatic approaches was occurring simultaneously. For example, when Dr. Swindell observed that 3-keto-steroids accumulated in the absence of either added or endogenous NADPH, he predicted that the next enzyme in the process must be NADPH-dependent, because 3-keto-4-methyl sterols were not further demethylated prior to reduction. 3-Ketosteroid reductase seemed to be the next likely enzyme in the sequence. Similarly, when Dr. Miller observed that NAD$^+$ was required for metabolism of the 4α-carboxylic acid, he established conditions for the assay of the NAD$^+$-dependent decarboxylase (Miller and Gaylor, 1970a,b) that appeared to be the first enzyme to act on carboxylic acid. These predictions of sequence of enzymatic activities arose from inspection of *conditions* used for incubation during the organic approach. Therefore, examination of Fig. 2 on an angle from the lower left- to the upper right-hand corner illustrates the development and use of the *enzymatic approach*. With the enzymatic approach, the predicted NAD$^+$-dependent decarboxylase and the NADPH-dependent 3-ketosteroid reductase have now been solubilized from liver microsomes by Dr. Rahimtula in this laboratory (Rahimtula and Gaylor, 1971).

II. Solubilization of Microsomal Enzymes

A. ESSENTIAL PRELIMINARY INFORMATION

1. *Evidence for the Existence of Enzyme*

Before setting out to isolate microsomal enzymes, the investigator must demonstrate that each enzyme-catalyzed reaction occurs, and conditions for a valid assay of the enzymatic activity must be obtained. As pointed out above, examination of the conditions under which a given intermediate is formed but not further metabolized affords considerable information about both the enzymatic processes of formation and metabolism, as well as evidence for the existence of the enzyme. This evidence for each enzyme is essential. The evidence based on observations of experimental conditions for formation and metabolism of an intermediate is far superior to basing "evidence" simply on analogy to other similar enzymatic processes. For example, we experienced a misleading delay that was based on analogy to other enzymatic processes rather than on the observation of conditions used in the organic approach. We had developed an assay for the initial part of demethylation that contained the mixed-function oxidation of the methyl to a hydroxymethyl group (Miller *et al.*, 1967):

$$R\text{---}CH_3 \xrightarrow[\text{O}_2]{\text{NAD(P)H}} R\text{---}CH_2OH \xrightarrow{B} R\text{---}CHO \xrightarrow{C} RCOOH.$$

The subsequent conversion of the hydroxymethyl compound to carboxylic acid was thought to occur by NAD$^+$-dependent alcohol (enzyme B) and aldehyde (enzyme C) dehydrogenase-catalyzed steps (Bloch, 1965; Olson, 1965; Clayton, 1965; Pudles and Bloch, 1960; Miller *et al.*, 1967). This assumption was based on the known conversions of similar alcohols and aldehydes. The analogy to NAD$^+$-dependent oxidation of alcohols to aldehydes guided our search for an alcohol dehydrogenase of liver microsomes that would catalyze the conversion of the hydroxymethyl compound to an aldehyde (i.e., enzyme B). We found an alcohol dehydrogenase associated with liver microsomes, and the enzyme was readily released from the particles by simply extracting the protein into dilute Tris-acetate buffer (Moir *et al.*, 1968). In further misleading us, the enzyme restored demethylase activity to Tris-acetate washed microsomes. However, the enzyme did not catalyze anaerobic dehydrogenation of the hydroxymethyl steroid to an aldehyde. Alternatively, when this work was done in 1967, if we had known the conditions under which the carboxylic acid was formed (worked out by 1969, see Miller and Gaylor, 1970a,b), the possibility of an alcohol dehydrogenase would have been eliminated because carboxylic acid subsequently was shown to be formed from 4α-methyl sterols under conditions in which an alcohol dehydrogenase would not be expected to be active, i.e., in the absence of NAD$^+$ (and NADP$^+$). Rather, carboxylic acid formation from 4-methyl sterol required oxygen and reduced pyridine nucleotide, which are conditions characteristic of a mixed-function oxidative conversion of alcohol to aldehyde rather than by a dehydrogenase. Furthermore, in a more recent study, mixed-function oxidative formation of carboxylic acid from hydroxymethyl substrate was demonstrated directly (Miller *et al.*, 1971). These observations correspond to analogous work in other laboratories on microsomal conversion of ethanol to acetaldehyde in which ethanol is oxidized by a mixed-function oxidase and not by an alcohol dehydrogenase of microsomes (Lieber *et al.*, 1970). (We did not have that analogy in 1967.) Therefore, the importance of basing further work on observations and not arguing by analogy cannot be stressed too much. In other words, we deserved our experience.

During these studies, properties of the oxidative system that catalyzes formation of carboxylic acid from hydroxymethyl substrates were found to be identical to properties of the methyl sterol oxidase that catalyzes formation of carboxylic acid from methyl sterols. Thus, the resulting aldehyde apparently is oxidized by the same enzymatic system[8] that catalyzes the first reaction and reaction B above. Accordingly, the isolation of enzymes responsible for carboxylic acid formation has been greatly simplified because a single mixed-function oxidase apparently catalyzes each of the three steps in the sequence of methyl sterol oxidase as shown above. Thus, combination of the mixed-function oxidative activity with the NAD$^+$-dependent decarboxylase and NADPH-dependent 3-ketoreductase apparently completes the process of complete demethyla-

---

[8] D. R. Brady and J. L. Gaylor (unpublished observations).

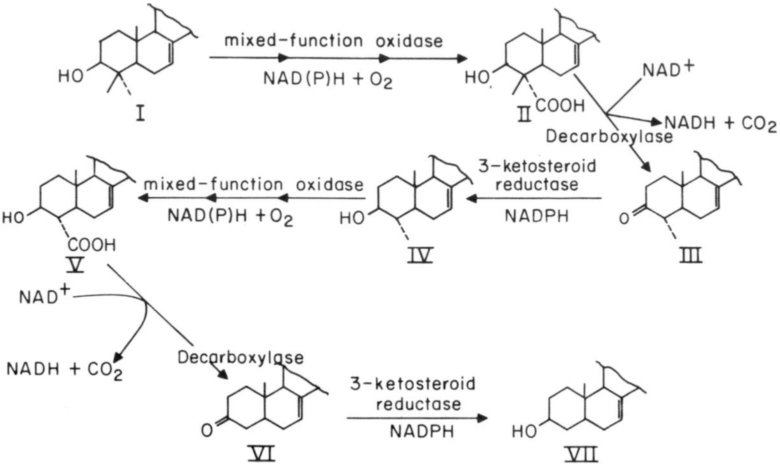

FIG. 3.   Reactions of methyl sterol demethylase.

tion of a 4,4-dimethyl sterol (Fig. 3). Although evidence for the stepwise formation of 4-hydroxymethyl and 4-formyl intermediates would complete the argument for the existence of each intermediate as we envision it now, the velocity increases approximately five- to tenfold with each oxidation. Interruption of the process appears unlikely. Finally, all of the enzymes appear to act on 4,4-dimethyl as well as on 4α-methyl steroid substrates; the only isolable steroid product of decarboxylation of the disubstituted substrate (Fig. 3, II) is the 4α-methyl ketone (Fig. 3, III; Rahimtula and Gaylor, 1971).

Evidence for the existence of enzymes and the elucidation of enzymatic type-reactions in sequence has been developed well by Dempsey and co-workers who have used various inhibitors to interrupt selectively some of the microsomal enzymes. By inspecting reactions that are known to occur in the presence of inhibitor, the cofactor and oxygen requirements of the enzyme, as well as the families of similar products formed with a single inhibitor, this group has successfully delineated many of the steps of cholesterol biosynthesis (see Dempsey, 1968). Further comments on the simultaneous use of inhibitors and other approaches follow later (Sections II,A,2 and III,C).

2. Assay

In general, the criteria of valid assays of microsomal enzymes are not substantially different from those used for assays of soluble enzymes: constant initial velocities; adequate cofactor supply; proportionality of velocity to concentration of enzyme and substrate; etc. However, assay of microsomal enzymes of sterol biosynthesis presents some additional special problems that must be handled.

If a single assay is used, it must be valid for the enzyme while it is particle-bound, as well as following solubilization if the total enzymatic activity in the soluble form is to be related to total activity of microsomes. Occasionally, more than one assay will have to be developed and proportionality of the two methods then must be established following isolation and purification of the enzyme. For example, prenol pyrophosphate pyrophosphohydrolase was readily assayed by measuring the rate of release of inorganic pyrophosphate (Tsai and Gaylor, 1966). Facile measurement of inorganic phosphate formation was possible because microsomes contain an inorganic pyrophosphate pyrophosphohydrolase that catalyzes the further breakdown of inorganic pyrophosphate that was released from prenol pyrophosphate; assay of the microsomal bound enzyme, based on the rate of release of inorganic pyrophosphate, was made impossible by the action of another enzyme acting on one of the products, in sequence. When the enzyme was solubilized and purified free of the inorganic pyrophosphate pyrophosphohydrolase, assay of the solubilized enzyme was carried out by measuring the release of [^{14}C]prenol pyrophosphate. After isolation and purification of the enzyme free of inorganic pyrophosphatase, the assays were related stoichiometrically. Thus, total activities of bound and solubilized enzyme were related (see Table IV,B).

Another example of complicating factors of enzyme assay is the need to prevent the effect of a second microsomal enzyme acting *sequentially* on one of the products formed by the sought-for enzyme; a good example was reported recently by Yamamoto and Bloch (1970b). Microsomal 2,3-oxidosqualene-lanosterol cyclase was found to be heat-sensitive relative to squalene epoxidase; thus, these workers were able to study the properties of the oxidase in the absence of the complicating cyclase activity.

Another situation encountered frequently is the unwanted *concomitant* action of two microsomal enzymes on the same sterol substrate. Most of the work on demethylation in this laboratory has been carried out with Δ^7-sterols because Δ^8-sterols, likely the quantitatively more significant intermediates, are isomerized to Δ^7-sterols by a microsomal-bound isomerase (Gaylor *et al.*, 1966b; Wilton *et al.*, 1969). Unfortunately, no method of inhibition of the isomerase (such as heat, drugs, mercurials, etc.) has been found that does not also reduce the rate of demethylase. Conversely, preventing demethylase action during the study of other enzymes was achieved relatively simply by carrying out the study of the other enzyme under anaerobic conditions. The decarboxylase, 3-ketosteroid reductase, and isomerase (Fig. 3), have been studied primarily under anaerobic conditions. Addition of glucose and glucose oxidase has been found to yield anaerobic conditions without requiring extensive exchange of air for other gases in the buffers (Miller *et al.*, 1967). Use of selective inhibitors of unwanted enzymatic activities has been very helpful. For example, Dempsey and co-workers have developed conditions for the specific inhibitions of the steroidal Δ^7- and Δ^{24}-ene reductases such as by Triparanol (for a summary, see Dempsey, 1967).

Finally, in addition to other microsomal enzymes acting either *concomitantly* on the same substrate or *sequentially* on one of the products in the multienzymatic microsomes, an additional special complication of assay of microsomal enzymes may be encountered; the assay may be complicated by interference produced by endogenous sterols. Cholesterol is found in microsomal lipids of liver, and microsomes from other sources contain many sterols in addition to cholesterol (Moore and Gaylor, 1968; Gaylor and Tsai, 1964; Gaylor *et al.*, 1966a). Accordingly, there may be an additive effect of the endogenous sterol to the assay of observed enzymatic rate on the one hand, or endogenous sterols may reduce the observed rate by serving as inhibitors in a second possibility. There is no simple solution to this problem because extraction of endogenous sterols is impractical, and, as we will observe later (see Section II,B,2,*b*), altering the microsomal lipids frequently reduces the rates of these processes drastically. Furthermore, the enzymes may be damaged by the conditions selected for extraction of the lipid. The situation is pointed out here to alert the worker to the problem and to make him aware of the possibility of both inhibition and observed stimulation. We know that we have encountered each effect of endogenous sterols: (1) a contribution of endogenous sterols to the rate of demethylation observed using preparations of microsomes from rat skin resulted in observed inhibition (Gaylor *et al.*, 1966a); and (2) an effect of endogenous zymosterol of yeast microsomes added both to the observed rate (see Table V), and a possibility of end-product inhibition by zymosterol was encountered, too (Moore and Gaylor, 1968, 1969, 1970). A similar possibility of end-product inhibition was reached quite separately by Katsuki and Bloch (1967).

3. Suspension of Insoluble Substrates

A suitable exposure of hydrophobic substrates to microsomal enzymes (see footnote 5) must be worked out for each enzyme assayed. Several alternatives are available for suspension of steroid substrates. In general, each worker tends to continue to use the same method of suspension in all of the investigations in his laboratory. A variety of treatments used to suspend substrates may be cited from a recent volume of *Methods in Enzymology* (Clayton, 1969). Some specific citations from this single volume are recorded for convenience because frequently the authors commented on their choice of method, and the reader should be aware that, although a single procedure generally is continued within a laboratory, the conditions in many cases were optimized by examining a variety of techniques. For example, a water-miscible solvent, such as acetone, may be used to prepare solutions of the substrate, and small volumes of the solution are added to the incubation mixture (Berséus *et al.*, 1969). Other miscible organic solvents such as propylene glycol have been used (Forchielli, 1969; Dempsey, 1969). Although others have reported the use of sonic suspensions and preparations stabilized with bovine serum albumin, the most commonly used stabilizer of suspensions of sterol subtrate in the aqueous medium has been detergents such as Tween 20 (Steinberg and Avigan, 1969; Staple, 1969) and Tween 80 (Dean, 1969; Doering, 1969). In our laboratory, most substrate suspensions have been prepared using nonionic detergents. Initially, Tween 80 was used (wt detergent/wt steroid = 20 to 100), but more recently, Triton WR-1339 has been the dispersing agent of choice because substantially higher concentrations of Triton may be used without observing toxic effects on the initial velocities (Swindell and Gaylor, 1968). There are several advantages of using detergents: (1) concentrations of substrate high enough to fully saturate the enzymes are obtained, whereas the limit of solubility of steroid without detergent (i.e., added in solvent) may be low; (2) the concentration in the incubation flask is known because precipitation of the steroid does not occur, thus Lineweaver-Burk plots may be constructed; and (3) in our hands, *initial* velocity measurements are much more rapid than with the addition of the same amount of steroid in solvent. Thus, with aqueous suspensions of substrate, investigations of relative rates have been possible, and enzymes may be isolated using assays in which saturating levels of substrate may be employed.

On the other hand, detergent may be a complicating factor, and results must be reported with appropriate reservations (see footnote 5). Interestingly, the 4α-carboxylic acid (II, Fig. 3) substrate is adequately soluble in water, and detergent was not needed to suspend the substrate for assay of decarboxylase (Fig. 3, II → III; Rahimtula and Gaylor, 1971). The K'_m for decarboxylase was the smallest value observed for any of these microsomal enzymes (approximately 7 μM), and suspension of the substrate with Triton WR-1339 altered neither the maximal velocity nor the Michaelis constant.

Finally, stimulation by detergents has been reported. For example, Bloch and co-workers showed that 2,3-oxidosqualene-lanosterol cyclase isolated from liver microsomes requires deoxycholic acid for activity (Yamamoto *et al.*, 1969), and the soluble cyclase isolated from yeast is stimulated by Triton X-100 (Schechter *et al.*, 1970).

Restated, the choice of method of preparation of substrate solutions is an open-ended problem. As long as the worker demonstrates that valid initial velocity measurements may be made with a given condition of exposure of substrate to enzyme, then the method of suspension may be used. Unfortunately, far too many studies have been carried out without the preliminary inspection of this aspect of working with hydrophobic substrates.

4. Before Going Ahead . . . .

It may seem too trivial to mention, but once the sought-for enzymatic activity has been established and a suitable assay has been developed, the worker should examine the length of time required for each assay of enzymatic activity. Obviously, an assay that requires saponification, extraction, and chromatography of the steroid substrate or products may be valid but inappropriate for an enzyme isolation unless the assay may be carried out within a short interval of time. Perhaps time may be saved eventually if an alternate method of assay that is more rapid is found. Furthermore, a severe limitation may be imparted if the sought-for enzyme is labile, especially under some of the extreme conditions employed for solubilization and purification (see below). Labile enzymes must be investigated, too. Various methods of stabilizing labile enzymes from microsomes have been used, such as the addition of glycerol (Miyake *et al.*, 1968), adjustment of pH or salt concentration (Yamamoto *et al.*, 1969), and addition of reducing substances such as glutathione (Gaylor and Mason, 1968) or dithiothreitol (Lu and Coon, 1968). However, if the enzyme is still labile under conditions needed for either solubilization or purification, a rapid assay is probably the only sound answer. For example, the two-step assay of methyl sterol oxidase (Miller *et al.*, 1967) has been reproducible and valid, but eight samples carried through an assay required 2 to 3 hours. The half-life of the oxidase under conditions of solubilization and chromatography is only about 3 hours (Gaylor *et al.*, 1970a). Accordingly, an alternate assay (20 minutes, total) was developed with a model substrate (Fig. 4) in which the second step (decarboxylation) had been eliminated by using the 3-ketosteroid substrate. Development of the alternate assay delayed the study initially, but purification of a labile enzyme with the use of an assay that required one half-life of the enzyme was impossible!

Now, you are ready to attempt solubilization; do you have a readily available source of microsomes?

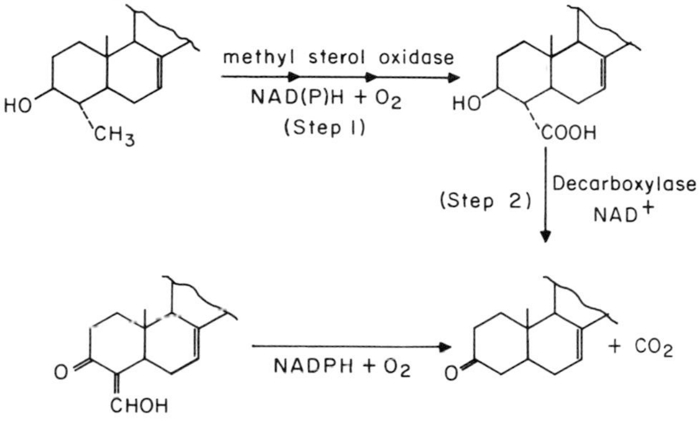

FIG. 4.   One-step assay of methyl sterol oxidase.

B. SOLUBILIZATION METHODS

Two principles should be kept in mind. First, the enzyme must be reasonably stable under conditions of solubilization and purification. Accordingly, substantial amounts of time are well spent in preliminary experiments that are designed to establish the limits of conditions. For example, the effect of bile salts on microsomal methyl sterol demethylation was studied extensively (Miller and Gaylor, 1967) by varying concentrations of the different compounds, incubating for different lengths of time at various temperatures, and studying the effect of exposure of bile salts under various buffer conditions before solubilization of the oxidase of demethylase was attempted with deoxycholic acid (Gaylor and Mason, 1968). The second principle is even more obvious; the method selected should be the most gentle procedure that adequately effects solubilization. Each of these principles requires considerable time-consuming, trial-and-error work to establish conditions through experimentation; therefore, as a reasonable alternative, a method of intermediate severity in which the enzymes for a particular segment of the pathway are found to be stable may be selected for initial studies. Deoxycholate treatment now occupies this intermediate position for investigation of demethylase in this laboratory. Each newly attempted solubilization now starts with deoxycholate treatment (e.g., as described in Gaylor *et al.*, 1970a), and severity of the treatment is altered according to stability and solubility of the enzyme. This short-cut to the laborious approach of investigating all procedures from gentle to harsh is illustrated below (Section II,B,1,*b*).

For ease of presentation, the description of solubilization is divided according to types of treatment: enzymatic and nonenzymatic. Within each type, a range of treatments from mild to severe is given. However, because lability may vary markedly between enzymatic systems, the reader should not consider this listing of severities as absolute; use them as guidelines. Features of some methods apart from solubilization per se are pointed out for certain merits (e.g., a procedure that generally leads to stability, simplicity, or ease of increasing the scale of operation).

1. Nonenzymatic Methods

a. Direct Extraction into Buffer. *From fresh microsomes.* Procedures that yield extraction of enzymes from microsomes in the absence of solubilizing agents are most attractive because mild conditions may be used, there is no solubilizing agent that must be removed subsequently, there is no possibility of the extracted enzyme returning to a particulate form as there is when a solubilizing agent is used, and the procedures are amenable to marked scaling-up.

Suspension of rat liver microsomes in cold Tris-acetate buffer (pH 7.4 and containing 2 mM glutathione and 30 mM nicotinamide) followed by centrifugation, led to a loss of specific activity of methyl sterol demethylase in the Tris-acetate washed microsomes (Moir et al., 1968). Repetition of the washing process was continued two more times until more than 90% of the demethylase activity was abolished (Table II). Addition of the supernatant fraction collected from the first Tris-acetate washing restored activity. Following purification and characterization of the active component of the supernatant fraction as an alcohol dehydrogenase, it was shown that addition of crystalline alcohol dehydrogenase could restore activity, too (Table II). Other buffers (e.g., phosphate, Tris-HCl) of various strengths were investigated, and these were

Table II

REDUCTION OF MICROSOMAL DEMETHYLASE BY TRIS-ACETATE EXTRACTION
OF A LOOSELY BOUND ALCOHOL DEHYDROGENASE[a]

Microsomes	Addition	Demethylase[b] (nmoles/mg protein)
Control	None	0.80
3-Times extracted	None	0.06
3-Times extracted	Supernatant fraction from extraction[c]	0.56
3-Times extracted	0.13 EU liver alcohol dehydrogenase	0.57

[a] Reproduced, in part, with kind permission of Academic Press; see Moir et al. (1968).
[b] Approximately 20 mg of microsomal protein was incubated for 10 minutes with [^{14}C]4,4-dimethyl-5α-cholest-7-en-3β-ol and NAD$^+$.
[c] Approximately 1.0 mg of protein.

found to be ineffective for the extraction of the microsomal alcohol dehydrogenase.

The extraction with dilute buffer was easy, carried out in high yield, and readily scaled-up when it was observed that frozen, stored microsomes could serve as a source of the dehydrogenase. (However, frozen microsomes could not be used as the source of washed microsomes that were needed for the assay and the reconstitution experiments shown in Table II.) Similarly, Krishna *et al.* (1966) extracted a squalene synthetase from pig liver microsomes simply by stirring a suspension of the microsomes in phosphate-bicarbonate buffer for 6 hours at 4°. Extrapolating to a general situation, extraction of microsomes with dilute buffer is probably the mildest of procedures, the most versatile because of a wide choice of buffer and salt solutions of various pH and ionic strengths, and probably the most *easily overlooked* of all procedures.

Drastic changes in buffer strength, pH, or salt additions may effect solubilizations that have been resistant to the direct extraction conditions described above. Voigt *et al.* (1968) reported that a clear suspension of liver microsomes in $1\,M$ phosphate buffer contained the complete 6β-hydroxylating system of chenodeoxycholic acid when microsomes were prepared from rat liver by homogenization in $0.01\,M$ phosphate buffer. Identical conditions yielded extraction of a steroidal aldehyde oxidase in our laboratory (see footnote 8) (Fig. 5b). Although the complete aldehyde oxidative system remained in the supernatant fraction following high-speed centrifugation of the extract, protein and the oxidase precipitated upon dialysis or dilution of the strong phosphate buffer. Thus, although the enzymatic system was very stable in the strong buffer, attempts to minimize precipitation were fruitless (e.g., addition of glycerol, slow filtration on Sephadex G-25), and the method of extraction was abandoned as an initial step in a purification study. In other words, as an extraction procedure, there was promise; as an initial step toward purification, there was no simple solution of the difficulty. [Actually, as it appears now, the aldehyde oxidase and methyl sterol oxidase are identical (see Figs. 3 and 4), and we would not expect to be able to work with this multienzyme system without the aid of a detergent (Gaylor *et al.*, 1970a).]

From desiccated microsomes. Several workers have reported successful isolation of enzymes from preparations of desiccated microsomes. Two methods of desiccation have been used successfully, lyophilization and preparations of acetone-dry powder. The former is likely to be more gentle and not complicated by the extraction of some of the microsomal lipid. Thus, Scholan and Boyd (1968) extracted cholesterol 7α-hydroxylase from lyophilized liver microsomes. The enzymatic activity remained in the supernatant fraction after high-speed centrifugation.

Microsomal acyl-coenzyme A desaturase (Fig. 6) of liver is a mixed-function oxidase that has many properties in common with methyl sterol oxidase (Oshino *et al.*, 1966; Gaylor and Mason, 1968). Thus, more recently, when workers reported the extraction of acyl-coenzyme A desaturase from preparations of lyophilized microsomes (Tietz and Stern, 1969; Gurr *et al.*, 1968; Gurr and Robinson, 1970) we attempted to use a similar extraction for methyl sterol oxidase.[9] The first preparation of oxidase was extracted from lyophilized microsomes that were prepared

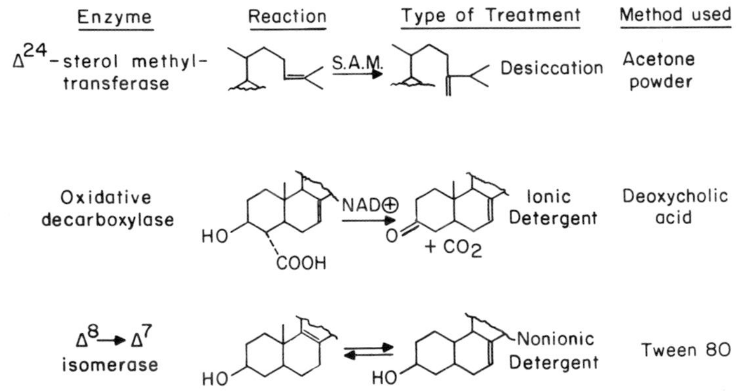

FIG. 5a.   Treatments used to obtain soluble microsomal enzymes, I.

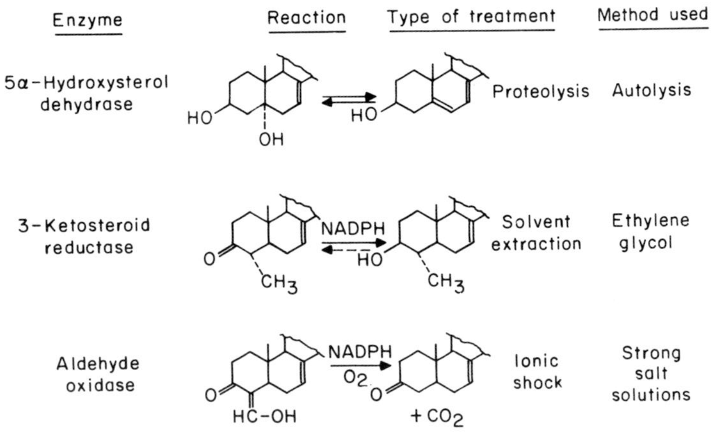

FIG. 5b.   Treatments used to obtain soluble microsomal enzymes, II.

[9] G. E. Opar and J. L. Gaylor (unpublished observations).

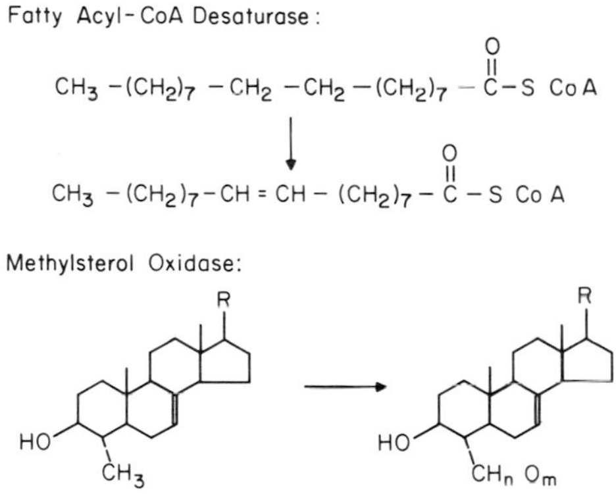

Fatty Acyl- CoA Desaturase :

$$CH_3 -(CH_2)_7 -CH_2 -CH_2 -(CH_2)_7 -\overset{\overset{\displaystyle O}{\|}}{C} -S\ CoA$$

$$\downarrow$$

$$CH_3 -(CH_2)_7 -CH = CH -(CH_2)_7 -\overset{\overset{\displaystyle O}{\|}}{C} -S\ CoA$$

Methylsterol Oxidase:

FIG. 6. Microsomal mixed-function oxidations of acyl-coenzyme A and methyl sterols.

from rat liver. Two marked advantages of using lyophilized microsomes were obvious immediately: the dry microsomes may be prepared when convenient and stored for long periods of time without loss of activity; and there is a *very* significant advantage in starting with a homogeneous source of enzymes when the following work entails making judgments on trial-and-error experimental data. Accordingly, we spent considerable time simply studying the preparation and properties of the lyophilized microsomes; in addition, we found that commercially available chicken liver was a cheap source of microsomal demethylase. Thus, the following digression is inserted. The lyophilization resulted in a loss of some activity, but demethylase was stable for more than a month in the dry preparation (Table III). The demethylase was dependent upon the addition of oxygen and cofactors as reported earlier for freshly prepared rat liver microsomes (Miller *et al.*, 1967). The rate of demethylation was reduced markedly by additions of cyanide (Table III), and the sensitivity to inhibition by cyanide was somewhat greater than that observed for fresh, rat liver microsomes (Gaylor and Mason, 1968). Velocity was constant through 15 minutes of incubation, and the rate was proportional to enzyme concentration which was varied from 2 through 14 mg of protein per milliliter. Accordingly, the Michaelis constant for 4,4-dimethyl-5α-cholest-7-en-3β-ol was calculated and found to be an invariable $2.2 \times 10^{-5}\ M$. This value agreed well with earlier measurements performed with rat liver microsomes (Gaylor, 1964). Furthermore, the V'_{max} was relatively constant for each homogeneous batch of lyophilized microsomes.

These observations illustrate some of the many advantages of using lyophilized microsomes mentioned above, in addition to the convenience

Table III

PROPERTIES OF METHYL STEROL DEMETHYLASE IN LYOPHILIZED PREPARATIONS
OF CHICKEN LIVER MICROSOMES[a]

Source of microsomes	Conditions of storage	Conditions of assay	Demethylase[b] (nmoles/mg protein)
Chicken, fresh	None	Complete[c]	0.32
Chicken, lyophilized	1 Day	Complete[c]	0.19
Chicken, lyophilized	33 Days	Complete[c]	0.18
Chicken, lyophilized	>1 Week	Complete minus oxygen	0.02
Chicken, lyophilized	>1 Week	Complete minus NAD$^+$	0.01
Chicken, lyophilized	>1 Week	Complete plus 0.1 mM CN$^-$	0.06
Chicken, lyophilized	>1 Week	Complete plus 0.25 mM CN$^-$	0.03

[a] From G. E. Opar and J. L. Gaylor (unpublished observations).

[b] Each incubation was carried out aerobically with about 20 mg of microsomal protein incubated with 100 nmoles of [^{14}C]4,4-dimethyl-5α-cholest-7-en-3β-ol for 10 minutes at 37°; final volume = 2.0 ml.

[c] Complete incubation mixtures contained 1 μmole of NAD$^+$ for each 20 mg of microsomal protein.

of preparation of material prior to extraction by buffer. Certainly, the advantages are so impressive that the worker should examine the stability of his microsomal enzyme under conditions of lyophilization and storage regardless of the procedure selected ultimately for solubilization. That is, detergent solubilizations could be carried out with lyophilized as well as with fresh microsomes.

Preparation and storage of acetone-dry powders has the advantages described for lyophilized preparations with the additional possibility that membranous phospholipids are either altered or removed to an extent that extraction may be facilitated. Linn (1967) extracted hydroxymethylglutaryl-coenzyme A reductase from acetone powders of rat liver microsomes. Although Scallen et al. (1968) described the preparation of an acetone powder of rat liver microsomes that will catalyze the conversion of squalene to cholesterol, we have not successfully extracted any enzymes of demethylase from the acetone-dry powder of liver microsomes.

From acetone powders of microsomes obtained from yeast and testicular tissue, we have isolated two enzymes that resisted other methods of solubilization. An S-adenosylmethionine:Δ^{24}-sterol methyltransferase (Fig. 5a) was isolated from acetone-dry particles that were prepared from yeast microsomes (Moore and Gaylor, 1969). The preparation of acetone powder required no special procedure, and the preparation could be stored at $-15°$ for months without appreciable loss of enzymatic activity. Solubilization into dilute Tris-HCl buffer was accomplished routinely. The purification table is reproduced as part A of Table IV. Possible complications in enzyme assays produced by endogenous sterols were discussed above (Section II,A,2). When the transmethylase was assayed with freshly prepared microsomes, there was a pronounced rate observed even in the absence of added zymosterol, the Δ^{24}-sterol substrate, and the increment of rate increase upon addition of substrate was only fivefold (Table V). However, following treatment with acetone, endogenous sterol was removed, and the activity ascribed to endogenous sterol was reduced to 5% of the rate measured with zymosterol. Accordingly, the activity was dependent upon added substrate in contrast to the earlier work of Katsuki and Bloch (1967), who relied upon an en-

Table IV

A. Purification of a Yeast Sterol Methyltransferase[a]

Stage of purification	Total activity (nmoles/hr)	Protein (mg)	Specific activity (nmoles/hr/ mg protein)	Purification
II. Dialyzed crude supernatant fraction	38.0	800.0	0.0475	1.0
III. Microsomes	59.0	62.5	0.944	20.0
IV. Acetone powder extract	62.0	30.8	2.02	42.1
V. 45 to 55% $(NH_4)_2SO_4$ precipitate	80.0	3.91	20.5	430.0
VI. Alumina C_γ gel	41.3	1.30	31.8	670.0

B. Release of Prenol-PP Pyrophosphohydrolase from Microsomes[b]

Treatment	Total activity (μg P_i/hr)	Total protein (mg)	Specific activity (μg Pi/hr/mg protein)	Purification
1. Supernatant fraction	72,000	2,340	30.8	1.0
2. Microsomes[c]	32,600	675	48.3	1.6
3. Washed microsomes[d]	32,900	248	132.0	4.3
4. Acetone powder	97,000	183	530.0	17.2
5. Extract of powder	81,000	117	693.0	22.5

[a] Reproduced with kind permission of the *Journal of Biological Chemistry;* Moore and Gaylor (1969).

[b] Reproduced with kind permission of the *Journal of Biological Chemistry;* Tsai and Gaylor (1966).

[c] The microsomes were washed and suspended in 0.1 M Tris-HCl buffer.

[d] The microsomal pellet from 2 was suspended in 2 volumes of 0.3 M Tris-HCl buffer (pH 7.4, 4 mmoles GSH). The suspension was centrifuged. The pellet was suspended in 0.1 M Tris-HCl buffer.

Table V

EFFECT OF ACETONE TREATMENT ON YEAST PARTICULATE TRANSMETHYLASE

	Rate with zymosterol (R_1) (nmoles/mg protein)[a]	Rate without zymosterol (R_2) (nmoles/mg protein)[a]	R_1/R_2
Fresh microsomes	0.22	0.04	5
Acetone powder	0.56	0.03	19

[a] 30-minute incubation (see Moore and Gaylor, 1969).

dogenous sterol acceptor of the methyl group. Thus, an additional advantage of acetone treatment was obvious, neutral lipids such as sterols may be removed.

The extraction of prenol pyrophosphate pyrophosphohydrolase (Tsai and Gaylor, 1966) from an acetone powder of rat testicular microsomes was similar to the preparation of methyltransferase described above with one notable exception. As shown in the purification table (Table IV), the microsomes were washed with 0.3 M Tris-HCl buffer prior to extraction of the enzyme. Considerable protein was removed without any loss of enzymatic activity; obviously, an increase in specific activity resulted. However, there was a more important aspect of this treatment. Omission of the washing step led to very poor yields of enzyme extracted from the acetone powder. Thus, the worker is encouraged to investigate similar washing procedures that may enhance the specific activity of the particle-bound enzyme and that may facilitate the extraction of the enzyme following the preparation of the acetone powder.

A reproducible effect was observed with both preparations of acetone powder. Upon treatment with acetone, the observed total activity of the enzyme increased in each case (Table IV). There is no simple explanation for this very welcome observation; "buried" enzyme may be exposed during the procedure; perhaps removal of bound substrate or inhibitor may be a factor as in the case of the methyltransferase assay.

Solvent fractionations. Others have used solvent fractionation procedures to effect dissection of liver microsomal particles (e.g., see the use of *tert*-amyl alcohol; Maclennan *et al.,* 1967); butanol solutions have been used to release phosphohydrolases from subcellular particles (Morton, 1954). Neither of the enzymes that we extracted from acetone powders remained reasonably active during solvent extraction treatments, and neither was found to be extractable under conditions of aqueous alcohol treatments. Although in Fig. 5b the 3-ketosteroid reductase is shown to be extracted into aqueous ethylene glycol, detergent was finally used in conjunction with ethylene glycol because the reductase returned to a particulate form when the ethylene glycol was removed in the absence of detergent (see Section II,B,4).

Soluble enzymes. To complete this subsection, mention should be made of a sterol-binding protein that, although it is obtained in the supernatant fraction following removal of microsomes by high-speed centrifugation, the protein stimulates many of the microsomal enzymatic steps of cholesterol biosynthesis. The protein has been studied primarily in two laboratories (Ritter and Dempsey, 1971; Scallen *et al.*, 1971). Whether or not the protein is derived from endoplasmic reticulum and appears in the supernatant fraction upon disruption of the liver cells remains to be established. However, obtaining the protein in a soluble form unassociated with particles greatly facilitated the investigation.

Comment. Many mild, simple techniques are available in which enzymes may be extracted directly from microsomes without the aid of an added detergent or other agent. The worker should investigate this type of treatment extensively before turning to less desirable options. Furthermore, there are several important advantages such as ease of increasing the quantities, storage of homogeneous starting material, etc.

b. Extraction with the Aid of Ionic Detergents. As mentioned above (Section II,B), treatment with deoxycholic acid occupies a central position in our current work. The reasons for selecting a single, useful method are several (in no particular order): (1) time is saved by avoiding extensive trial-and-error experiments with other solubilization methods; (2) one can develop a "minimal solubilization scheme" with which he shows that the enzymes that catalyze a *segment* of the biosynthesis are stable, and then the scheme may be attempted with the individual enzymes of that segment; (3) there is an advantage that accrues in the use of a single treatment repeatedly in one laboratory over the course of years; during a period of time, different people add different innovations (I feel that this point should be underscored); and (4) it costs less in dollars and time; for example, the solubilization and purification of microsomal cyanide-binding protein (Gaylor *et al.*, 1970a) yields 4α-carboxylic acid decarboxylase (Rahimtula and Gaylor, 1971) as a by-product. These points are made to the critic who feels that there is nothing innovative in the repeated use of the ionic detergent methods; perhaps it is the most expedient advance to the immediate goal of solubilizing enzymes.

Many ionic detergents are commercially available, and treatments using these detergents alone and in combination have been highly successful. However, deoxycholic acid will be used as a working example in this subsection because it has been used most extensively in this laboratory. Most of these investigations could have been carried out with other detergents substituted for deoxycholate. Deoxycholic acid treatment has been used to solubilize many microsomal enzymes of sterol biosynthesis: hydroxymethylglutaryl-coenzyme A reductase (Kawachi and Rudney, 1970); 2,3-oxidosqualene-lanosterol cyclase (Dean et al., 1967; Yamamoto et al., 1969); methyl sterol oxidase (Gaylor and Mason, 1968); sterol 4α-carboxylic acid decarboxylase (Rahimtula and Gaylor, 1971); and the cyanide-binding protein (Gaylor et al., 1970a). In addition, cyto-chrome P-450 and NADPH-dependent cytochrome P-450-reductase of the related microsomal electron transport process have been solubilized from microsomes by deoxycholic acid (Lu and Coon, 1968; Lu et al., 1969). Before turning to specific examples in this laboratory, it might be helpful to examine some of the variables in the use of an ionic detergent first. The sequence of steps in each of these investigations was essen-tially as outlined previously (see Section II,A,1 through 4). An assay was developed, the stability of each enzyme was studied under condi-tions necessary for solubilization, and the solubilized enzyme was puri-fied. However, the actual conditions have been quite variable.

Dean et al. (1967) added a solution of sodium deoxycholate to hog liver microsomes that were suspended in a minimal buffer (0.1 M phos-phate, pH 7.4) at 4°; the final concentration was about 800 mg of sodium deoxycholate added to 10 gm of microsomes, wet weight (approximately 1100 mg of protein according to Dean et al., 1967). After 15 minutes, a solution of calcium chloride was added to remove the deoxycholate as the insoluble salt, and the cyclase was purified by differential treatment with ammonium sulfate. Lipid bound to the partially purified enzyme was extracted from the protein as one of the terminal steps in purifica-tion. In a larger scale preparation of the cyclase, Yamamoto et al. (1969) used approximately 1 mg of sodium deoxycholate per milligram of pro-tein, and they omitted the treatment with calcium chloride; rather, pro-tein was precipitated with solid ammonium sulfate, leaving a soluble salt of deoxycholate in solution. Although the standard assay of cyclase included addition of 0.4 M potassium chloride (Yamamoto et al., 1969), neither potassium chloride nor any other stabilizing agent was added to the mixture at the time of exposure of microsomes to sodium deoxy-cholate. Thus, the reader should see some of the variables unfolding, and some of the reasons for examining the variables should be obvious (Table VI).

For example, contrast these relatively minimal conditions with the complex media and procedure published by Lu and Coon (1968), who used deoxycholate to solubilize cytochrome P-450 and cytochrome P-450-reductase from rabbit liver microsomes. Microsomes were suspended in 0.25 M sucrose solution to which glycerol, citrate buffer, potassium

Table VI

Some Categories of Variables Used to Obtain Maximal Yield of Active
Enzyme by Treatment with Sodium Deoxycholate

Variable to study	Reason for studying variable
1. Medium in which microsomes are suspended prior to exposure to deoxycholate.	To maximize stability during exposure to deoxycholate.
2. Amount of deoxycholate used.	To balance between amount needed for solubilization and excessive amount that leads to lability.
3. Time and temperature of exposure to deoxycholate.	Needed for balance as above; e.g., solubilization may be achieved with less deoxycholate when the temperature is raised to 15°.
4. The extent to which purification is carried before removing deoxycholate.	Detergent may facilitate initial stages of purification; the goal is to obtain purified enzymes—not just solubilized proteins.

chloride, and dithiothreitol were added before exposure of the microsomes to sodium deoxycholate (0.4 mg of sodium deoxycholate per 1.0 mg of protein). (One of my students reports that even the sequence of additions before deoxycholate treatment is important in this procedure.) The treatment was carried out for 20 minutes at 4°. The mixture was centrifuged to remove residual particles. The clarified suspension was transferred to a diethylaminoethyl-cellulose column; a gradient of potassium chloride in Tris-HCl buffer was used to elute the proteins. In addition, the eluting solvents contained dithiothreitol and 0.05% of deoxycholate; thus, the enzymes were not separated from detergent prior to the first purification step. Modifications of the basic procedure have been carried out subsequently by Dr. Lu and Dr. Coon, but in each case, the changes have generally dealt with alteration of chromatographic conditions; solubilization has been achieved as originally described (Lu et al., 1969). For example, slight modification of the chromatographic procedure (longer column and slower KCl gradient) allowed Rikans and Van Dyke (1971) to use this procedure for resolution, from rat liver microsomes, of a novel cytochrome that had properties that distinguished it from cytochromes P-450, P-420, and b_5.

With examples from work in our own laboratory, perhaps more of the reasons for varying the different conditions will become obvious. In addition to the decarboxylase indicated in Fig. 5a, methyl sterol oxidase (Fig. 3, I to II, and IV to V), acyl-coenzyme A desaturase (Fig. 6), and the microsomal cyanide-binding protein have been isolated from rat liver microsomes using deoxycholate solubilization.

Methyl sterol demethylase, a segment of the synthetic pathway (either

I → III or IV → VI of Fig. 3), withstands exposure to 0.3 mg of deoxycholate per milligram of protein for more than 1 hour at 4° (Table VII). When the concentration of deoxycholate (DOC) was doubled, the rate of demethylase was reduced. However, when similar preparations of microsomes were suspended in Tris-HCl buffer containing 2 mM GSH and treated at room temperature with 0.5 mg of deoxycholate per milligram of protein for 20 minutes, enzyme of high specific activity was collected when deoxycholate was removed by filtration on Sephadex G-25. The filtration was carried out at room temperature, too. After cooling to 4° and adding buffer, centrifugation at 105,000g for 90 minutes yielded a supernatant fraction of even higher specific activity (Table VII). The methyl sterol oxidase in the resulting supernatant fraction was adequately stable to be fractionated further (Gaylor and Mason, 1968). In the fractions that contained the enriched oxidase (5 and 6 of Table VII), the activity of overall demethylase activity (Fig. 3, I → III) was almost immeasurable. Thus, if demethylase is composed of the oxidase and decarboxylase, these conditions of solubilization were suitable for the oxidase but not for decarboxylase. Thus, when solubilization of decarboxylase was attempted with deoxycholate (Rahimtula and Gaylor, 1971), the initial investigation dealt with attempts to find conditions under which the decarboxylase would be stable in the presence of the approximately 0.5 mg of deoxycholate per milligram of protein required

Table VII

EFFECT OF DEOXYCHOLATE TREATMENT ON METHYL STEROL DEMETHYLASE
AND METHYL STEROL OXIDASE

Assay	Treatment	Time	Activity (nmoles/ mg protein)	Reference[a]
1. Methyl sterol demethylase[b]	None	—	0.70[c]	1
2. Methyl sterol demethylase	0.3 mg DOC/mg protein	75 min	0.73	1
3. Methyl sterol demethylase	0.6 mg DOC/mg protein	75 min	0.27	1
4. Methyl sterol oxidase	None	—	0.37	1
5. Methyl sterol oxidase	0.5 mg DOC/mg protein, 20°, then G-25	20 min	0.74	1
6. Methyl sterol oxidase	Supernatant fraction from 5	—	1.54	1
7. Decarboxylase	None	—	5.8	2
8. Decarboxylase	Same as 5 plus 10% glycerol	—	18.5	2

[a] References: (1) Gaylor and Mason (1968); (2) Rahimtula and Gaylor (1971).
[b] Carried out in 0.1 M Tris-HCl buffer containing 1 mM GSH (glutathione).
[c] 10-minute incubation.

for solubilization. We observed that addition of 10% of glycerol to the 0.1 M Tris-HCl buffer (containing 2 mM GSH) afforded complete stabilization. Furthermore, deoxycholate treatment to release decarboxylase could be carried out at room temperature. We have found that deoxycholate (measured by thin-layer chromatography; Gregg, 1966) may be resolved from the main bulk of protein by filtration at 25° on Sephadex G-25. As mentioned above, deoxycholate is removed from the enzyme suspension immediately to minimize lability (point 4 of Table VI, and line 3 versus 2 in Table VII).

To this point, very little reference to the criteria of solubility has been made. Generally, the worker is satisfied with an operational definition (see footnote 2) to investigate the effect of variables such as those indicated in Table VI. Retention of activity in the supernatant fraction following centrifugation at 105,000g for periods in excess of 1 hour and retention of clarity of the suspension following either dilution, dialysis, or gel filtration are used routinely as criteria of solubilization.

In 1968, work on isolation of acyl-coenzyme A desaturase and further resolution of the methyl sterol oxidase was in progress in our laboratory when the initial report of the method of Lu and Coon (1968) was published. We used their method with liver microsomes from rats and assayed for enzymatic activities of sterol demethylation instead of cytochrome P-450 and NADPH-cytochrome P-450-reductase. The isolation was highly successful (Gaylor *et al.*, 1970a), and we have employed an essentially unmodified method ever since. The solubilized methyl sterol oxidase obtained chromatographically has properties (Table VIII) that are essentially identical to the properties of the microsomal-bound oxi-

Table VIII

ASSAY OF METHYL STEROL OXIDASE ISOLATED BY DEOXYCHOLATE TREATMENT

	Specific activity	
Additions	nmoles/mg protein[a]	%
Complete[b]	1.5	100
Minus O$_2$	0.1	7
Minus NADH	0.2	13
Plus 0.05 mM CN$^-$	1.0	67
Plus 0.2 mM CN$^-$	0.6	40

[a] 10-minute incubation.

[b] Isolated enzyme was collected following chromatography on DEAE-cellulose (Gaylor *et al.*, 1970a). The complete system included: approximately 4 mg of protein; 4 μmoles of NADH; 9 μmoles of GSH; 40 μmoles of nicotinamide; and 100 nmoles of [30-^{14}C]4α-methyl-5α-cholest-7-en-3β-ol in a final volume of 4 ml. The incubation at 37° was carried out under air.

dase (Gaylor and Mason, 1968) in that reduced pyridine nucleotide and oxygen are required for activity, and the system retained sensitivity to inhibition by cyanide. However, as pointed out above, in the method of Lu and Coon deoxycholate is present at all stages and in all buffers. Lability of the cyanide-binding protein was observed (half-life of about 3 hours), and attempts to prevent lability by addition of glycerol or reducing substances, removal of oxygen, and keeping the materials in the dark (suggested by Rikans and Van Dyke, 1971) were not successful. Alternatively, simply removing the salt and deoxycholate, following chromatography on diethylaminoethyl-cellulose, by filtration on Sephadex G-25 yielded a preparation that remained fully active for more than 24 hours.[10] In addition to imparting lability, deoxycholate at higher concentrations, such as that in the elution solution, was shown to inhibit methyl sterol oxidase and acyl-coenzyme A desaturase. Thus, when proportionality of enzymatic activity and concentration of enzyme that was collected from the column and containing 0.05% deoxycholate were measured, with the larger amounts of added enzyme (and added deoxycholate) inhibition of methyl sterol oxidase was observed (Fig. 7). Therefore, removal of the deoxycholate before assay of the methyl sterol oxidase has been carried out routinely; the acyl-coenzyme A desaturase has been measured directly.

Comment. At first appearance, the number of variables in the use of an ionic detergent such as deoxycholic acid as a solubilizing agent seems to be very much smaller than the options described in subsection *a* above. However, from the list of variables (Table VI) and the specific examples, the reader should have the impression that this general method of solubilization is rather attractive.

c. Extraction with the Aid of Nonionic Detergents. With the availability of many nonionic detergents from commercial sources, there will be frequent use of nonionic detergents for solubilization of particle-bound enzymes. In many respects, treatments with nonionic detergents are very gentle. However, there is one substantial disadvantage; the detergents tend to accompany proteins during fractionations, and removal of these solubilizing agents may be difficult.

The examples of the specific use of nonionic detergents to solubilize microsomal enzymes of sterol metabolism are limited. Christophe and Popják (1961) reported that an attempt to solubilize prenol pyrophosphate pyrophosphohydrolase from liver microsomes with Lubrol W was not successful. In a related microsomal system, Kusunose *et al.* (1970) were able to solubilize and fractionate an omega-hydroxylating enzyme

---

[10] K. Comai and J. L. Gaylor (unpublished observations).

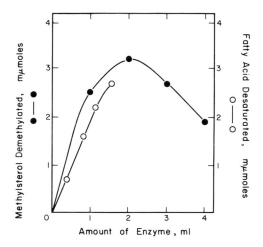

FIG. 7. Oxidation of methyl sterol and acyl-coenzyme A by partially purified system containing the microsomal cyanide-binding protein. Preparation of the cyanide-binding protein was carried out as described previously (Gaylor *et al.*, 1970a). Stearyl-coenzyme A desaturase was measured according to the methods outlined by Oshino *et al.* (1966). Specifically, for stearyl-coenzyme A desaturase, 60 nmoles of [1-^{14}C]stearyl-coenzyme A (2.5 × 10^5 dpm, purchased from New England Nuclear), 1.2 μmoles each of NADH and NADPH, and enzyme were incubated aerobically at 37° for 5 minutes in a final volume of 1.0 ml. Carrier oleic and stearic acids were added; conversion was calculated following thin-layer chromatographic resolution of the methyl esters of the fatty acids. Methyl sterol oxidase was determined as described previously (Gaylor and Mason, 1968). In 4-ml final volume, 4 μmoles of NADH, 9 μmoles of glutathione, 40 μmoles of nicotinamide, and 100 nmoles of [30-^{14}C]4α-methyl-5α-cholest-7-en-3β-ol were incubated aerobically for 10 minutes at 37°.

system by treating rat liver microsomes with Triton X-100. The more closely related microsomal stearyl-coenzyme A desaturase has been prepared in an apparently soluble form by treatment of chicken liver microsomes with Triton X-100 (Gurr and Robinson, 1970).

When rat liver microsomes were incubated anaerobically with sterol biosynthetic intermediates that have double bonds in the $\Delta^{8(9)}$-position, the compounds were converted into the corresponding Δ^7-sterol isomers (see Fig. 5a; Gaylor *et al.*, 1966b). Earlier attempts to solubilize the enzyme were unsuccessful. Recently, however, a student in this laboratory observed that the isomerase remained active after the addition of Tween 80 to a suspension of microsomes.[11] When the mitochondria-free supernatant fraction of rat liver homogenate was treated by gentle homogenization with 0.1 to 0.5% of Tween 80 (w/v) and centrifuged at 105,000g

---

[11] J. B. Yanni and J. L. Gaylor (unpublished observations).

for 1.5 hours, isomerase activity remained in the resulting supernatant fraction. No further purification has been attempted. The NADPH-dependent 3-ketosteroid reductase of liver microsomes (Fig. 5b) has been liberated from microsomes and partially purified with the aid of Lubrol WX (see Section II,B,4).

Nonionic detergents have been used more successfully to solubilize other microsomal proteins such as cytochromes and cytochrome-reducing systems. For example, Miyake *et al.* (1968) treated a suspension of rabbit liver microsomes in 25% glycerol with a 1% solution of Lubrol WX[12] and obtained a supernatant fraction from high-speed centrifugation that contained most of the cytochromes P-450 and b_5. The two cytochromes were resolved by chromatography on diethylaminoethyl-Sephadex A-50; elution was carried out in the presence of the Lubrol. The preparation of cytochrome P-450 by this procedure was shown to be in a native state by investigating the effect of ligands on the spectral and electronic properties of the isolated cytochrome P-450 (Miyake *et al.*, 1968; Jefcoate *et al.*, 1969). The use of Lubrol to the extent of obtaining solubilization appears to be advantageous. Similar preparations obtained from rat liver microsomes by Lubrol treatment contained methyl sterol oxidase (Gaylor and Mason, 1968), but purification of this solubilized form of the oxidase has not been achieved.

Similarly, Ito and Sato (1968) reported the solubilization of cytochrome b_5 from rabbit liver microsomes by using a mixture of 1% of Triton X-100 and 1% of deoxycholic acid. The cytochrome was collected and partially purified from detergent by precipitation of the protein with ammonium sulfate; the cytochrome has been further purified to homogeneity.

Generally, in most of these studies microsomes were suspended in dilute solutions of the detergents and the mixtures were homogenized gently. Resistant microsomal particulate material then is removed by high-speed centrifugation, and protein is recovered from the resulting supernatant fraction. As pointed out above, the detergents generally accompany proteins during the purification; they are difficult to remove, and this property limits the use of nonionic detergents as solubilizing agents. We were able to develop a chromatographic method in which the greater affinity of Sephadex LH-20 for nonionic detergent relative to the filtration of protein on the gel resulted in separation of detergent from protein (Gaylor and Delwiche, 1969). Briefly, to the suspension of micro-

---

[12] Lubrol WX is the ether of cetyl alcohol and polyoxyethylene; the average molecular weight is 947.

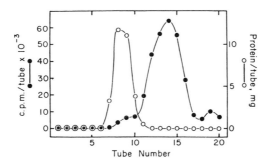

Fig. 8. Separation of liver microsomes and Lubrol by chromatography on Sephadex LH-20. Suspension of rat liver microsomes (45.9 mg protein) in 3 ml of ethylene glycol/0.01 M phosphate buffer solution (1:1) was homogenized with 49.2 mg of Lubrol (790,000 cpm). A sample of the suspension (2 ml containing 30.6 mg of protein and 32.9 mg of Lubrol [527,000 cpm]) was transferred to a column of Sephadex LH-20 (4.7 × 13.0 cm) that was equilibrated with the 50% ethylene glycol-buffer solution. Protein and Lubrol were eluted with the same solvent mixture. Fractions of 10 ml each were collected. Recovery of protein was complete, 30.5 mg; 42% of the [³H]Lubrol (about 224,000 cpm) remained tightly bound to the column and was not eluted with 50% ethylene glycol. Reproduced with kind permission of Academic Press, Inc.; see Gaylor and Delwiche (1969).

somes in detergent solution, ethylene glycol was added to a final concentration of 20 to 50% (v/v). The mixture was transferred to a column of Sephadex LH-20 that had been equilibrated with the same solution of aqueous ethylene glycol. Protein emerged from the column with the void volume (Fig. 8), and the Lubrol was retained in two forms; approximately 25-fold enrichment in the ratio of protein to Lubrol was achieved. Approximately one-half of the retained Lubrol emerged as an approximately tetrameric species with an apparent molecular weight of about 4000, and the remaining retained Lubrol was bound tightly to the column. Acetone was needed to release the latter species of Lubrol from Sephadex LH-20. In our hands, columns of greater size increased the fraction of Lubrol that remained tenaciously bound to the column. The Sephadex LH-20 is regenerated for subsequent use simply by washing with warm acetone and equilibrating again with the eluting solvent. An application of use of this procedure is described below (Section II,B,4).

Comment. The use of nonionic detergents is just starting. With suitable methods for removing the detergent, solubilization with nonionic detergent will become more attractive. One precautionary note, many commercial detergents have been oxidized upon storage; removal of oxidation products may be achieved according to the methods generally used to free lipids of peroxides (Privett *et al.*, 1953).

2. Enzymatic Methods

a. Partial Proteolysis. As we turn to additional solubilization techniques, there are many fewer examples in general, and outside of work in this laboratory there are almost no reports of the use of enzymatic methods to free microsomal enzymes of sterol metabolism. Part of the situation results because the initial successes in microdissection of microsomal vesicles by selective enzymatic digestion has just been reported (Ito and Sato, 1969), and as we find out from the same workers, use of partial proteolysis to effect release of microsomal enzymes may lead to a partially proteolyzed enzyme. Further information on this point follows below. On the other hand, limited use of partial proteolysis has been made in this laboratory. One example illustrates partial proteolysis to effect solubilization and, in the other example, partial proteolysis was used to remove a readily accessible contaminating protein of microsomes prior to solubilization of the sought-for enzyme.

Anaerobic incubation of broken-cell preparations of yeast with ergosta-7,22-diene-3β,5α-diol resulted in the net formation of ergosterol (Topham and Gaylor, 1967). Different methods of disruption of the yeast cells lead to differences in the partitioning of the dehydrating enzyme between the particles and supernatant fraction that result from centrifugation at 105,000g (Topham and Gaylor, 1970). As indicated in Fig. 5b, a limited amount of evidence led us to the conclusion that release of the dehydrase from particles was the result of partial proteolysis that occurred during autolysis of yeast. If sonic disruption or a pressure cell was used to make the cell-free preparation, essentially all of the enzyme was retained as a particulate form. Subsequent experiments to mimic the effect of autolysis by treating sonically prepared microsomes with trypsin were not successful.

The preparation of cyanide-binding protein obtained by deoxycholate treatment of liver microsomes is contaminated with microsomal cytochrome b_5 (Gaylor *et al.*, 1970a). Earlier, we had shown that upon mild trypsin digestion of microsomes, methyl sterol demethylase remained active, and much of the cytochrome b_5 could be removed with trypsin without substantial inactivation of demethylase (Gaylor and Mason, 1968). Conditions needed for complete removal of cytochrome b_5 generally yielded enzymatically inactive preparations. Accordingly, when Ito and Sato published their work on dissection of microsomal hemoproteins and enzymes using Nagarse, a bacterial protease obtained from *Bacillus subtilus* N', we incubated preparations of rat liver microsomes with Nagarse to remove cytochrome b_5 selectively (Gaylor *et al.*, 1970a). Almost complete removal of cytochrome b_5 and no loss of cyanide-binding protein was achieved by incubating Nagarse with liver micro-somes that were suspended in solutions containing 20% of glycerol. Changes in time, temperature, and Nagarse concentration were used to obtain selectivity. The preparation of cyanide-binding protein from these particles was free of contaminating cytochrome b_5 (Gaylor *et al.*, 1970a).

Caution must be used when proteolysis is selected for solubilization of an enzyme; the enzyme may be partially degraded during solubiliza-tion. Ito and Sato (1968) found that cytochrome b_5 prepared by deter-gent treatment (see Section II,B,1,*c*) had a molecular weight of 25,000. Cytochrome b_5 that exhibits the same spectral properties was prepared by treatment of microsomes with trypsin; the latter had a molecular weight of 12,000. Furthermore, Ito and Sato found that upon tryptic digestion of the cytochrome obtained by detergent treatment, the molec-ular weight of the protein was reduced to about 12,000. They suggested that very selective, partial proteolysis of cytochrome b_5 yielded an altered protein when trypsin was used. Parallel studies were reported recently by Spatz and Strittmatter (1971), who obtained a product of 16,000 molecular weight when they used a combination of ionic and non-ionic detergents for solubilization of cytochrome b_5. Thus, precautions must be taken in guarding against the generation of partially digested proteins. This method may best be limited to removal of contaminating proteins or to use in pretreatment of microsomes before detergent, etc., solubilization.

b. Partial Digestion of Lipids. Microsomal lipids are attacked by phos-pholipases A, C, and D (Graham and Wood, 1969; Lumper *et al.*, 1969). In addition, soluble proteins have been obtained following digestion of microsomes with lipase (Williams and Kamin, 1962). Thus, use of partial digestion of microsomal lipids to facilitate extraction of particulate en-zymes has remained very attractive. The shortcoming of partial proteo-lysis is avoided if phospholipase or lipase preparations are free of proteases.

Recently, we found that treatment of 50 mg of rat liver microsomes with either 25 μg of crude snake venom or 1 μg of purified phospholipase A resulted in the loss of methyl sterol demethylase activities (Fig. 9). When the fully digested particles (i.e., 15 minutes on Fig. 9) were in-cubated with supernatant fraction recovered from the phospholipase A treatment, activity was fully restored. Heat or trypsin treatment of the supernatant fraction before reconstitution negated the effect of addition of supernatant fraction on the activity. The supernatant fraction was shown to contain both an essential heat-stable and a heat-labile factor. An enzyme that apparently functions in methyl sterol demethylase is being purified from the supernatant fraction. It is premature to speculate

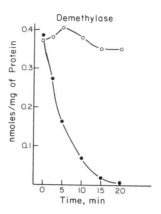

Fig. 9. Effect of phospholipase A on methyl sterol demethylase. Rat liver micro-somes (50 mg of protein) were suspended in 2 ml of 0.1 M Tris-HCl buffer (pH 7.4 and containing 2 mM GSH and 10 mM nicotinamide) and incubated with 25 μg of snake venom (*Crotalus adamanteus,* Ross Allen Reptile Institute, Silver Springs, Florida) for the indicated lengths of time at 37° with 5 mM Ca^{++}. The phospholipase A action was stopped by adding 25 mM EDTA, and the partially digested microsomes were collected by centrifugation and assayed as described previously (Table III). Values obtained without added snake venom, O——O.

about the nature of the enzymatic process, but with this example, we have our first solid indication that partial digestion of phospholipid may render certain of the enzymes either soluble or readily extractable.

Apart from the use of phospholipase to yield soluble enzyme, from the work of others it is clear that phospholipids are essential for some cata-lytic processes of microsomes. Observations such as the effect of phos-pholipases on microsomal enzymatic activities described above, as well as work on microsomal drug metabolism (e.g., see effect of phospho-lipase C described by Chaplin and Mannering, 1970), indicate that phos-pholipase action may be used to unravel some of the possible functions of microsomal lipids in sterol biosynthesis. Two very detailed reports that may serve as bases for both experimental methods and explanations have been published recently on the effects of phospholipase action on microsomal glucose-6-phosphatase activity (Zakim, 1970; Trump *et al.,* 1970). Some additional comments on phospholipids of microsomal mem-branes follow later (Section III,A).

3. Combinations of Methods

The effectiveness of the simultaneous use of more than one method should be obvious to the reader at this point. Several examples have been given without making particular mention. For example, the cyanide-binding protein (Gaylor *et al.,* 1970a) was isolated free of cytochrome

b_5 by treatment of liver microsomes with deoxycholate (Section II,B,1,*b*) after cytochrome b_5 was removed by Nagarse treatment (Section II,B,2,*a*). The prenol pyrophosphate pyrophosphohydrolase (Tsai and Gaylor, 1966) was isolated from an acetone powder of microsomes (Section II,B,1,*a*) after the microsomes were treated with strong Tris buffer to remove more readily solubilized proteins (Section II,B,1,*a*; Table IV). Both Ito and Sato (1968) and Spatz and Strittmatter (1971) used combinations of ionic and nonionic detergents to isolate cytochrome b_5 from liver microsomes (Section II,B,2). The example described below (Section II,B,4) illustrates that solubilization of the 3-ketosteroid reductase (Fig. 3) was accomplished by a combination of solvent (Section II,B,1,*a*) and nonionic detergent treatment (Section II,B,1,*c*). The purpose of this brief subsection is to expand the possibilities of combinations of methods to procedures not hitherto described. Two of these are identified: the use of different sources of the enzyme; and the use of novel purification methods in conjunction with solubilization techniques.

a. With Biological Variations. There is understandable resistance to seeking an enzyme from an alternate source such as from a different tissue or a different organism. However, there may be significant advantages. The worker should consider these advantages as seriously as he considers the combination of any two of the techniques described above in this section.

The enzyme may be more easily solubilized from broken-cell preparations of tissue from a different source. There is a platitude that many enzymes that are particle-bound in broken-cell preparations of mammalian tissues (e.g., liver) may be obtained as soluble enzymes from homogenates of simpler organisms. An excellent example within the investigation of sterol biosynthesis has been mentioned (Schechter *et al.*, 1970). These workers reported that 2,3-oxidosqualene-lanosterol cyclase is found in the soluble fraction of broken-cell preparations of yeast, whereas the same enzyme is bound to microsomes in liver homogenates (Yamamoto *et al.*, 1969). Notably, certain properties of the enzyme from the two sources are different, but the ease of obtaining purified cyclase from yeast is impressive. Another elegant example of obtaining an enzyme in a soluble form from microorganisms rather than from mammalian liver microsomes is the isolation, purification, and characterization of cytochrome P-450 that has been carried out by Gunsalus and co-workers (Katagiri *et al.*, 1968; Gunsalus, 1968). Investigations of the structure of the purified cytochrome P-450 from *Pseudomonas putida* will make a significant contribution to understanding the nature of the microsomal hemoprotein (Tsai *et al.*, 1970). A third example, and one closer to sterol biosynthesis, β-hydroxy-β-methylglutaryl-coenzyme A reductase, illustrates the point, too. Only recently, Kawachi and Rudney (1970) reported the successful solubilization and purification of the microsomal enzyme from rat liver. However, in the same laboratory, the yeast enzyme had been isolated and purified 10 years earlier (Durr and Rudney, 1960). The 5α-hydroxysterol dehydrase of yeast was in the supernatant fraction of autolyzed cells after high-speed centrifugation (Topham and Gaylor, 1970).

A synthetic system free of complicating enzymes may be obtained from tissue other than liver or preparations of liver from different species. For example, when we were collecting evidence against the possible participation of cytochrome P-450 in methyl sterol oxidase, examination of the comparative biochemistry of distribution of cytochrome P-450 (Garfinkel, 1963) and cholesterol biosynthetic enzymes (Kritchevsky, 1958) in various organisms led to the finding of enzymes from many sources that are essentially free of cytochrome P-450. Similarly, acyl-coenzyme A desaturase is abundant in microsomes from adipose tissue,[13] but this source of desaturase is essentially free of methyl sterol oxidase.[14] Thus, the desaturase may be studied in the absence of sterol demethylase activity. The investigation of acyl-coenzyme A desaturase of rat liver microsomes is complicated by a particularly active microsomal acyl-coenzyme A hydrolase; hen liver microsomes have a much more favorable relative rate of desaturation compared to hydrolysis (Gurr and Robinson, 1970). Similarly, the prenol pyrophosphate pyrophosphohydrolase in microsomes from testicular tissue was about three times as active as the enzyme of liver microsomes (Nightingale et al., 1967); thus, the former was used as the better source of the enzyme (Tsai and Gaylor, 1966). Equilibria between high- and low-spin forms of cytochrome P-450 were measured with particles from adrenal mitochondria (Jefcoate and Gaylor, 1970) because shifts in equilibria upon ligand additions to cytochrome P-450 of rabbit liver microsomes occurred too slowly for measurements to be carried out within practical time limits (Jefcoate et al., 1969).

A parallel argument exists for attempting solubilizations of enzymes that have been enriched by changes in physiological or nutritional status. For example, Oshino et al. (1971) used fasting and refeeding to increase the specific activity of acyl-coenzyme A desaturase of liver microsomes at least tenfold over the control value. Treatment of rats with dietary cholestyramine enhanced microsomal methyl sterol oxidase to about 300%

---

[13] S. J. Odell and J. L. Gaylor (unpublished observations).
[14] C. V. Delwiche and J. L. Gaylor (unpublished observations).

of the rates observed with liver from control rats (Moir *et al.*, 1970). Altering culture conditions of yeast may be used similarly. This list could be extended considerably, but the point should be obvious.

Finally, use of yeast and mutant strains of yeasts to study the sequence of reactions of sterol biosynthesis presents an exciting possibility. Recently, Thompon *et al.* (1971) reported the isolation of a mutant strain of *Saccharomyces cerevisiae* that exhibits normal growth but in which ergosterol is replaced by a different C_{28}-sterol.

b. With Purification Procedures. Some mention of purification procedures needs to be made. As Kawachi and Rudney (1970) put it, the β-hydroxy-β-methylglutaryl-coenzyme A reductase was purified by "standard methods" after isolation from liver microsomes with deoxycholic acid. Only conventional methods of enzyme purification have been used in this laboratory, too. However, some more novel methods may be developed in the future for use with enzymes that have been solubilized from particles.

In addition, certain advantages in even conventional purifications may be obtained because of the membranous origin of the enzymes. For example, the 5α-hydroxysterol dehydrase (Topham and Gaylor, 1970), as isolated, contained phospholipid. Gel filtration on Sephadex G-100 yielded enzyme that was eluted with the void volume breakthrough; smaller proteins were removed. The enzyme was treated with phospholipase A to remove phospholipid and filtered again on Sephadex G-100; the enzyme was retained on the column, thereby purifying it from larger proteins.

Affinity labeling (see Muldoon and Warren, 1969, for interesting possibilities; also Ganguly and Warren, 1971) of the microsomal enzymes has special appeal because steroids with reactive functional groups should be able to penetrate microsomal lipids and react with specific microsomal enzymes. Labeling would facilitate the trial-and-error experiments of solubilization as well as purification procedures. Affinity chromatography may become a useful technique for purification. Electrofocusing of microsomal subparticle preparations has just been achieved by using Triton N-101 in the medium.[15]

Comment. The investigator should be as willing to try superimposition of biological or innovative purification methods onto a solubilization procedure as he is to attempt to use two methods of solubilization simultaneously.

---

[15] W. Levin, R. Kuntzman, A. Y. H. Lu, and A. H. Conney (private communication).

4. *An Example of Trial-and-Error Steps in an Attempted Solubilization: NADPH-3-Ketosteroid Reductase* (with Dr. A. D. Rahimtula)

a. Evidence for Existence of Enzyme. Extensive evidence has been presented earlier (Section I,B; and Fig. 3). Briefly, Lindberg *et al.* (1963) proposed that 3-ketosteroids were formed as intermediates during methyl sterol demethylation (Fig. 2). 3-Ketosteroid products of 4-methyl sterol demethylation were identified (Swindell and Gaylor, 1968) and it was shown that the 4α-methyl group of 3-keto-4α-methyl sterols was not attacked oxidatively prior to reduction of the 3-ketone to a 3β-alcohol. Decarboxylation of 4α-carboxylic acids (II and V of Fig. 3) yielded stoichiometric amounts of 3-ketosteroids and carbon dioxide (III and VI of Fig. 3; Miller and Gaylor, 1970a,b).

b. Assay. The 3-ketosteroids accumulated when pyridine nucleotides were removed from microsomes by Triton treatment and NAD⁺ was the only pyridine nucleotide added to the incubation. Further metabolism of the 3-ketosteroids required NADPH (Swindell and Gaylor, 1968). Thus, for the assay of 3-ketosteroid reductase, NADPH was added to the medium. Finally, incubations were carried out anaerobically to prevent oxidative attack of the product(s), and the substrate contained only one double bond in the $\Delta^{7(8)}$-position to eliminate concomitant isomerization.

[¹⁴C]4,4-Dimethyl-5α-cholest-7-en-3-one was prepared by oxidation of the synthetic 3β-alcohol with *tert*-butyl chromate (Menini and Norymberski, 1962). Following incubation in 2 ml of 1 μmole of NADPH and 100 nmoles of the substrate with the equivalent of 5 mg of rat liver microsomal protein, carrier 3β-hydroxy- and 3-ketosteroid was added, and the mixture was saponified. The steroids were extracted, the extracting solvent was evaporated, and the residue containing the steroids was transferred to an alumina column. From the [¹⁴C]radioactivity in the substrate and product and the specific activity of the substrate, the amount of 3β-alcohol formed was calculated.

c. Preliminary Experiments. The rate of conversion of ketone to alcohol was shown to be proportional to the enzyme concentration over the range from 1 to 5 mg of protein, a constant initial velocity was observed for 30 minutes of incubation at 37°, and the velocity increased with increasing concentration of substrate.

In the summer of 1967, we set out to isolate the reductase. The specific activity of the microsomal-bound enzyme was 1.84 nmoles of ketone reduced per milligram of protein (30-minute incubation). An acetone-dry powder was prepared as described for another microsomal enzyme isolation in this laboratory (Tsai and Gaylor, 1966). The reductase was active in the powder (2.29 nmoles per milligram of protein). The activity was stable on storage of the powder. The remainder of the work appeared to be routine!

Initial attempts to extract the reductase from the acetone powder were unsuccessful. Various conditions were tried (i.e., dilute and strong buffers; different buffers; buffers plus KCl of various concentrations; buffers plus miscible solvents, e.g., ethylene glycol). Alternatively, the microsomes were washed with strong buffer and salt solutions prior to preparation of the acetone powder (see Table IV). The reductase was not readily released into dilute buffer from the acetone powder of the residue. A series of experiments was initiated in which the acetone powder was treated with stronger methods (Section II,B,1,2) to release the enzyme. Accordingly, deoxycholate (Section II,B,1,b) was added over the range of 0.1 to 1.0 mg of bile salt per milligram of protein. Solubilization by sonic disruption was attempted. Extractions with solutions of 0.5 to 1.0% of either Triton WR-1339 or Tween 80 (Section II,B,1,c) were carried out with no success. Finally, partial tryptic hydrolysis (Section II,B,2,a) was investigated, with the hope that inert protein (perhaps acting like "glue") could be removed first, thus rendering the 3-ketosteroid reductase more accessible. Activity was lost rapidly in the presence of trypsin (Fig. 10, ●—●). However, simultaneous extraction of inert protein by combining solvent extractions with trypsin treatment at least yielded particles that contained active enzyme following various intervals of digestion (Fig. 10, ○—○). Thus, extensive experiments were carried

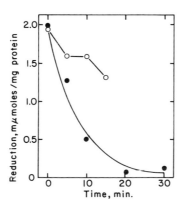

Fig. 10. Effect of trypsin treatment on 3-ketosteroid reductase. A suspension of 50 mg of microsomes was suspended in Tris-HCl buffer (pH 7.4 and containing 2 mM GSH). The suspension was incubated with 1 mg of trypsin (Sigma Chemical Company, lot 97B-8000) at 25° for the times indicated. When samples of 10 mg of microsomes were withdrawn, 2 mg of crystalline trypsin inhibitor was added (Sigma Chemical Company, Type I-S, lot 47B-0330). The samples were incubated with 3-ketosteroid. Without 20% ethylene glycol, ●—●; with 20% ethylene glycol, ○—○.

out with ethylene glycol (trypsin was omitted) to remove the inert protein prior to attempting extraction of reductase with the use of other procedures (Section II,B,1,a). Although conditions for the extraction of the enzyme following partial proteolysis by trypsin were never obtained (the enzyme, if active, always remained associated with the particulate fraction following highspeed centrifugation), the stabilizing effect of ethylene glycol on the reductase proved valuable for future experiments. (A simple admission—we were still thinking of ethylene glycol as an extracting solvent at this point, not as a stabilizing agent.) By the spring of 1969, five people had attempted to solubilize the reductase from the easily prepared, stable acetone powder.[16] Work with the acetone powder finally was abandoned; we had exhausted our options.

By late 1970, with the purification of the decarboxylase (Rahimtula and Gaylor, 1971) and progress on the further resolution of methyl sterol oxidase (Gaylor et al., 1970a), the ultimate need for purified 3-ketosteroid reductase to carry out reconstitution experiments became obvious and discomforting. With the knowledge of previous lack of success, Dr. Rahimtula initiated a thorough study of solubilization of the reductase.

d. *Subsequent Solubilization Attempts.* (Numbers in parentheses correspond to numbers in first column of Table IX.) (1) With the abandonment of acetone powder preparations, lyophilization (Section II,B,1,a) was used to prepare large quantities of stable, homogeneous microsomes. Microsomes from chicken liver proved to be a rich source of reductase (specific activity = 1 to 2 nmoles of steroid reduced per milligram of protein). From the earlier work with the effect of trypsin on acetone powder (Fig. 10; and Section II,B,4,c, above), a suspension of the lyophilized microsomes was treated with 1% of trypsin (w/v) at room temperature for 2 hours. Tryptic activity was arrested with trypsin inhibitor (Gaylor and Mason, 1968). Both the digested suspension (before centrifugation) and the supernatant fraction (after centrifugation) were inactive (Table IX).

(2) Rat liver microsomes were treated similarly with reduction of time and temperature for tryptic treatments. 3-Ketosteroid reductase in suspension was completely inactivated.

(3) Nagarse had been found to release cytochrome b_5 completely from rat liver microsomes under even milder conditions than those used with trypsin (Gaylor et al., 1970a): 5 mg of Nagarse per 130 mg of lyoph-

---

[16] These experiments were carried out by John Donelson, Archie Swindell, Donna Vanderpool, Connie Delwiche, and J. L. Gaylor.

ilized rat liver microsomes was incubated for 12 hours at 4°. Although under these conditions we had found retention of methyl sterol oxidase activity (e.g., I → II, Fig. 3), the reductase appeared to be too labile. Thus, perhaps the 3-ketosteroid reductase is very exposed in microsomes and it is attacked rapidly by trypsin (after all, a rapid time-course of loss of activity was observed with acetone powder preparations; see Fig. 10). Therefore, reasoning that the reductase is exposed, then the entire attack was changed *away* from removing extraneous protein, and once again attempts were made to free the enzyme directly from the microsomes. Only, unlike work reported above (subsection *c*), lyoph-ilized microsomes were substituted for the acetone powder preparation.

(4) Gentle hydrolysis of phospholipids by treatment with phospho-lipase A (Section II,B,2,*b*) was attempted first because others in the laboratory had found that microsomal methyl sterol oxidase remained active when treated similarly, and turbidity of the suspension of micro-somes decreased markedly upon treatment of the particles with phos-pholipase A. Whereas trypsin treatment destroyed activity in the sus-pension of particles (Table IX, lines 1 and 2), the reductase in the suspension remained active; however, it was not released. This appeared to be a step in the right direction, only perhaps the step was too large. Reduction of the amount of phospholipase A was attempted (Table IX, 4b); no conditions were found in which activity remained in the super-natant fraction. On the other hand, the particles following digestion with phospholipase A retained activity. Because the specific activity of the reductase in digested particles was about one-half that in the undigested controls, we argued that perhaps some enzyme was being released and inactivated following release. Thus, nonenzymatic (Section II,B,1) methods of gentle extraction were tried.

(5) Extraction with strong Tris-HCl (1 *M*, pH 7.4) yielded consider-able protein and no activity in the supernatant fraction, but the specific activity of reductase in recovered particles was equal to that in controls. At last a condition had been found under which total activity was not lost—the enzyme just was not extracted into the supernatant fraction.

(6) A final concentration of 1% of Tween 80 was tried first. The en-zyme was inhibited somewhat. However, microsomes collected after treatment with Tween 80 were fully active. (The normal psychological response to these frustrations is to expand the number of variables within any experiment with the hope that the right combination will result.)

(7) Thus, we will remove easily dissolved enzymes with Tris-acetate buffer (Moir *et al.*, 1968), more resistant proteins will be extracted with solvent (20% ethylene glycol, Fig. 10), and we will put in Tween 80 (at three concentrations) to facilitate everything. The composite result was

Table IX

SEQUENCE OF STEPS IN SOLUBILIZATION OF MICROSOMAL 3-KETOSTEROID REDUCTASE

Method	Reason	Result	Conclusion
(1) 1% Trypsin treatment of lyophilized microsomes from chickens, 2 hr at 25°.	Trypsin may be used to remove inert protein to allow extraction.	Inactive enzyme in treated suspension and particles and supernatant fraction from centrifugation.	Preparation was too sensitive to trypsin.
(2) Same as 1 above, only rat liver and 30 min at 20°.	Milder than in 1.	Inactive preparation. Considerable protein was released.	Perhaps conditions are still too strong.
(3) 5 mg of Nagarse, 12 hr at 4°.	Nagarse treatment had been shown to be milder than conditions in 2 above.	Inactive. About 50% of protein was released.	Perhaps partial proteolysis should be abandoned. Reductase may be too exposed.
(4a) 1 mg of phospholipase A, 10 min at 37°.	Assume reductase exposed on surface. Remove lipid to facilitate extraction of enzyme.	No active reductase in supernatant fraction, but digested suspension was 50% as active as controls.	Too strong. Some hope, though, because activity in suspension of particles was not destroyed.
(4b) 0.5 mg → less phospholipase A.	—	Same as 4a.	Try some other "gentle" method.
(5) Extract lyophilized microsomes with strong Tris buffer.	Perhaps enzyme is extracted by gentle means, but trypsin, Nagarse, or phospholipase A inactivated the extracted enzyme.	Inactive supernatant fraction—*fully* active particles recovered from centrifugation.	Try *mild* detergent to free enzyme. At least particle-bound enzyme remained fully active.
(6) 1% Tween 80 with lyophilized microsomes.	This is a mild detergent treatment.	Inactive supernatant fraction; active particles; Some direct inhibition by Tween.	Try combination of Tween and strong buffer next. Forget about inhibition—we can try to get rid of Tween before enzymatic assay. Therefore, use more Tween.

(7) Tris-acetate buffer ± 1, 2, and 5% Tween 80 and ±20% ethylene glycol. Fresh microsomes used.	See text. Argument is if one treatment does not work perhaps some clue from 3 simultaneous treatments (that do not inactivate particle-bound enzyme) may work.	In all cases, the residue collected by centrifugation was fully active. No activity in supernatant fraction, but some activity was found in suspension that contained 1% of Tween 80.	Grandiose experiment no better than predecessors.
(8) Ionic shock with 0.01 to 1.0 M phosphate. Used fresh microsomes.	This is gentle, and evidence still for enzyme on "outside" of microsome. Freshly prepared microsomes were used.	Same as above. Collected microsomes fully active.	No release, but activity of collected microsomes remained high. Try other methods with fresh microsomes (see reason in text).
(9) Phospholipase A—25 µg per 50 mg of protein, 10 min at 37°. Fresh microsomes were used.	Try fresh microsomes again.	Supernatant fraction inactive.	Keep trying.
(10) Deoxycholate, Lu and Coon (1968) method.[a]	Try fresh microsomes.	Supernatant fraction inactive. However, *in contrast* to earlier experiments with deoxycholate, the particles were fully active.	Deoxycholate not useful. Questioned why the particles were active this time but could not answer question. (Now we know that glycerol of the Lu and Coon method protected the reductase.)
(11) Sonic treatment of acetone powder in Tris-acetate. Time course, 30 sec to 4 min, of sonic treatment.	May be able to reduce size of particle to facilitate extraction.	Particles active. Supernatant fraction inactive.	Forget sonic treatment.
(12)–(13) Repeat trypsin (1%, 20 min, 20°, Tris-acetate buffer ± ethylene glycol).[a]	We had extra acetone powder.	Activity of particles remained high with ethylene glycol. Activity was lost without added ethylene glycol.	Ethylene glycol may solubilize enzyme. Repeat earlier attempts only do everything in the presence of ethylene glycol.
(14) 2% Lubrol WX in 20% ethylene glycol.	We may have been extracting the enzyme all along, and the extracted enzyme was labile. Protection of extracted enzyme may be required.	Supernatant fraction slightly active with Lubrol present, fully active when Lubrol was removed chromatographically.	Success!

[a] Along in here somewhere, at a seminar, someone said, "Why don't you try 8 M urea?" We did. It did not work either.

no better. Clarification resulted upon addition of Tween 80 to samples containing ethylene glycol. Go back to simple experiments.

(8) Microsomes were prepared with dilute (0.01 to 0.1 M) phosphate buffer, and proteins were extracted from the resulting microsomes with 1.0 M phosphate. The supernatant fraction was inactive. Also, lyophilized microsomes were abandoned simultaneously. Reason: perhaps whatever change renders the enzyme unextractable from acetone powders also occurs when microsomes are lyophilized. Although the experiments were unsuccessful, it was concluded that other methods should be investigated again with freshly prepared microsomes.

(9) Very little phospholipase A was incubated with fresh microsomes; no activity was released into the supernatant fraction.

(10) We tried deoxycholate with fresh microsomes. (You will recall, as mentioned in subsection c, that deoxycholate completely destroyed activity in acetone powder; deoxycholate had not been reinvestigated for some time. Perhaps the inactivity resulted earlier because an acetone powder was used.) No such luck. However, glycerol was added to the microsomal suspension because, between 1968 and 1971, we had switched to the deoxycholate solubilization method of Lu and Coon (1968) in which glycerol is used. Unlike the earlier work with deoxycholate, the particles remained fully active. We did not assign the difference to a protective action of glycerol, though, and subsequent experiments were carried out without added ethylene glycol or glycerol. We returned to acetone powder for a brief pause from preparing microsomes every day. (You might be surprised to know how many times substitutions for the one-half day preparation of microsomes are made.)

(11) We have never had success with sonic treatment apart from reducing the size of particles. (It simply takes longer to sediment the fragments at 105,000g.) But, we tried again, only this time Tris-acetate buffer and a time-course of sonic treatment was investigated.

(12) As long as we had a large preparation of acetone powder, some of the year's earlier experiments were repeated.

(13) Trypsin treatment (only in Tris-acetate) ± ethylene glycol was repeated. The retention of activity in the presence of ethylene glycol (Fig. 10) was observed again. *Perhaps* ethylene glycol is protecting the enzyme and not extracting it; once again, as shown in Fig. 5b which was drawn a year before, we thought that the solvent was extracting the enzyme. Therefore, go back and do everything ± ethylene glycol!

(14) Other than optimizing the conditions, little else was done before partial purification of the extracted enzyme was achieved.

e. Purification. (See Table X.) June, 1971—Livers from three male adult rats were homogenized in 3 volumes of 0.1 M Tris-HCl buffer con-

Table X

SOLUBILIZATION OF MICROSOMAL 3-KETOSTEROID REDUCTASE

Enzyme fraction	Total protein (mg)	Total activity[a] (nmoles of product formed)	Recovery (%)	Specific activity (nmoles of product formed/30 min per mg protein)	-Fold purifica- tion
Microsomes	650	16,350	100.0	0.84	1.0
Supernatant fraction after Sephadex LH-20 and centrifugation	365	14,600	89.4	1.33	1.6
After DEAE-cellulose chromatography	73	5,590	34.2	2.55	3.2
0 to 40% Ammonium sulfate fraction	25	5,500	33.7	7.35	8.8

[a] Each incubation flask contained 212 nmoles of [^{14}C]4,4-dimethyl-5α-cholest-7-en-3-one, 330 nmoles of glucose, 50 μl of glucose oxidase (Calbiochem, 1500 units/ml, lot 800019), 115 μmoles of isocitrate, 50 μl of isocitric dehydrogenase (Calbiochem, 29 IU/ml, lot 000722), 1.35 μmoles of NADP$^+$ and the appropriate enzyme fraction in a total volume of 2.25 ml of 0.1 M Tris-HCl buffer, pH 7.4. Incubation time was 30 minutes at 37°.

taining 2 mM GSH and 10 mM nicotinamide. Microsomes were collected and homogenized in 30 ml of 0.1 M Tris-HCl buffer containing 20% of ethylene glycol and 1% (v/v) of Lubrol ($\sim$14 mg of protein per milliliter). The mixture was centrifuged for 2 hours at 105,000g. The supernatant fraction was poured onto a column of Sephadex LH-20 (8 × 4.5 cm), and protein containing reductase activity was eluted with 0.1 M Tris-HCl buffer plus 20% of ethylene glycol. The colored eluate was collected ($\sim$30 ml) and centrifuged for 2 hours at 105,000g. The clear supernatant fraction ($\sim$25 ml; with a small amount of lipid floating on top) was removed with a pipette and transferred to a column of diethylaminoethyl-cellulose that was equilibrated with 0.1 M Tris-HCl buffer (pH 7.5 at 25°) plus 1 mM GSH. Protein was fully eluted with 200 ml of the same buffer (10-ml fractions were collected). Fractions 7 to 11 containing colored material were combined ($\sim$60 ml), and the solution was concentrated to about 13 to 15 ml by the use of an Amicon Ultrafiltrator equipped with an XM-50 membrane. The concentrated solution was treated with a saturated ammonium sulfate solution (adjusted to pH 7.4) to give 40% of saturation; the mixture was centrifuged at 18,000 rpm (Servall centrifuge, r = 4.25 inches) for 20 minutes. The protein fraction floating on the surface of the resulting solution was removed, dissolved in 5 ml of 0.1 M Tris-HCl buffer (containing 20% of ethylene glycol), and the solution was poured onto a small column of Sephadex LH-20 (10 × 1 cm). Protein was eluted with the same buffer. The eluted protein was dialyzed twice against 1 liter of 0.1 M Tris-HCl buffer.

Now, if you had read that synopsis is a journal article without first hearing of points (1) through (14) of Table IX, and the preliminary work in subsection c, you might be misled enough to think that we are either brilliant or lucky experimentalists. Actually, we are neither; perhaps only persistent.

III. Other Aspects of Purification of Microsomal Enzymes

A. MICROSOMAL MEMBRANES

The membranes of the endoplasmic reticulum and the resulting microsomes should not be viewed naïvely as homogeneous structures. Many lines of evidence support the conclusion that even after the disruptive preparation of microsomes, discrete, identifiable components of the membranes exist. The purpose of this subsection is simply to inform the experimentalist who is attempting to isolate microsomal enzymes that he is working with a heterogeneous population of components, and he should attempt to use this information to his advantage. Others have developed the evidence quite well. For example, the reader is encouraged to study the brief review of microsomal oxidases by Schenkman (1970). Glaumann (1970, 1971) has published excellent summaries that contain references to the development of the concept of microsomal heterogeneity, as well as extensive citations of published work and reviews. In a recent review of membrane structural proteins by Kaplan and Criddle (1971), the authors report work on the structural proteins of microsomes that appear to be a family of species that are associated with the lipid components. Mention has been made of the work of Trump et al. (1970) on the association of lipids and protein in microsomal membranes. More generally, the association of lipid and protein was related in a study of red blood cell membrane disruption using deoxycholate (Philippot, 1971). Finally, the modern understanding of biological membranes was reviewed very well by Rothfield and Finkelstein (1968).

Study of these well-written articles in addition to the known effects of removal of microsomal lipids on specific enzymatic processes (see paragraph above; also included in Jones and Armstrong, 1965; Jones

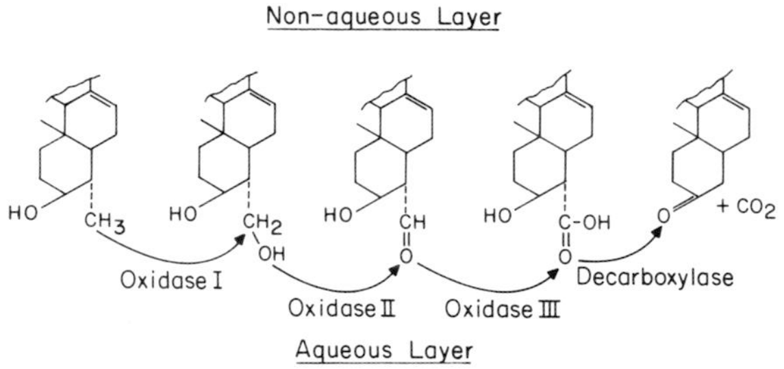

Non-aqueous Layer

FIG. 11.   Possible role of membrane in demethylase.

and Wakil, 1967; Jones *et al.*, 1969; Holloway and Wakil, 1970; Holloway, 1971) leads to an interesting possibility. Perhaps, in addition to direct effects of lipids upon single enzymes of microsomal sterol biosynthesis, the phospholipids of microsomal membranes may serve an additional function of fixing spatial arrangement of the separate enzymes with each other, with substrate, or with both. An oversimplified diagram of this idea is shown (Fig. 11). However, experiments are underway in this laboratory in which the hypothesis is being tested by assaying both component enzymatic activities and composite methyl sterol demethylase during the course of removal of phospholipids by treatment with phospholipase A (Section II,B,2,*b*). Clearly, these experiments must be carried out before proceeding to attempts to reconstitute the overall process from the purified enzymes and lipids.

B. PITFALLS

Many of the major objections to the enzymatic approach may be countered by successfully carrying out reconstitution experiments. In reconstitution it is possible to: demonstrate the essential nature of each enzyme added; exclude other suggested enzymes; and confirm that the isolated enzymes have not been altered to the extent of remaining enzymatically active but not suitable for reconstitution. Furthermore, reconstitution experiments will allow each component to be examined for contributions to specificity such as in the experiments on cytochrome P-450 that were reported recently by Lu *et al.* (1971). Specificity for the lipids associated either with individual enzymes or, if essential, with the multienzyme system may be studied, too. Factors affecting the control of the rate of the process may be elucidated by this means. Reconstitution experiments may require more intimate mixing than that simply achieved by combining the solubilized proteins and suspensions of lipid. Partial reconstitution with lipids may require mixing of lipids and enzymes with deoxycholate, followed by slow removal of the detergent.

Isolated phospholipids may be replaced by enzymatically facilitating exchange of phospholipids (Wirtz and Zilversmit, 1968).

Experiments that are not carried through to reconstitution may suffer from additional pitfalls. The enzymes may be altered subtly upon isolation, and the alteration may be undetected. The partially hydrolyzed cytochrome b_5 obtained by trypsin treatment exhibited characteristic spectral properties of native cytochrome b_5 (pointed out by Ito and Sato, 1968). Furthermore, properties may unavoidably change upon isolation. This possibility makes the relating of enzymatic properties of the solubilized protein to the microsomal-bound enzyme impossible. The latter still must be attempted to show that the worker has isolated not just one stable species of a family of enzymes, but one that quantitatively accounts for the enzymatic activity of microsomes. For example, a point was made in Section II,B,1,b and Table VIII that the properties of the soluble methyl sterol oxidase and the microsomal oxidase were found to be similar.

All of the problems associated with working with membranous systems may be inherent in these studies. For example, peroxidation of an essential lipid may occur. Assay of the extent of peroxidation of the phospholipid should accompany solubilization studies (for a method, see Glavind and Hartmann, 1955).

Of course, the worker must remember one more possibility. The sought-for enzyme may require the intact membrane for activity, and it will not be isolable in a lipid-free, active form.

C. Use of Soluble Enzymes

To end positively, throughout this chapter there has been the assumption that investigation of properties of component enzymes of a multienzymatic process will yield information that could not be obtained with other approaches. A few examples may illustrate some advantages.

In the biosynthesis of ergosterol by yeast, the "extra" methyl group of the side chain is transferred to the 24-C position of the molecule (Fig. 5a). When we had purified the methyltransferase of yeast (Moore and Gaylor, 1969), we were in a position to resolve an enigma in the assignment of the sequence of biosynthetic reactions of ergosterol formation. Others had suggested that the extra methyl group may be transferred to the side chain before complete demethylation of the 4α-, 4β-, and 14α-methyl groups of lanosterol (Akhtar et al., 1966; Barton et al., 1968). Investigation of substrate specificity of the purified enzyme clearly showed that zymosterol ($R_1=R_2=R_3=H$ of Fig. 12) was by far the best

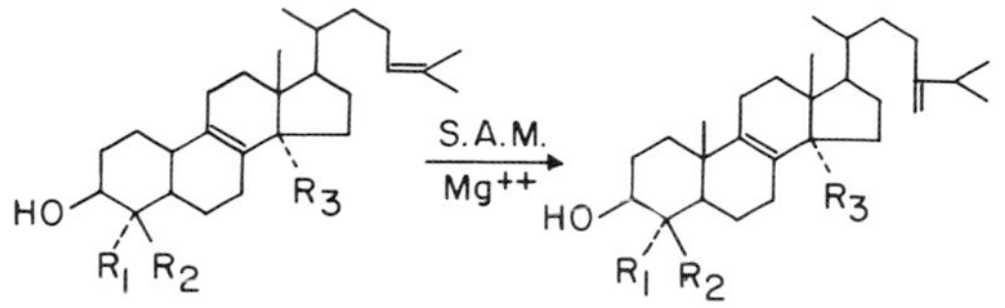

	R₁	R₂	R₃	nmoles*	%
	CH_3	CH_3	CH_3	0	0
	CH_3	CH_3	H	0.2	2
	CH_3	H	H	0.6	5
	H	H	H	12	100

* per mg of protein; 30 min incubation

Fig. 12. Substrate specificity of yeast Δ^{24}-sterol methyltransferase.

substrate (Moore and Gaylor, 1970). If the isolated methyltransferase is the enzyme responsible for this reaction *in vivo*, the extra methyl group appears to be added after complete demethylation of lanosterol. Thus, problems related to sequence of chemical reactions in the biosynthesis may be solved.

The extensive work of Dempsey and her co-workers on the inhibition of cholesterol biosynthesis has been described briefly (see also Witiak *et al*, 1971). Examination of the interaction of inhibitors with specific enzymes isolated from microsomes may yield information on factors that affect the rate of sterol synthesis. Furthermore, additional knowledge about the interaction of various drugs may lead to the design of more specific and efficacious inhibitors. Thus, such studies could result in the development of drugs that are used to slow the rate of cholesterol formation.

A third achievement may lie in related areas that have been cited extensively in this chapter, but each is a problem that has not been solved. For example, the relationship of microsomal electron transport of methyl sterol oxidase to other microsomal oxidases such as mammalian acyl-coenzyme A desaturase (Bloch, 1969) or cytochrome P-450-dependent oxidations of xenobiotics (Mason *et al.*, 1965) would be an important contribution.

Finally, the author hopes that these methods will be found useful to other "microsomologists" in attacking a wide variety of problems.

Comment. I welcome comments and inquiries about these procedures.

ACKNOWLEDGMENTS

I am very much indebted to Mrs. C. V. Delwiche, Mrs. P. L. MacIntyre, and Dr. A. D. Rahimtula, who helped to prepare this manuscript. I am equally indebted to those students who worked out most of the details summarized in this chapter. Notably, those students who stuck with frustrating and unsuccessful attempts (you will find their names in footnotes citing unpublished observations) taught us as much as those who were apparently more successful (you will find their names in the list of references).

References

Akhtar, M., Hunt, P. F., and Parvez, M. A. (1966). *Chem. Commun.* p. 565.

Barton, D. H. R., Harrison, D. M., and Widdowson, D. A. (1968). *Chem. Commun.* p. 17.

Battersby, A. R. (1963). *Proc. Chem. Soc., London* p. 189.

Battersby, A. R. (1967). *Pure Appl. Chem.* **14**, 117.

Berséus, O., Danielsson, H., and Einarsson, K. (1969). *In* "Steroids and Terpenoids" (R. B. Clayton, ed.), Methods in Enzymology, Vol. 15, pp. 551–562. Academic Press, New York.

Bloch, K. (1965). *Science* **150**, 19.

Bloch, K. (1969). *Accounts Chem. Res.* **2**, 193.

Brunner, G., and Bygrave, F. L. (1969). *Eur. J. Biochem.* **8**, 530.

Chaplin, M. D., and Mannering, G. J. (1970). *Mol. Pharmacol.* **6**, 631.

Chesterton, C. J. (1968). *J. Biol. Chem.* **243**, 1147.

Chevallier, F. (1964). *Biochim. Biophys. Acta* **84**, 316.

Christophe, J., and Popják, G. (1961). *J. Lipid Res.* **2**, 244.

Clayton, R. B. (1965). *Quart. Rev. Chem. Soc.* **19**, 168.

Clayton, R. B., ed. (1969). "Steroids and Terpenoids," Methods in Enzymology, Vol. 15. Academic Press, New York.

Dean, P. D. G. (1969). *In* "Steroids and Terpenoids," (R. B. Clayton, ed.), Methods in Enzymology, Vol. 15, pp. 495–501. Academic Press, New York.

Dean, P. D. G., Ortiz de Montellano, P. R., and Bloch, K. (1967). *J. Biol. Chem.* **242**, 3014.

Dempsey, M. E. (1967). *Progr. Biochem. Pharmacol.* **2**, 21.

Dempsey, M. E. (1968). *Ann. N. Y. Acad. Sci.* **148**, 631.

Dempsey, M. E. (1969). *In* "Steroids and Terpenoids" (R. B. Clayton, ed.), Methods in Enzymology, Vol. 15, pp. 501–514. Academic Press, New York.

Doering, C. H. (1969). *In* "Steroids and Terpenoids" (R. B. Clayton, ed.), Methods in Enzymology, Vol. 15, pp. 591–596. Academic Press, New York.

Durr, I. F., and Rudney, H. (1960). *J. Biol. Chem.* **235**, 2572.

Ernster, L., and Orrenius, S. (1965). *Fed. Proc., Fed. Amer. Soc. Exp. Biol.* **24**, 1190.

Fleischer, S., Fleischer, B., Azzi, A., and Chance, B. (1971). *Biochim. Biophys. Acta* **225**, 194.

Forchielli, E. (1969). *In* "Steroids and Terpenoids" (R. B. Clayton, ed.), Methods in Enzymology, Vol. 15, pp. 585–591. Academic Press, New York.

Frantz, I. D., Jr., and Schroepfer, G. J., Jr. (1967). *Annu. Rev. Biochem.* **36**, 691.

Frantz, I. D., Jr., Grev, J. E., and Ener, M. (1969). *Progr. Biochem. Pharmacol.* **5**, 24.

Ganguly, M., and Warren, J. C. (1971). *J. Biol. Chem.* **246**, 3646.

Garfinkel, D. (1963). *Comp. Biochem. Physiol.* **8**, 367.

Gaylor, J. L. (1964). *J. Biol. Chem.* **239**, 756.

Gaylor, J. L., and Delwiche, C. V. (1969). *Anal. Biochem.* **28**, 361.

Gaylor, J. L., and Mason, H. S. (1968). *J. Biol. Chem.* **243**, 4966.

Gaylor, J. L., and Tsai, S.-C. (1964). *Biochim. Biophys. Acta* **84**, 739.

Gaylor, J. L., Chang, Y.-J., Nightingale, M. S., Recio, E., and Ying, B. P. (1965). *Biochemistry* **4**, 1144.

Gaylor, J. L., Delwiche, C. V., Brady, D. R., and Green, A. J. (1966a). *J. Lipid Res.* **7**, 501.

Gaylor, J. L., Delwiche, C. V., and Swindell, A. C. (1966b). *Steroids* **8**, 353.

Gaylor, J. L., Moir, N. J., Seifried, H. E., and Jefcoate, C. R. E. (1970a). *J. Biol. Chem.* **245**, 5511.

Gaylor, J L., Moir, N. J., Topham, R. W., and Miller, W. L. (1970b). *Amer. Oil Chem. Soc., Annu. Meet., New Orleans* Paper No. 78.

Glaumann, H. (1970). *Chem.-Biol. Interactions* **2**, 369.

Glaumann, H. (1971). "Structural and Functional Heterogeneity of the Endoplasmic Reticulum in the Liver Cell." Dep. Pathol., Sabbatsberg Hosp., Karolinska Inst., Stockholm. Balder, Stockholm.

Glavind, J., and Hartmann, S. (1955). *Acta Chem. Scand.* **9**, 497.

Graham, A. B., and Wood, G. C. (1969). *Biochem. Biophys. Res. Commun.* **37**, 567.

Gregg, J. A. (1966). *J. Lipid Res.* **7**, 579.

Gunsalus, I. C. (1968). *Hoppe-Seyler's Z. Physiol. Chem.* **349**, 1610.

Gurr, M. I., and Robinson, M. P. (1970). *Eur. J. Biochem.* **15**, 335.

Gurr, M. I., Davey, K. W., and James, A. T. (1968). *FEBS (Fed. Eur. Biochem. Soc.), Lett.* **1**, 320.

Holloway, P. W. (1971). *Biochemistry* **10**, 1556.

Holloway, P. W., and Wakil, S. J. (1970). *J. Biol. Chem.* **245**, 1862.

Ito, A., and Sato, R. (1968). *J. Biol. Chem.* **243**, 4922.

Ito, A., and Sato, R. (1969). *J. Cell. Biol.* **40**, 179.

Jefcoate, C. R. E., and Gaylor, J. L. (1970). *Biochemistry* **9**, 3816.

Jefcoate, C. R. E., Calabrese, R. L., and Gaylor, J. L. (1969). *Biochemistry* **8**, 3455.

Jones, A. L., and Armstrong, D. T. (1965). *Proc. Soc. Exp. Biol. Med.* **119**, 1136.

Jones, P. D., and Wakil, S. J. (1967). *J. Biol. Chem.* **242**, 5267.

Jones, P. D., Holloway, P. W., Peluffo, R. O., and Wakil, S. J. (1969). *J. Biol. Chem.* **244**, 744.

Kaplan, D. M., and Criddle, R. S. (1971). *Physiol. Rev.* **51**, 249.

Katagiri, M., Ganguli, B. N., and Gunsalus, I. C. (1968). *J. Biol. Chem.* **243**, 3543.

Katsuki, H., and Bloch, K. (1967). *J. Biol. Chem.* **242**, 222.

Kawachi, T., and Rudney, H. (1970). *Biochemistry* **9**, 1700.

Krishna, G., Whitlock, H., Feldbruegge, D. H., and Porter, J. W. (1966). *Arch. Biochem. Biophys.* **114**, 200.

Kritchevsky, D. (1958). "Cholesterol." Wiley, New York.

Kusunose, E., Ichihara, K., and Kusunose, M. (1970). *FEBS (Fed. Eur. Biochem. Soc.), Lett.* **11**, 23.

Lee, T. P., and Gaylor, J. L. (1968). *Steroids* **11**, 699.

Lieber, C. S., Rubin, E., and DeCarli, L. M. (1970). *Biochem. Biophys. Res. Commun.* **40**, 858.

Lindberg, M., Gautschi, F., and Bloch, K. (1963). *J. Biol. Chem.* **238**, 1661.

Linn, T. C. (1967). *J. Biol. Chem.* **242**, 984.

Lu, A. Y. H., and Coon, M. J. (1968). *J. Biol. Chem.* **243**, 1331.

Lu, A. Y. H., Junk, K. W., and Coon, M. J. (1969). *J. Biol. Chem.* **244**, 3714.

Lu, A. Y. H., Kuntzman, R., West, S., and Conney, A. H. (1971). *Biochem. Biophys. Res. Commun.* **42**, 1200.

Lumper, L., Zubrzycki, Z., and Staudinger, H. (1969). *Hoppe-Seyler's Z. Physiol. Chem.* **350**, 163.

Maclennan, D. H., Tzagoloff, A., and McConnell, D. G. (1967). *Biochim. Biophys. Acta* **131**, 59.

Mason, H. S., North, J. C., and Vanneste, M. (1965). *Fed. Proc., Fed. Amer. Soc. Exp. Biol.* **24**, 1172.

Menini, E., and Norymberski, J. K. (1962). *Biochem. J.* **84**, 195.

Miller, W. L., and Gaylor, J. L. (1967). *Biochim. Biophys. Acta* **137**, 399.

Miller, W. L., and Gaylor, J. L. (1970a). *J. Biol. Chem.* **245**, 5369.

Miller, W. L., and Gaylor, J. L. (1970b). *J. Biol. Chem.* **245**, 5375.

Miller, W. L., Kalafer, M. E., Gaylor, J. L., and Delwiche, C. V. (1967). *Biochemistry* **6**, 2673.

Miller, W. L., Brady, D. R., and Gaylor, J. L. (1971). *J. Biol. Chem.* **246**, 5147.

Miyake, Y., Gaylor, J. L., and Mason, H. S. (1968). *J. Biol. Chem.* **243**, 5788.

Moir, N. J., Miller, W. L., and Gaylor, J. L. (1968). *Biochem. Biophys. Res. Commun.* **33**, 916.

Moir, N. J., Gaylor, J. L., and Yanni, J. B. (1970). *Arch. Biochem. Biophys.* **141**, 465.

Moller, M. L., and Tchen, T. T. (1961). *J. Lipid Res.* **2**, 342.

Moore, J. T., Jr., and Gaylor, J. L. (1968). *Arch. Biochem. Biophys.* **124**, 167.

Moore, J. T., Jr., and Gaylor, J. L. (1969). *J. Biol. Chem.* **244**, 6334.

Moore, J. T., Jr., and Gaylor, J. L. (1970). *J. Biol. Chem.* **245**, 4684.

Morton, R. K. (1954). *Biochem. J.* **57**, 595.

Muldoon, T. G., and Warren, J. C. (1969). *J. Biol. Chem.* **244**, 5430.

Nightingale, M. S., Tsai, S.-C., and Gaylor, J. L. (1967). *J. Biol. Chem.* **242**, 341.

Olson, J. A., Jr. (1965). *Ergeb. Physiol. Biol. Chem. Exp. Pharmakol.* **56**, 173.

Olson, J. A., Jr., Lindberg, M., and Bloch, K. (1957). *J. Biol. Chem.* **226**, 941.

Oshino, N., Imai, Y., and Sato, R. (1966). *Biochim. Biophys. Acta* **128**, 13.

Oshino, N., Imai, Y., and Sato, R. (1971). *J. Biochem. (Tokyo)* **69**, 155.

Philippot, J. (1971). *Biochim. Biophys. Acta* **225**, 201.

Privett, O. S., Lundberg, W. O., Khan, N. A., Tolberg, W. E., and Wheeler, D. H. (1953). *J. Amer. Oil Chem. Soc.* **30**, 61.

Pudles, J., and Bloch, K. (1960). *J. Biol. Chem.* **235**, 3417.

Rahimtula, A. D., and Gaylor, J. L. (1972). *J. Biol. Chem.* **247**, 9.

Rikans, L. E., and Van Dyke, R. A. (1971). *Biochem. Pharmacol.* **20**, 15.

Ritter, M. C., and Dempsey, M. E. (1971). *J. Biol. Chem.* **246**, 1536.

Rothfield, L., and Finkelstein, A. (1968). *Annu. Rev. Biochem.* **37**, 463.

Scallen, T. J., Dean, W. J., and Schuster, M. W. (1968). *J. Biol. Chem.* **243**, 5202.

Scallen, T. J., Schuster, M. W., and Dhar, A. K. (1971). *J. Biol. Chem.* **246**, 224.

Schechter, I., Sweat, F. W., and Bloch, K. (1970). *Biochim. Biophys. Acta* **220**, 463.

Schenkman, J. B. (1970). *Science* **168**, 612.

Scholan, N. A., and Boyd, G. S. (1968). *Hoppe-Seyler's Z. Physiol. Chem.* **349**, 1628.

Siekevitz, P. (1965). *Fed. Proc., Fed. Amer. Soc. Exp. Biol.* **24**, 1153.

Sih, C. J., and Whitlock, H. W., Jr. (1968). *Annu. Rev. Biochem.* **37**, 661.

Spatz, L., and Strittmatter, P. (1971). *Fed. Proc., Fed. Amer. Soc. Exp. Biol.* **30**, 1144.

Staple, E. (1969). *In* "Steroids and Terpenoids" (R. B. Clayton, ed.), Methods in Enzymology, Vol. 15, pp. 562–582. Academic Press, New York.

Staunton, J. (1969). *Annu. Rep. Progr. Chem.* **66**, 555.

Steinberg, D., and Avigan, J. (1969). *In* "Steroids and Terpenoids" (R. B. Clayton, ed.), Methods in Enzymology, Vol. 15, pp. 514–522. Academic Press, New York.

Swindell, A. C., and Gaylor, J. L. (1968). *J. Biol. Chem.* **243**, 5546.

Thompson, E. D., Stari, P. R., and Parks, L. W. (1971). *Biochem. Biophys. Res. Commun.* **43**, 1304.

Tietz, A., and Stern, N. (1969). *FEBS (Fed. Eur. Biochem. Soc.), Lett.* **2**, 286.

Topham, R. W., and Gaylor, J. L. (1967). *Biochem. Biophys. Res. Commun.* **27**, 644.

Topham, R. W., and Gaylor, J. L. (1970). *J. Biol. Chem.* **245**, 2319.

Trump, B. F., Duttera, S. M., Byrne, W. L., and Arstila, A. U. (1970). *Proc. Nat. Acad. Sci. U. S.* **66**, 433.

Tsai, R., Yu, C. A., Gunsalus, I. C., Peisach, J., Blumberg, W., Orme-Johnson, W. H., and Beinert, H. (1970). *Proc. Nat. Acad. Sci. U. S.* **66**, 1157.

Tsai, S.-C., and Gaylor, J. L. (1966). *J. Biol. Chem.* **241**, 4043.

Van Tol, A. (1970). *Biochim. Biophys. Acta* **219**, 227.

Voigt, W., Thomas, P. J., and Hsia, S. L. (1968). *J. Biol. Chem.* **243**, 3493.

Voigt, W., Fernandez, E. P., and Hsia, S. L. (1970). *J. Biol. Chem.* **245**, 5594.

Williams, C. H., Jr., and Kamin, H. (1962). *J. Biol. Chem.* **237**, 587.

Wilton, D. C., Rahimtula, A. D., and Akhtar, M. (1969). *Biochem. J.* **114**, 71.

Wirtz, K. W. A., and Zilversmit, D. B. (1968). *J. Biol. Chem.* **243**, 3596.

Witiak, D. T., Parker, R. A., Brann, D. R., Dempsey, M. E., Ritter, M. C., Connor, W. E., and Brahmankar, D. M. (1971). *J. Med. Chem.* **14**, 216.

Yamamoto, S., and Bloch, K. (1970a). *Biochem. Soc. Symp.* **29**, 35.

Yamamoto, S., and Bloch, K. (1970b). *J. Biol. Chem.* **245**, 1670.

Yamamoto, S., Lin, K., and Bloch, K. (1969). *Proc. Nat. Acad. Sci. U. S.* **63**, 110.

Zakim, D. (1970). *J. Biol. Chem.* **245**, 4953.

Brain Lipids

ROBERT B. RAMSEY AND HAROLD J. NICHOLAS

*Institute of Medical Education and Research and Department
of Biochemistry, St. Louis University School of Medicine,
St. Louis, Missouri*

I. Introduction

Several excellent reviews on lipids and lipid metabolism of the brain have appeared within the past 5 years. Some of these have concentrated on specialized aspects (e.g., cholesterol: Kabara, 1967; myelin lipids: Smith, 1967), and at least two of them have been general in nature (Eichberg, *et al.*, 1969; Davison, 1970a). The excellent *Handbook of Neurochemistry Series* (Lajtha, 1969–1970) and *Progress in Brain Research Series* (1968) contain chapters which cover almost all aspects of the chemistry, metabolism, and methods of determination of the major lipids of the brain and spinal cord. More recently, excellent coverage of recent data plus many original observations in certain areas of brain lipid research have been presented for selected brain lipids, in *Chemistry and Brain Development* (Paoletti and Davison, 1971). Himwich (1970) in a comprehensive survey has discussed the physiology of the neonatal central nervous system. Such a review inevitably encompasses many physiological aspects, which cannot be intrinsically separated from biochemical phenomena. Martin (1970) has also covered some aspects of brain lipid biochemistry.

In view of the magnitude of coverage presented in these reviews, bridging the gaps for the present manuscript has been especially challenging. Our interest has been to ·duplicate past coverage as little as possible, present a comprehensive summary of work during the years from 1968 to the spring of 1971, and place special emphasis on some aspects not stressed in prior reviews. The literature reflects the tremendous interest in lipids with relation to diseased states, and we have therefore attempted to stress this aspect, especially with respect to the lipoidoses. The authors have utilized the service of the Medlars Section, University of Colorado Medical Center, Denver, Colorado, and Brain Research Institute of Los Angeles, and the Biochemical Section of *Chemical Abstracts* extensively for this survey. No attempt has been made to make the coverage encyclopedic, and the authors apologize for omissions of manuscripts which individual investigators may feel to be key references. We have hopefully covered such research in cross-references. Finally, in any review of this type there will be inevitable cross-coverage, as, for example, in discussing brain fatty acids independently of the many lipid classes which contain these compounds.

II. Fatty Acids

The metabolism of brain hydroxy fatty acids was reviewed in this series in 1968 (Bowen and Radin, 1968b) and more recently fatty acid metabolism in the central nervous system in general has been discussed in detail by D'Adamo (1970). Both reviews cover the major contributions to the field up to the latter portions of the '60 decade.

A. Normal Brain Values and Methods of Determination

Although free fatty acids are present only in small amount in central nervous tissue, in combination, mainly as long-chain fatty acids (C_{16} to C_{20}) they constitute a large portion of the major lipids of the brain and spinal cord. A prominent reference for the type of fatty acid and percentage composition of the fatty acid content of most brain lipids has been compiled by Eichberg *et al.* (1969). There would be little merit in repeating these extensive data here. Since then only a few references to normal brain fatty acid composition have appeared. Fatty acids of the human fetal brain were investigated by Hansen and Clausen (1968). The predominant acids were palmitic, stearic, and oleic in brain as a whole, and in fetal brain lecithin, phosphatidylethanolamine, and phosphatidylserine. In adult brain oleic was dominant in all of these phospholipid fractions. Linoleic acid was practically absent in fetal brain but represented 4.5% of the total fatty acids present in adult brain. This work was prompted by the idea that the dietary content of polyunsaturated fatty acids in infancy may play a role in the etiology of such diseases as multiple sclerosis and encephalomyelitis.

The fatty acid composition of individual phospholipids of the sockeye salmon, *Oncorhynchus nerka*, has been examined. While differences were found in muscle and liver phospholipid fatty acids of "marine" and "fresh-water periods" of life for the fish, brain values were found to be almost identical for both periods of growth (Kreps *et al.*, 1969a). The contents of saturated and unsaturated fatty acids ranging in length from C_{14} to C_{22} are tabulated in an additional manuscript (Akulin *et al.*, 1969).

A detailed investigation involving the structural determination of the trimethylsilyl ether derivatives of the hydroxy fatty acids of cerebrosides of beef brain by mass spectra has been reported by Capella *et al.* (1968).

B. Subcellular Content

Despite extensive analyses of the general lipid content of the subcellular fractions of brain (Eichberg et al., 1969), few values are recorded for the individual fatty acid content of these fractions. This situation now appears about to be modified. All of the methods currently utilized for analysis are dependent on GLC (gas-liquid chromatography) of the methyl esters, and the importance of "purity" of the fractions investigated is discussed by almost all reports. In a study of the phospholipid content of brain subcellular fractions (Pomazanskaya et al., 1967) the complexity of distribution was indicated. In lecithin from all fractions the fatty acid composition was about the same, with palmitic, stearic, and polyeneoleic acids constituting, as in all other subcellular organelles, the principal acids. Polyunsaturated acids were low in these fractions. Phosphatidyl ethanolamine and phosphatidyl serine fatty acids were also almost the same in all subcellular organelles except for myelin. In the sphingomyelins from all fractions stearic acid was predominant. In fact, unsaturated fatty acids were almost completely absent. In myelin sphingomyelin, 50% of the saturated fatty acid was neuronic acid. In a later manuscript from the same laboratory (Pravdina and Chebotareva, 1971) the fatty acids from phospholipids of brain myelin and mitochondria of several widely variant vertebrate species have been recorded, but since that original manuscript was not available to the authors the reader is referred to the original manuscript for details.

Indication of the complexity of fatty acid composition of brain subcellular fractions (in rat brain) was presented by Kishimoto et al. (1969). Among the important observations presented, some of them verifying previous preliminary observations from other laboratories, were marked differences in fatty acid patterns of the phosphatidylethanolamine and phosphatidyl serine from myelin and subcellular fractions of gray matter, with the microsomes of white matter maintaining an intermediate composition. It was suggested from these observations that brain microsomes, probably the major site of synthesis of the fatty acid-containing lipids, furnish characteristic lipids for the synthesis or renewal of specific membranes. These lipids may accumulate before being released. The mechanism of the transfer process which must be involved appears a promising area for research. The fatty acid composition of cerebrosides from mouse brain microsomes and myelin has also been studied (Blass, 1970). Eighty percent of the fatty acids in myelin cerebrosides and 55% in both light and heavy microsomes consisted of 2-hydroxy fatty acids. The majority of fatty acids in myelin, both normal and hydroxy, were of chain length greater than C_{20}, whereas in microsomes, acids of chain length C_{16} to C_{20} predominated.

C. Biosynthesis, Degradation, and Utilization

Fatty acids can be synthesized *de novo* or by chain elongation from acetate (see Bowen and Radin, 1968b, for discussion and previous pertinent references). This process, the utilization of malonyl-CoA (coenzyme A) and the subcellular localization of the enzymes responsible have been discussed in detail by D'Adamo (1970). Most recent investigations have tended to concentrate and expand on details associated with biosynthesis at the subcellular level. Unesterified fatty acids in mouse brain vary markedly in quantity and type of distribution depending upon whether the analyses are conducted on fresh tissue, tissue frozen *in situ,* or tissue incubated at low (0°) or high (37°) temperature (Lunt and Rowe, 1968). The combined yield of free fatty acids from subcellular fractions of rat brain was greater than that from fresh tissue. The exact origin of the increased quantity, where found, was not clear; both *de novo* synthesis and potential origin from the hydrolysis of esters was suggested. In the same investigation, sodium acetate-1-^{14}C was found to be incorporated into free fatty acids of all subcellular fractions, following incubation of the labeled precursor with brain slices.

Fatty acid biosynthesis in developing brain microsomes was studied by Aeberhard *et al.* (1969). Using both acetyl-1-^{14}C-CoA and malonyl-1, 3-^{14}C-CoA as precursors, it was found that total fatty acid synthesis was maximal at 15–16 days of age, the period of most rapid myelination in the rat. This total fatty acid synthesis, however, was due primarily to the biosynthesis of saturated fatty acids. The incorporation of malonyl-CoA polyunsaturated fatty acids did not change significantly from 15 days to maturation. Fatty acid chain elongation, therefore, which does not occur with polyunsaturated fatty acids, appears to correlate closely with the period of rapid myelination. Bourre *et al.* (1970) incubated mouse brain microsomes with malonyl-CoA-1,3-^{14}C and either palmityl-CoA or stearyl-CoA and found that chain elongation occurred at different pH values for both acids, implying different enzyme systems for each process.

An additional study on the relationship between acetate transfer into brain as determined by the "blood-brain barrier" has recently been made (Dhopeshwarkar *et al.,* 1969). When sodium acetate-1-^{14}C was injected intraperitoneally into weanling and adult rats respectively, incorporation into long-chain fatty acids of the adult brain was low as compared to analogous fractions in the weanling rats. In both cases palmitic acid had the highest specific activity. Despite the decreased penetration of acetate into adult brain, irrespective of whether or not one considers the "barrier" to be anatomical or physiological, acetate was utilized for both *de novo* synthesis and chain elongation. These observations have a particular bearing on the significance of acetate transport and the blood-brain barrier, as indicated in earlier studies by another laboratory (Nicholas and Thomas, 1961).

A fatty acid elongation system has been localized in 21-day-old rat brain mitochondria (Boone and Wakil, 1970). The system localized in the organelle can elongate many saturated and unsaturated acyl coenzymes ranging in chain length from C_{12} to C_{22}. The components required for the synthesis were acyl-CoA, acetyl-CoA, NADH (nicotinamide-adenine dinucleotide), and NADPH (nicotinamide-adenine dinucleotide phosphate). Acetyl-CoA and not malonyl-CoA was the immediate precursor of the C_2 unit taking apart in the elongation process.

While it has been adequately established that glucose represents the principal (if not sole) energy source for normal brain metabolism, other substances *can* be metabolized for this purpose. Palmitic acid, for example, can be oxidized and metabolized by rat brain minces for this purpose (Openshaw and Bortz, 1968), even in severely ketotic rats, where glucose was the preferred substrate. The determination of oxygen consumption by the slices was the method utilized to draw this conclusion. The pathway or extent of degradation of the palmitic acid was not investigated. The enzymatic system in brain microsomes responsible for decarboxylation of 2-hydroxy stearic acid *in vitro* has been described (Lippel and Mead, 1968). The solubilized enzyme, requiring Fe^{2+} and O_2, was stimulated by a peroxide-generating system, and had a pH optimum of 6.1 in phosphate buffer and pH 6.9 in Tris buffer. Since *p*-chloromercuric benzoate inhibited the release of CO_2 during incubation, sulfhydryl groups may be present at the active site of the enzyme.

When tracer amounts of palmitic acid-1-^{14}C were infused into the subarachnoid space of anesthetized dogs, [14]CO_2 appeared in the cortical subarachnoid fluid (Little *et al.*, 1969). The results provided additional evidence that fatty acids can be oxidized by brain tissue. Volatile fatty acids can also be utilized by brain tissue as energy sources in dog (nonruminant), and goat (ruminant) (Oyler *et al.*, 1970). This conclusion was reached by measuring the arteriovenous differences between acetate, propionate, and butyrate administered surgically to dogs. Glucose was still the major source of energy in both species investigated.

Two enzymes of the fatty acid oxidizing system are β-hydroxyacyl dehydrogenase and β-ketoacyl thiolase (Lynen, 1954), but the activity of these enzymes has only recently been studied with respect to long-chain fatty acids. The extrahepatic distribution of an additional enzyme required for long-chain fatty acid degradation, fatty acyl-CoA synthetase (acid: CoA ligase (AMP), EC 6.2.1.3), has been studied by Pande and Mead (1968). On a specific activity basis, liver was most active, testes and serum least active, and brain somewhere in between.

D. ABSORPTION AND TRANSPORT INTO BRAIN

Since long-chain fatty acids are needed continuously for the integrity of membrane structure (essentially quoted from Dhopeshwarkar and Mead, 1970), detailed knowledge of how they are provided to the central nervous system (CNS) is of considerable importance. Citing a number of earlier references, D'Amado (1970) has indicated that fatty acids in the central nervous system can arise by synthesis *in situ* and by transport from the bloodstream. A number of recent studies have again indicated that both possibilities exist.

Utilizing the autoradiographic technique, it was shown that in the *Brachydanio rerio* (Zebra fish), ^{3}H-labeled palmitic acid injected intraperitoneally was incorporated into the fibrous part and perikarya of nervous tissue lipids (Rahmann and Korfsmeier, 1968). There appeared to be no transport of labeled lipids comparable to that occurring with neuronal proteins. Palmitic acid-1-^{14}C was found to be incorporated into brain lipids to the extent of 0.02% of the oral dose in adult rats (Dhopeshwarkar, *et al.,* 1969). All brain tissue lipid components examined, including lecithin, phosphatidylethanolamine, phosphatidylserine, and cerebrosides were labeled. The ^{14}C values indicated clearly that palmitic acid was incorporated unchanged into the lipids, rather than having been oxidized to acetate, which in turn could serve as the label.

1-^{14}C-Oleic acid administered either orally or intravenously to adult rats was found to be incorporated into brain lipids, after either 4 or 24 hours, by direct uptake (Dhopeshwarkar and Mead, 1970). This was substantiated by the fact that 84% of the label was still present in the carboxyl carbon, after isolation from brain tissue. When 1-^{14}C-acetate was similarly administered, only 30% of the radioactivity was present in the carboxyl of the oleic acid isolated from brain tissue, and 23% after 24 hours, again clearly substantiating the direct uptake of oleic acid from the bloodstream without prior degradation.

Although palmitic and oleic acids in brain can be synthesized *in situ* and can reach the organ from the bloodstream the question of the origin of linoleic acid origin is more critical, since this essential fatty acid as well as linolenic and arachidonic acids, cannot be synthesized by animal tissues from acetate. Dhopeshwarkar *et al.* (1971) have now shown that

1-^{14}C-linoleic acid administered to adult rats orally can also be incorporated intact into brain lipids. This conclusion was based on the distribution of label ^{14}C into the linoleic acid isolated from the brain, where 88% of the total radioactivity was retained in the carboxyl carbon after 24 hours. This percentage would not have remained at this level had prior degradation to acetate occurred. These same investigators also showed that arachidonic acid obtained from the brain following the feeding of 1-^{14}C-linoleic acid arose by desaturation and chain elongation as in liver.

When palmitic acid-1-^{14}C was injected intracerebrally into the mouse, it was rapidly incorporated into several groups of brain lipids (Sun and Horrocks, 1969a). After 12 hours, 78% of the ^{14}C-label was present in phospholipids, 15% in triacylglycerols, 1% each in free fatty acids and galactolipids, and the remainder in neutral glycerides. More than 65% of the label in the phospholipids was present in the choline phosphoglycerides, but this amount decreased with time. At longer time periods, increasing amounts of label were present in the monounsaturated acyl and alkenyl groups, but no label was found in cholesterol or polyunsaturated acyl groups. The results were interpreted to indicate that most of the extensive recycling of ^{14}C occurred without oxidative degradation of the palmitoyl groups. In a somewhat similar study with 1-^{14}C-linoleic acid administered intracisternally to adult cats (Bernsohn et al., 1971), it was found that about 1% of the injected label was incorporated into CNS lipids. The conclusion was reached, by careful analysis of data collected over several time periods, that adult CNS tissue can carry out de novo fatty acid synthesis, acyl transferase, elongation, saturation, desaturation to a limited extent under the experimental conditions. Most of the label was incorporated into phosphoglycerides, with both choline and ethanolamine glycerophosphatides equally labeled. It is obvious from these collective experiments that long-chain fatty acids, including the essential fatty acids, can be obtained from the diet of both immature and adult animals if necessary, the blood-brain barrier imposing no critical blockage.

E. Fatty Acid Variation in Certain Pathological Conditions
(See also Section XIII)

1. Encephalomalacia

Although several earlier reports (e.g., Witting and Horwitt, 1967) indicated changes in the fatty acid content of various tissues in vitamin E deficiency, two recent manuscripts tend to indicate that the changes have little significance with respect to brain tissue. For example Lee and Barnes (1969) subjected hooded rats to a vitamin E-deficient diet and found no consistent pattern of changes in total fatty acid of several tissues, including brain after 7 months on the dietary regime. After 14 months there were decreases in the total fatty acids of phospholipids in the same tissues, with the pattern similar to that found in essential fatty acid deficiency. Changes in the brain fatty acid composition were not outstandingly different from those in other tissues. Pfeifer and Barnes (1969) in a similar study found support for the concept (Witting, 1967) that in the vitamin E-deficient chick there is a homostatic response whereby, despite an overall decrease in fatty acid synthesis, the rate of synthesis of polyunsaturated fatty acids, including those in the brain, rises relative to that of saturated and monoenoic acids.

2. Essential Fatty Acid Deficiency

As summarized by Galli *et al.* (1971), the major biochemical changes detected in the tissues of animals on an essential fatty acid-deficient diet are a decrease in polyunsaturated essential fatty acids (PEFA) of the linoleate (18:2 ω6) and linolenate (18:3 ω3) families and a corresponding increase in trienes, especially 20:3 (a review of contributions by others is given in this manuscript). The Paoletti group, in studying changes in rat brain fatty acids from animals subjected to essential fatty acid-deficient diets for long periods, or in animals from pregnant rats similarly treated, found that considerable changes in brain fatty acids were induced during early periods of life. However, despite alterations in brain fatty acid composition, the existence of a regulatory mechanism for the maintenance of membrane constituents was apparent. A dynamic process for the metabolism of nervous membrane fatty acid constituents was implied. Essentially the same principles were expressed in an earlier report by the same group (C. Galli *et al.*, 1970). In a prior manuscript, Walker (1968) found that following the feeding of male rats for 25 weeks on a diet containing 10% hydrogenated cocoanut oil and subsequent transfer to a diet containing 10% corn oil, changes in brain fatty acids were slow. Docosahexaenoic acid concentration in brain, normally relatively high, was independent of the initial diet or of the supplemental corn oil diet. His data also were interpreted as reflecting the slow metabolic turnover of fatty acids in brain.

3. Alloxan Diabetes

In contrast to marked changes occurring in the lipid composition of peripheral nerve of rats subjected to production of alloxan diabetes, brain lipids, including fatty acids, of both adult and young animals were unaffected by the experimental disease (Pratt *et al.*, 1969). Brain weights and total crude lipids in young rats were reduced, however. This was due in young rats to decrease in cholesterol phosphatidylethanolamine and cerebrosides. The data again illustrate the comparative insulation of the central nervous system to some challenges that readily affect the peripheral nervous system.

4. Scrapie

The long-chain fatty acid composition of whole brain and myelin from normal and scrapie-affected mice has been examined (Heitzman and Skipworth, 1969). The only significant difference in the normal and diseased tissues was a lower total fatty acid value for the diseased brains. The fatty acid distribution was the same for both normal and diseased tissue.

5. Multiple Sclerosis

The idea that an abnormality in fatty acid composition in the brain during maturation, or otherwise, is not new [see Bernsohn and Stephanides (1967), also Hansen and Clausen (1968) for discussion]. In a follow-up of previous work, Clarke and Gittens (1968) have reported that rat cerebral cortex slices incubated in a buffered medium containing serum from multiple sclerosis (MS) patients, but not serum from normal humans, released a considerable amount of free fatty acid into the medium. They attribute the increase to some neurotoxic agent in the MS serum, somewhat analogous to the findings of Bornstein (Bornstein and Crain, 1965). The globulin fraction of MS serum seemed the source of the agent(s) responsible for the production of the free fatty acids.

6. Short-Chain Fatty Acid-Inducted Coma

Evidence linking short-chain fatty acids (SCFA) of 4 to 8 carbons and the induction of hepatic coma has been summarized by Walker et al. (1970). Included in the evidence is the fact that administration of short-chain fatty acids can induce comas in experimental animals. Walker et al. were able to demonstrate that in animals developing acute SCFA-induced coma the phenomenon was not due to decreased cerebral energy metabolism. Dahl (1968) considered the possibility that the short-chain fatty acids might inhibit the sodium-potassium activated adenosine triphosphatase (ATPase) of brain. Partial inhibition was indeed found, but the exact relationship between this phenomenon and the induced narcosis was not clear. The precise reason for the induced narcosis must still be considered unknown.

7. Electroconvulsive Shock and Ischemia

Following post-decapitation ischemia and after electroconvulsive shock in rats, Bazan (1970) found that a striking rise in the total free acid pool in brain occurred. This was mainly the result of increased arachidonic, stearic, oleic, and palmitic acids. The phenomenon was believed to be due to activation of brain phospholipase A enzyme. Essentially the same results were reported by Bazan and Rakowski (1970).

III. Galactosyl Mono- and Diglycerides

A glycolipid having the chromatographic properties of digalactosyl diglyceride was reported present in human brain by Rouser *et al.* (1967). A detailed study of the biosynthesis (Wenger *et al.*, 1970) and degradation (Rao *et al.*, 1970) of such a diglyceride has now been reported, using particulate preparations from rat brain. The monogalactosyl diglyceride, 1,2-di-*O*-acyl-3-*O*-(β-D-galactopyranosyl)-*sn*-glycerol had previously been shown to be formed from uridine diphosphate galactose (UDP-galactose) and 1,2-diglyceride by rat brain microsome fractions (Wenger *et al.*, 1968). In the studies of Wenger *et al.* (1970) this substance was implicated as an intermediate in the biosynthesis of digalactosyl diglyceride. Sodium deoxycholate was essential for the microsomal reaction, appearing to function as a surface-active adjuvant promoting the reaction between UDP-galactose, enzyme, and endogenous monogalactosyl diglyceride. By using specific α- and β-galactosidases it was shown that the anomeric carbon of the galactose-to-galactose bond has the α-configuration. Of particular interest was the fact that the biosynthetic enzyme activity was low or nonexistent before 11 days, *increasing* sharply after this time and reaching a peak at 16 to 18 days postpartum. When biosynthetically prepared monogalactosyl-U-^{14}C-diglyceride was incubated with brain mitochondria hydrolysis to ^{14}C-galactose occurred (Rao *et al.*, 1970). With brain microsomal preparations, hydrolysis to monogalactosyl-U-^{14}C glycerol occurred (at different pH values). Biosynthesized digalactosyl-U-^{14}C diglyceride was similarly degraded. The galactolipase activity was notably depressed in brains from rats 10 to 20 days old. The implications of these phenomena for myelination are obvious.

IV. Phospholipids: Introduction

The importance of phosphorus-containing lipids of the central nervous system, presumably dependent upon their role as membrane constituents, has been stressed in several of the general reviews previously cited. The following recent summaries are recommended for additional important aspects on the biosynthesis, degradation, and probable function of these compounds: sphingolipids (Rosenberg, 1970; Gatt, 1970; Kanfer, 1970;

Karlsson, 1970); phosphoglycerides (Rossiter and Strickland, 1970); phospholipid metabolism (Thompson, 1970; Davison, 1970a; Ansell, 1971; Rouser et al., 1971). Although not necessarily directly germane to studies on the biochemistry of phospholipids, an excellent treatise on the chemistry of phospholipids has recently been published (Slotboom and Bonsen, 1970).

A. PHOSPHATIDYL GLYCEROL AND RELATED COMPOUNDS

Phosphatidyl glycerol is only a minor component of cerebral lipids, but interest continues in its biosynthesis and metabolic function. Kiyasu et al. (1963) first established that the compound is biosynthesized in chicken and rat liver organelles by the following reactions:

1. CPD-diacylglycerol + sn-glycero-3-phosphoric acid → 3-sn-phosphatidyl-1'-glycerol -3'-phosphate + CMP.
2. 3-sn-phosphatidyl-1'-glycero-3'-phosphate → phosphatidylglycerol + P_1.

Confirmation that this same reaction occurs in brain was obtained independently by Stanacev et al. (1968) in a preliminary communication and by Possmayer et al. (1968). Stanacev et al. established that 3-sn-phosphatidyl-1'-sn-glycerol could be biosynthesized by sheep brain homogenates, with the activity located largely in the mitochondria. Possmayer et al. (1968) incubated rat brain homogenates with ^{32}P-rac-glycero-3-phosphoric acid and CDP-diacylglycerol and identified (tentatively) phosphatidylglycerophosphate as a reaction product. ^{14}C-sn-Glycero-3-phosphoric acid in a similar incubation was incorporated into phosphatidylglycerol. In the presence of an acylating system, ^{32}P-rac-glycero-3-phosphoric acid was incorporated into phosphatidylglycerol, but in small amount. Glycerophosphorylglycerophosphate biosynthesis from phosphatidylglycerophosphate was also indicated in this work. In a more detailed study, Davidson and Stanacev (1970), using isolated sheep brain mitochondria, again established the pathway for reactions 1 and 2 (previously given). In addition, the enzymatic dephosphorylation of phosphatidylglycerophosphate to phosphatidylglycerol was observed. No biosynthesis of cardiolipin which would be formed by the following reaction was detected:

phosphatidylglycerol + CDP-D-diglyceride → cardiolipin + CMP

Several suggested reasons were given for this.

The stereospecificity of the reactions reported by the two groups was emphasized by the observation that the natural phospholipid precursor has the 3-sn-phosphatidyl-1'-sn-glycerol configuration (Haverkate and Van Deenen, 1965).

The wide variety of fatty acid composition of phospholipids raises the question of whether the variations result from enzyme specificity during phosphatidic acid biosynthesis or whether partial hydrolysis and re-acylation occur at a later step in the biosynthetic sequence. Sanchez De Jimenez and Cleland (1969) have presented kinetic studies indicating that the reaction occurs with direct acylation of L-glycerol-3-phosphate by two acyl-CoA molecules without the release of lysophosphatidic acid as an intermediate (no hydrolysis with subsequent reacylation). The reaction occurs in microsomes, but the data presented suggest that the microsomal enzymes use fatty acids rather than acyl-CoA's from the cytoplasm as their natural substrates. Zahler and Cleland (1969) have also studied the anomalous behavior of palmityl-CoA in the acyltransferase reaction in which L-glycerol-3-phosphate is esterified by palmitoyl-CoA by brain microsomes. The unusual kinetics appeared to be the result of palmitoyl-CoA occurring largely in micellar form at high concentration. Only the free monomeric molecules whose concentration is essentially constant above the critical micelle concentration are active in the enzymatic reaction. This is probably the reason for many observations showing the inhibition of enzymes by palmitoyl-CoA, in which the substance acts essentially as a detergent (see references quoted in Zahler and Cleland, 1969).

A partially purified enzyme system that catalyzes acylation of L-glycerol-3-phosphate to phosphatidic acid has been described by Martensson and Kanfer (1968). The activity was found in the 100,000g supernatant. With the addition of boiled, dialyzed 100,000g supernatant an almost sixfold stimulation of activity was found. On a dry tissue weight basis, the phosphatidic acid content of 3-day postnatal brain is higher than in adult brain, although the rate of incorporation of ^{32}P into this compound is higher in the young than in adult brain (Smirnov and Chirkovskaya, 1969).

B. PHOSPHATIDYL CHOLINE

A discussion of the fundamental facets of phosphatidyl choline (lecithin) biosynthesis, including origin of the diglyceride moiety from phosphatidic acid and the incorporation of phosphorylcholine as a unit via the cytidine diphosphate choline pathway, has been given by Rossiter and Strickland (1970). A direct approach via intracerebral injection of CH_3-^{14}C-choline, has been studied recently by Ansell and Spanner (1968b). Using adult rats, it was concluded that the base was incorporated exclusively into choline-containing brain lipids. The initial phosphorylation of the free choline followed by the formation of CDP-choline and the transfer of the phosphorylcholine to a diglyceride appeared to be one of the principal routes for lecithin formation in brain.

For unknown reasons, the injected ^{14}C-choline underwent a rapid disappearance from the brain, in contrast to the findings in previous work by the same investigators with ^{14}C-ethanolamine. From the observations reported and other data it was concluded that choline is supplied to the brain from the liver. This has been partially established by Diamond (1971), who injected ^{14}C-labeled choline intravenously into mice. The choline was rapidly metabolized to phosphoryl choline and within 30 minutes 52% of the radioactivity was in a "membrane-localized" chloroform-soluble derivative.

Lapetina et al. (1970) have observed that, in vivo, Me-^{14}C choline in various subcellular fractions of rat brain undergoes a different rate of turnover. The shortest half-life was exhibited in the mitochondrial fraction with microsomes and synaptic vesicles similar in turnover rates. Turnover of the labeled choline in the nerve ending membranes was slowest. Previous work from the same laboratory (Lapetina et al., 1968) had indicated that each subcellular organelle or rat cerebral cortex has a characteristic lipid composition which may reflect its widely divergent functions. Although it was found that ^{32}P-phosphate was incorporated in vivo into total phospholipids of all organelles at the same rate (Lapetina and Rodriques De Lores Arnaiz, 1969), it was considered unlikely by the investigators that each membrane "was able to synthesize intact phospholipid at the same rate but rather that each membrane had the capacity to exchange the various moieties of its phospholipid molecules in situ" (quoted from Lunt and Lapetina, 1970a). This conclusion was based also in part on additional observations from the same laboratory (Lapetina et al., 1969) in which it was found that with 1-^{14}C-acetate, ^{14}C-glycerol, and ^{32}P-phosphate respectively as precursors, the different moieties of the phospholipids of rat cerebral cortex had different half-lives. In a later study in which Me-^{14}C-choline was incubated with rat cerebral cortex (for 2 hours) followed by preparation of subcellular membranes, it was indeed concluded (Lunt and Lapetina, 1970b) that each membrane has the capacity to incorporate choline into phosphatidyl choline in vitro, and that the incorporation does result from exchange in situ of the choline residue of phosphatidyl choline. The complexity of interpreting such data was indicated by the fact that the investigators could not exclude the possibility of translocaion of labeled intact phospholipid from one organelle to another. This complexity is bound to occur when more than one organelle is capable of synthesizing appreciable metabolites from added labeled substrate. Although not necessarily germane to the brain itself, it should be noted that phosphorylcholine-1,2-^{14}C and choline-1,2-^{14}C-labeled-cytidine diphosphate were found to be incorporated into whole homogenates and microsomal fractions of rat retina (Swartz and Mitchell, 1970). A factor stimulating incorporation of label and release of P_i was indicated present in the cytosol. Mg^{++} was required for optimal incorporation of the labeled compounds in the presence of added diglyceride. Retina is therefore capable of *de novo* synthesis of phospholipids.

By injecting ^{14}C-choline, ^{14}C-glycerol, and ^{32}P-orthophosphate intracerebrally into rats during the period of most active myelination (12–18 days), Abdel-Latif and Smith (1970) also obtained data indicating that the metabolism of phospholipids is a complex, heterogeneous process in brain. All the organelles studied were found to incorporate the three labeled precursors into their respective major phospholipids, with the microsomes possessing the greatest capacity to form lecithin.

C. PHOSPHATIDYL ETHANOLAMINES

As indicated by Rossiter and Strickland (1970), the experiments on phosphatidylethanolamine biosynthesis have paralleled those conducted with lecithin. As usual the experiments were first performed with liver, and the conversion of phosphorylethanolamine to phosphatidylethanolamine via the participation of cytidine diphosphate ethanolamine (CDPE) was soon established. Following intracerebral injection of ^{14}C-ethanolamine into rats, the ethanolamine is rapidly converted to phosphorylethanolamine also, transformed into cytidine 5'-diphosphate ethanolamine, and then incorporated into the ethanolamine phosphoglycerides of all subcellular organelles examined (Ansell and Spanner, 1967). However, the process is largely microsomal, as has been emphasized by recent *in vitro* studies of Porcellati *et al.* (1970a) (see, for previous reference to *in vitro* work, Porcellati *et al.*, 1970b). Using chicken brain microsomes, it was found that the synthesis of ethanolamine phosphoglycerides was considerably more efficient from CDPE than from phosphorylethanolamine. It was suggested by the investigators that the conversion of phosphorylcholine to cytidine diphosphate phosphorylcholine (via PE/CTP cytidyltransferase enzyme EC 2.7.7.14) may represent a rate-limiting step in the biosynthesis of phosphorylethanolamines. The rate of synthesis of ethanolamine phosphoglyceride from CDPE in brain homogenates was increased fivefold on the addition of optimum concentration of diacyl glycerols. No other lipid was labeled after the addition of ^{14}C-ethanolamine cytidine diphosphate, suggesting that the ethanolamine moiety was not incorporated into other lipids.

Ansell and Spanner (1970) have suggested that since ethanolamine phospholipids constitute such a large portion of brain lipids (9% of the

dry weight of whole brain), their breakdown, particularly in pathological conditions where demyelination occurs, could be serious. Further
study was therefore suggested. On incubation of brain homogenates in
oxygenated Krebs-Ringer bicarbonate medium for short periods, there
was a breakdown of endogenous ethanolamine phospholipids resulting
in a rise in concentration of water-soluble ethanolamine compounds, particularly ethanolamine. Incubation of ethanolamine plasmalogen with an
undialyzed extract of brain acetone powder resulted in a loss of acyl
ester groups, vinyl ether groups, and lipid-bound phosphorus. The results are discussed in terms of the possible principal enzymes involved
(phospholipases A, C, and D) and are particularly interesting in view
of the difficulty encountered in studying such breakdown *in vivo*.

A report indicating the continuing difficulty in analyzing "total groups"
of brain lipids has been presented by Sun and Horrocks (1969b). From
mouse and ox brain the ethanolamine phosphoglycerides were prepared
from the respective tissue and cyclic acetate (1,3-dioxolane) derivatives
of the alk-1-enyl groups were made by treating the ethanolamine phosphoglycerides with 1,3-propanediol, after which separation was accomplished from the unchanged ethanolamine phosphoglycerides. After
alkaline hydrolysis the fatty acid moieties from both groups were analyzed
by GLC as the cyclic acetates or methyl esters. It was found that the
side chains from the 1-position of both groups were different in chain
length, unsaturation, and chemical bonding. The acyl groups from the
2-position of the alk-1-enyl acyl glycerophosphoryl ethanolamines were
predominantly saturated. The work illustrates well that individual components of glycerophosphorylethanolamines must be examined for pertinent differences to be verified, rather than analyzed as a single group of
compounds. These analyses may be the only significant way to evaluate
the complex turnover rates which the individual lipid entities may undergo. In a more recent study (Sun and Horrocks, 1970) the method was
applied to ox brain myelin and to mouse brain microsomal, mitochondrial,
and myelin major phospholipids, including glycerophosphorylethanolamines, and cardiolipin. Myelin acyl moieties were characteristically
different from those of the microsomal and mitochondrial fractions
(Ansell and Metcalfe, 1970).

D. PLASMALOGENS AND RELATED COMPOUNDS

Glycerolipids (containing an ether linkage) in plant and animal tissues
may have this linkage present in two basic forms (Snyder *et al.*, 1970a):

1. *O*-alkyl: (—C—O—CH$_2$—CH$_2$—R)
2. *O*-alkyl-1-enyl: (C—O—CH=CH—R)

The classical plasmalogens or phosphatidal derivatives contain unit 2.

While the basic principles in the formation of these compounds in brain have been formulated (see Rossiter and Strickland, 1970, for summary) the origin of the unique vinylic ether bond of the plasmalogens or even the ether linkage of the more simple alkyl ether phosphoglycerides has remained the principal point of interest. Many contributions to the general problem have recently been made by investigators working on tissues other than brain (Thompson, 1968; Snyder *et al.*, 1970a,b; Blank *et al.*, 1970; Wood and Healy, 1970; Wykle and Snyder, 1970). A comprehensive review of the chemistry and metabolism of the plasmalogens and related compounds has recently been presented by Piantadosi and Snyder (1970), and it thoroughly surveys the literature prior to 1968.

Insofar as the biosynthetic process for brain is concerned, Bickerstaffe and Mead (1968) injected ^{14}C-phosphatidylethanolamine and ^{3}H-chimyl alcohol intracerebrally into 18-day-old rats. No ^{14}C was found in the dimethyl acetate obtained from the alkenyl acyl ethanolamine phosphoglycerides, indicating that phosphatidyl ethanolamine was not a precursor of the phosphatidal ethanolamine (plasmalogen). On the other hand an increase in ^{3}H content of both the glyceryl ethers and dimethyl acetate indicated that chimyl alcohol (glyceryl ether) was a precursor of both types of phospholipid. The data did not establish whether or not reduction of the alkyl to the alkenyl group took place as the diglyceride or as phosphatidic acid.

Joffe (1969) in a detailed analysis of rat brains at periods from 17 to 22 days of age has shown that the fatty acid composition of the ethanolamine phosphatides is quite different when the alkyl glyceryl ethers and diacyl phosphatides (1 (3)-positions) are compared. The intraperitoneal injection of 1-^{14}C-acetate showed no clear-cut precursor-product relationship between the saturated and unsaturated ethanolamine ethers. Independent pathways were suggested (see Segal and Wysocki, 1970) for the biosynthesis of alkenyl ether, alkyl ether, and ester linkages.

Etzrodt and Debuch (1970) injected 1-^{14}C-acetate intracerebrally into 14-day-old rats and isolated the ^{14}C-labeled *O*-(1,2-diacyl)- and *O*-(1-alk-1'-enyl-*sn*-glycerol-3-phosphoryl) ethanolamines, and later (Debuch *et al.*, 1970) injected the latter two substances intracerebrally into 14-day-old rats. The results were in general agreement with those of Bickerstaffe and Mead (1968).

One source of a portion of the plasmalogen molecule appears to be the degradation products of sphinganine (dihydrosphingosine) (Stoffel *et al.*, 1970). The latter investigators injected 3-^{3}H-sphinganine intraperitoneally and intracerebrally into rats during the period of active myelination. The 1-^{3}H palmitaldehyde released during the biodegradation of the sphinganine was incorporated into plasmalogens. Similar injection of 3-^{3}H, 3-^{14}C-sphinganine led to the incorporation of doubly labeled palmitaldehyde into the plasmalogen molecule. The ^{3}H/^{14}C ratios led the investigators to conclude that the palmitaldehyde was reduced to hexadecanol, which in turn supplied the hexadecyl glycerol ether derivative which was subsequently dehydrogenated to the vinyl ether moiety. An alcohol dehydrogenase capable of reducing the palmitaldehyde to hexadecanol was found in the 100,000g supernatant of rat liver homogenate. Attention might here be called to recent recognition of an NADH-linked aldehyde reductase present in brain (Tabakoff and Erwin, 1970). More recently Stoffel and Lekim (1971) have firmly established that in rat brain, dehydrogenation of the alkyl groups leads to the vinyl ether group of plasmalogens. In a study of the stereochemistry of the introduction of the double bond it was found that a high degree of stereospecificity exists. In the formation of the double bond *cis* elimination of the hydrogens leads to the vinyl ether structure, in which the double bond has the *cis*-configuration, as previously shown by Warner and Lands (1963).

Both Stoffel *et al.* (1970) and Schmid and Takahashi (1970) conclude that hexadecanol rather than its oxidized analog palmitic acid is incorporated into alkyl, alk-1-enyl, and 1-acyl and 2-acyl moieties of the ethanolamine phosphatides of myelinating brain. Thus long-chain alcohols rather than aldehydes or acids appear to be the key intermediate for formation of both alkyl and alk-1-enyl glycerophosphatides.

Finally, conclusive evidence for the origin of the O-alk-1-enyl unsaturation and the source of oxygen in the glyceryl ethers has been obtained. Snyder *et al.* (1971) measured the β-alkyl glycerolipid synthesizing enzymes in the brains of fetal and postnatal rats and concluded that the β-alkyl lipids are the probable precursors of plasmalogens during myelination. The conclusion was based on the fact that liver at the same time of growth contains enzymes that cleave the O-alkyl moiety whereas the brain does not contain these enzymes at that period. This follows since plasmalogens are rapidly synthesized in brain during active myelination. Additional conclusive data for the later principle have been presented by Bell *et al.* (1971), who injected 1-^{14}C hexadecanol and ^{18}O-hexadecanol intracerebrally into 12-day-old rats. The data obtained indicated that the O-alkyl lipids were converted into the O-alk-1-enyl lipids of myelinating brain, and that the oxygen in both O-alkyl and O-alkyl-1-enyl lipids came from the alcohol used in the biosynthesis of the molecules.

A minor glycolipid containing an alkyl ether moiety (an alkyl ether analog of diacyl glycerol galactoside; monogalactosyl diglyceride), first detected in bovine brain (Norton and Brotz, 1963) has been reexamined by Rumsby and Rossiter (1968) and its identity further confirmed.

Thus most of the major previously unresolved problems in the biosynthesis of plasmalogens have been clarified. Probably the first report of the biosynthesis of plasmalogens in a cell-free system has been given by Wykle *et al.* (1970), using preparations from Ehrlich ascites cells. It is anticipated that these studies will be extended to brain preparations, with consequent considerable advancement in the general area of study.

E. PHOSPHOINOSITIDES

The excellent review by Hawthorne and Kai (1970) has summarized (to that period) most of the pertinent factors pertaining to phosphoinositide biosynthesis and catabolism, as well as such facets as the effects of cations and electrical stimulation of nerve tissue, on the metabolism of the compounds.

The biosynthesis of the monophosphoinositides has in general been delineated, and can be equated as follows (Hawthorne and Kai, 1970):

1. CTP + phosphatidic acid→CDP-diglyceride + pyrophosphate
2. CDP-diglyceride + inositol→phosphatidylinositol + CMP

Another biosynthetic route is indicated by 3 and 4 below:

3. Monoglyceride + ATP→lysophosphatidic acid + ADP
4. Lysophosphatidic acid + acyl CoA→phosphatidic acid + CoA

In addition, the following route also is known:

5. Lysophosphatidylinositol and oleoyl CoA→phosphatidylinositol + CoA

Biosynthesis of the di- and triphosphoinositides can then be described as follows:

6. Phosphatidylinositol + ATP→diphosphoinositide + ADP
7. Diphosphoinositide + ATP→triphosphoinositide + ADP

The catabolism of the phosphoinositides will not be discussed here (see Kai and Hawthorne, 1969), but it is well established that post-mortem changes are rapid and should be considered in interpreting experiments involving incubation, for long periods, of tissue or subcellular preparations.

Much interest in the biosynthesis of the phosphoinositides has been generated by the observation that $^{32}P_i$ is rapidly incorporated *in vivo* into triphosphoinositide, diphosphoinositide, and phosphatidylinositol of whole brain (see Hawthorne and Kai, 1970, for review). The detailed mechanisms involved in the biosynthesis of the di- and triphosphoinositides from the monophosphoinositide and efforts to establish the exact structure of the various species has also occupied much recent effort. Prottey *et al.* (1968) determined, for example, the structures of enzymatically synthesized diphosphoinositide and triphosphoinositide. Phosphatidylinositol kinase of rat brain produced diphosphoinositide having the inositol 1,4-diphosphate structure:

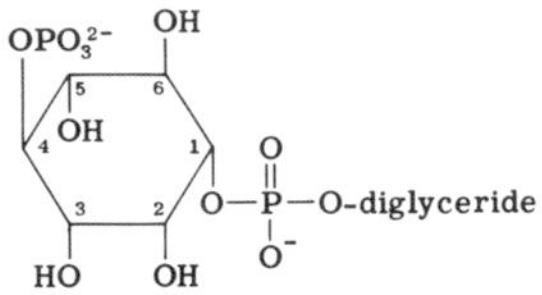

FIG. 1.   1-Phosphatidyl-L-myoinositol-4-phosphate.

This enzymatic work established that the inositoldiphosphate formed has the same structure as 1-phosphatidyl-L-myoinositol-4-phosphate isolated from ox brain postmortem by this group and earlier by Chang and Ballou (1967). Sheltawy and Dawson (1969) have studied the course of intraperitoneally injected ^{32}P into acid-soluble phosphorus, phosphoinositides, and total phospholipids of hen brain and sciatic nerve. On a per gram of tissue basis, the incorporation of ^{32}P into brain triphosphoinositide was three times that of sciatic nerves. This difference is discussed by the authors as possibly resulting from the greater amount of connective tissue in sciatic nerve than in brain, and to other factors.

Agranoff *et al.* (1969) have demonstrated that guinea pig microsomes show specificity for myoinositol, although inososes were weakly active as substrates also. Experiments from the same investigation uncovered a novel pathway of phosphatidic acid biosynthesis involving acyldihydroxy acetone phosphate. This involves the transfer of fatty acid from CoA to dihydroxyacetone phosphate, catalyzed by a mitochondrial preparation that reduces the product to lysophosphatidate in the presence of NADP. Accordingly, glycerophosphate may not be an obligatory intermediate in the formation of glycerolipids.

Bishop and Strickland (1970) have studied reaction 2 (see p. 161) with subcellular fractions of rat brain and found that the enzyme responsible, cytidine diphosphate diglyceride: inositol transferase, is located primarily in the microsomal fraction. Of several cytidine diphosphate diglycerides with different fatty acids in the 1- and 2-positions used as substrates, those containing oleic acid at the 2-position were more readily utilized than those containing palmitic or stearic acids (or at both 1- and 2-positions). These observations are consistent with the pattern of fatty acid distribution found for monophosphoinositide isolated from rat brain.

Holub *et al.* (1970) prepared the mono-, di-, and triphosphoinositides of bovine brain and observed that the distribution of fatty acid in each class was fairly specific. For example, the 1-stearate-2-arachidonate unit contributed more than 40% of the total of each inositide class. All the long-chain and polyunsaturated fatty acids were in the 2-position and were preferentially paired with stearic acid in the 1-position. Oleic acid in the 2-position was found to be equally divided between the species with palmitic and stearic acids in the 1-position. Dvorkin and Kiselev (1969) have also reported fractionation of brain phosphoinositides (of rats) but the manuscript was not available in translation for our evaluation.

These data and additional observations reported in this chapter on other brain lipid classes all tend to point to a nonrandom distribution of fatty acids in glycerophosphatides in brain (see also Thompson, 1969).

A method for quantitatively extracting di- and triphosphoinositides from guinea pig brain has been reported (Michell *et al.*, 1970). The method involves extraction with a chloroform, methanol, 2 M KCl mixture, and provides extracts which are colorless and not severely contaminated with chloroform-insoluble material or inorganic phosphate.

Two reviews by Kai and Hawthorne (1969) and Dawson (1969) have stressed the possible metabolic function(s) of the phosphoinositides. The former authors have evolved the hypothesis that the "metabolically active polyphosphoinositides are located in the excitable membrane of the neurone, particularly the axolemma." This distribution in brain of the enzymes responsible for the biosynthesis of the compounds and the influence of cations (e.g., Ca^{++}) on the enzymes suggests that the phosphorylation and dephosphorylation of *di*phosphoinositide is at least partially responsible for the regulation of axonal membrane permeability to Na^+ and K^+ ions. Therein may lie a principal metabolic function of the phosphoinositides. The hypothesis is consistent with the high concentration of di- and triphosphoinositides in the myelin sheath. An interesting visualization of the possible function of these compounds is shown in Fig. 2.

Dawson in 1969 still considered the metabolic function of the phosphoinositides to be still largely unknown. He suggested that the specific localization of the polyphosphoinositides in the myelin sheath, either on the surface bilayer in close contact with the axoplasm or extracellular fluid, or at a node or cleft in the sheath, may be intimately related to their rapid metabolism and thereby their physiological function.

In an additional thorough review, Durell and Garland (1969) sum-

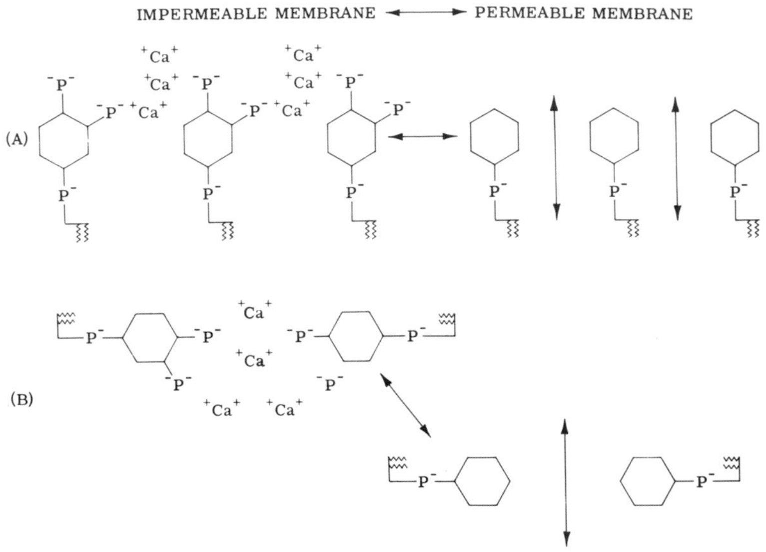

IMPERMEABLE MEMBRANE ◄────► PERMEABLE MEMBRANE

FIG. 2. Possible control of permeability of nerve cell membrane by polyphosphoinositides. Long axis of the inositide molecule is perpendicular to that of the membrane (A) or parallel to the membrane (B). Taken from Kai and Hawthorne (1969).

marized earlier interpretations on the phenomenon whereby cholinergic stimulation results in increased incorporation of $^{32}P_i$ into phospholipids, particularly phosphatidylinositol and phosphatidic acid, in neural and glandular tissues. Evidence was presented that acetylcholine stimulates the phosphodiesterotic cleavage of phosphoinositides, and they suggest that this may be the primary step leading to secondary increases in the synthesis of phosphatidic acid and phosphatidylinositol (in particular). It was accordingly suggested that this cleavage results in increased local membrane permeability, with subsequent influence on the nerve transmission phenomenon.

Larrabee (1968) has shown that an increase in ^{32}P labeling of phosphatidylinositol, previously reported to occur in excised sympathetic ganglia excited by preganglionic nerve impulses, also occurs in naturally stimulated (*in situ*) ganglia. Thus it appears that increased turnover of phosphatidylinositol is normally accompanied by synaptic transmission in these ganglia. In this same context Yagihara *et al.* (1969), on incubating rat sympathetic ganglia, vagus nerve, and sciatic nerve with ^{32}P had found that at all periods up to 3 hours, phosphatidylinositol was the most highly labeled lipid in ganglia. In vagus and sciatic nerve, triphosphoinositide was the most highly labeled lipid. Limitations in interpreting such incubation data are discussed by Yagihara *et al.* However, the data suggested that the more rapid labeling of triphosphoinositide in nerve trunks as compared with that in ganglia is in keeping with the prior suggestion that this polyphosphatide is important in controlling the permeability of the axonal membrane.

Lunt *et al.* (1971) have reviewed other recent work on this general phenomenon and have found that the effect of acetylcholine on phosphatidylinositol is associated with a "receptor" proteolipid from nerve ending membranes of cerebral cortex. They suggest that acetylcholine acts at two levels at the synapse, and that neurotransmission involves a complex interplay of these systems. We quote: "First, there is a direct action with the receptor proteolipid, producing a specific conformational change which induces ionic translocation. This we consider to be the primary event in synaptic transmission. Coincident with this is the secondary effect on the phosphatidylinositol pool associated with the receptor. This second system, probably involving membrane bound phospholipid hydrolases may provide a mechanism for modulating a particular synaptic pathway."

According to Formby (1968), monophosphoinositide obtained in pure form from bovine brain shows a high capacity to bind noradrenaline *in vitro*. The binding was strongly influenced by the presence of Ca^{++} and Mg^{++}. This phenomenon suggests a possible receptor function of monophosphoinositide for noradrenaline in synaptosomes.

F. Phospholipids: Miscellaneous

Roozemond (1970) has reported the phospholipid composition of various parts of the rat hypothalamus by histochemical methods, and histochemical methods have been applied to the distribution of phospholipids in the brains of certain teleostean fishes (Saxena, 1969). The distribution of neutral lipids (including phospholipids) in the finback whale brain have also been reported (Lesch and Bernhard, 1968).

Changes in the brain phospholipids of goldfish exposed to temperatures varying from 5° to 30° were examined by Roots (1968). Changes that were found were characteristic of particular lipids, and it was suggested that modification of the phospholipid species in acclimation to temperature changes assists in the maintenance of a specific membrane "fluidity" and membrane permeability properties. The changes were largely in fatty acid content of the phospholipids. At lower environmental temperatures there was a general tendency for a greater degree of unsaturation of the fatty acid components. These observations seem particularly pertinent to the potential role of phospholipids in membranes.

Two interesting manuscripts have suggested a possible physiological role for phospholipids. Palmer and Davenport (1969), for example, have suggested that phospholipids may be involved in the biochemical processes that mediate spinal reflexes in newborn rats. Wang (1970) has suggested that phospholipids may be instrumental in regulating ionic permeability of excitable membranes. Both propositions suggest promising further investigation.

Catabolic changes in phospholipids in rabbit brains during anesthesia have been examined by Hinzen *et al.* (1970).

Finally we wish to list several manuscripts concerning phospholipid metabolism in the central nervous system (CNS). These were available to us only as abstracts in English or otherwise unavailable, and the reader is referred to the original complete version for details. They include manuscripts by Ivanova *et al.* (1969), Gasteva and Raize (1970), Ovsepyan and Karagezyan (1969), Dvorkin (1969), Chetverikov *et al.* (1970), and Tesoriero *et al.* (1970).

V. Sphingolipids

A. CERAMIDES

The ceramides occupy a key position in the biosynthesis of the sphingomyelins, as shown in the following sequence (after Davison, 1968b)

$$CH_3-(CH_2)_{12}-CH=CH-\overset{\overset{\text{H}}{|}}{\underset{\underset{\text{HO}}{|}}{C}}-\overset{\overset{\text{H}}{|}}{\underset{\underset{\text{NH}_2}{|}}{C}}-CH_2OH$$

sphingosine (*trans*-4-erythro-1,3-dihydroxy-2-aminooctadecene-4)

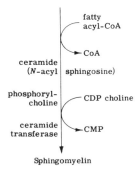

Since the biosynthesis of ceramide itself has been much clarified (Davison, 1968b), recent attention has been largely directed to steps leading from ceramide to the sphingomyelins. However, a recent detailed study by Morell and Radin (1970) has added much to our knowledge of the biosynthetic *control* involved. They found that the rate and extent of conversion of stearoyl-, lignoceryl-, palmitoyl-, and oleoyl- CoA to ceramide were of the order 60:12:3:1 respectively. This ratio resembles the relative distribution of these fatty acids in brain sphingolipids and suggested that the transferase plays an important part in controlling the distribution. Ceramide synthesis occurred primarily in microsomal membranes: ceramide hydrolysis was widely distributed in subcellular fractions, with the highest activity in lysosome-rich fractions.

Basu *et al.* (1968) (see also the cerebrosides) have detected two glycosyltransferases in 13-day-old embryonic chicken brain homogenates and microsomal preparations. One of these transfers glucose from UDP-glucose to ceramide to give ceramide-glucose. The other transfers galactose, further indication that sugars are added in a stepwise manner by specific glycosyltransferases, thus leading to the synthesis of disialoganglioside. Each enzyme requires a specific sugar nucleotide as glycose donor and a specific lipid as glycose acceptor. Systems of this type have been designated *multiglycosyl-transferase systems* (Roseman, 1968). Shah (1971) has shown that enzymes present in microsomal fractions of rat brain are capable of synthesizing both glucosyl and galactosyl ceramide from hydroxy fatty acid ceramide and hexose nucleotide. Both hydroxy fatty acid ceramide and nonhydroxy fatty acid ceramide were found to serve as acceptors for glucose, but only the hydroxy fatty acid ceramide was an acceptor for galactose. Glucose transferase activity was highest between birth and 15 days of age and declined slowly thereafter. Galactose transferase activity did not appear until the tenth postnatal day and reached a peak at 30 days. Galactose transferase activity was present principally in white matter microsomes, but glucose transferase activity was present in both white and gray microsome fractions. This, coupled with the changes occurring during development, suggested a correlation of development and distribution of cerebrosides and gangliosides respectively.

According to Behrens *et al.* (1971) dolichol monophosphate, believed to have a role in sugar transfer, is not an intermediate in the glucosylation of ceramide by brain extracts.

B. SPHINGOMYELIN AND RELATED COMPOUNDS

Accelerated interest in the sphingolipids has been emphasized by the publication of several excellent reviews on both the chemistry and the biochemistry of the compounds, e.g., Rosenberg (1970) and Stoffel (1970). The reader is referred especially to a collection of papers given at the International Symposium on the Chemistry and Metabolism of Sphingolipids (1970), dedicated to Dr. Herbert E. Carter. Only brief references can be made to some of the excellent manuscripts in this presentation.

The basic steps in the biosynthesis of sphingomyelin have been discussed by Rosenberg (1970) and summarized in the following series of equations (rearranged). Analogies with the biosynthesis of lecithin will be apparent.

1. Palmitoyl-CoA and L-serine + $\xrightarrow[\text{nicotinamide}]{\text{Mg}^{2+}}$ palmitoyl sphingosine[1]
   (ceramide)

2. N-Acyl sphingosine + CDP choline $\xrightarrow[\text{phosphorylcholine ceramide transferase}]{\text{Mg}^{2+}}$ sphingomyelin + CMP
   (ceramide)

Essential to this series of reactions is that palmitoyl serine is not an intermediate in the reaction, sphingosine first being synthesized *in toto*, then reacting with palmitoyl CoA to form ceramide. Essential to the above is the formation of ceramide, which can also be accomplished through hydrolysis of cerebroside as follows:

3. Sphingosine + UDPgal $\xrightarrow{\text{transferase I}}$ psychosine

4. Psychosine + fatty acyl-CoA $\xrightarrow{\text{transferase II}}$ cerebroside

5. Cerebroside + H_2O $\xrightarrow{\text{hydrolase}}$ galactose and ceramide

Sphingomyelin can also be synthesized from sphingosylphosphorylcholine (A. Rosenberg, 1970):

6. Stearoyl-CoA + sphingosylphosphorylcholine →
   N-acyl sphingosylphosphorylcholine + CoASH
   (sphingomyelin)

Early work delineating cofactor requirements, the particulate and soluble enzymes involved, etc., have been discussed in the Rosenberg review.

Recently, Fujino and Negishi (1968) have suggested that in spite of the fact that the naturally occurring sphingolipids have the *erythro* structure, in reaction 6 (above), the sphingosine base moiety of the active ceramide should have the *trans* double bond configuration and the

---

[1] One or more steps have been omitted from this reaction.

hydroxyl group at C-3 must possess the *threo* relationship to the amino group on C-2. Crude brain particulate fractions from 14-day-old mice, and *erythro-* and *threo-* type sphingosylphosphorylcholinases were incubated with 1-^{14}C-labeled acetyl-, palmitoyl-, stearoyl-, and oleyl-CoA respectively. Both types (*erythro* and *threo*) were active as fatty acyl-CoA acceptors. With ceramide as the precursor only the *threo* form is active in this alternative biosynthetic synthesis of sphingomyelin (see reference given by Fujino and Negishi).

An extensive group of *in vitro* experiments by Kanfer (1970) has established that a particulate fraction from the brains of young (10-day-old) rats can catalyze the following reactions:

UDP-glucose-^{14}C + sphingosine → glucosylceramide
UDP-galactose-^{14}C + sphingosine → galactosylsphingosine
Serine-^{14}C + palmitoyl-CoA → dihydrosphingosine + ceramide + cerebroside
CDP-choline-^{14}C → sphingomyelin

These multiple reactions, believed to be initial steps involved in the biosynthesis of sphingolipids, were accomplished by a brain preparation consisting of a "mixture of particles," but apparently containing few microsomes. According to the investigator, the preparation, as verified by electron microscopy, consisted of a populus of membranous sacs in which the biosynthesis of the sphingolipids can occur in an organized fashion with the sphingolipid perhaps not released until the final product was formed.

3-Keto-dihydrosphingosine in rat brain has been demonstrated as an intermediate in the reactions (Braun *et al.*, 1970):

1. L-Serine + palmitoyl-CoA → 3-keto-dihydrosphingosine and CO_2 + CoA
2. 3-Keto-dihydrosphingosine + NADP → dihydrosphingosine + NAD$^+$

Mouse brain microsomes were used to demonstrate the reaction in CNS tissue, and dihydrosphingosine was the major sphingolipid formed. Smaller amounts of N-acyldihydrosphingosine and N-acylsphingosine were also formed. Stearoyl-CoA produced the corresponding C_{20}-sphingolipids, whereas oleoyl- and lignoceroyl-CoA were inactive. Kanfer and Bates (1970) have found that by the addition of ethylenediamine tetraacetate (EDTA) to a partially purified enzyme system from rat brain, the product of the reaction was solely 3-keto-dihydrosphingosine. Neither myristoyl nor stearoyl-CoA was effective in replacing palmitoyl-CoA in the reaction.

Interrelationships between various phospholipids and their role in sphingolipid biosynthesis, and the degradation of the sphingolipids as well have been given increased attention. Segal and Wysocki (1970) presented [^{3}H]ethanolamine glycerophospholipids (prepared biosynthetically) to 13-day-old rats and, following isolation of various lipid classes, found that the alkyl groups of the ethanolamine plasmologens were better precursors of sphingomyelin and cerebroside than either the acyl groups of the phosphatidyl ethanolamine or free palmitic acid. Brain plasmalogenase increases rapidly during the myelinating period (Ansell, 1968). The relationship between sphingosine degradation, serine metabolism, and the biosynthesis of various phospholipids in liver has been examined by Henning and Stoffel (1969). Following parenteral administration to rats of [1-^{3}H$_2$]DL-erythrosphingosine and [3-^{14}C]DL-serine, the incorporation of ^{3}H into phospholipids was almost exclusively associated with phosphorylethanolamine and phosphorylcholine and exceeded the incorporation of ^{14}C by a considerable factor in both young and adult rats. The mechanism by which the liver cell prefers phosphorylethanolamine from sphingosine to that formed by the degradation of serine was discussed. These relationships also extend to the central nervous system, and Gatt (1970a) has made a detailed study of enzymes in brain which are responsible for the degradation of most spinal tissue sphingolipids. The enzymes include ceramidase, which hydrolyzes the amide bond of ceramide (N-acyl sphingosine), sphingomyelinase, which is a phospholipase of the "C" type which hydrolyzes the linkage between ceramide and phosphorylcholine of sphingomyelin, N-acetyl hexosaminodases, which hydrolyze both N-acetyl glucosaminides and N-acetyl galactosaminides, plus several other degradative enzymes, many of which also possess reverse biosynthetic capacity. The reactions involved in the hydrolysis of brain (and other organ) sphingolipids are shown in Fig. 3. Rosenberg (1970) has admirably summed up the literature on sphingomyelin degradation prior to 1968.

Gilliland and Moscatelli (1969) have recently studied the sphingosine base distribution in the whole brains of rat, chicken, turtle, frog, fish, and crayfish. A downward trend in lipid recovery was found in going to the lower species, presumably related to the myelin being richer in lipids in the higher species. Glycolipids were distinctly lower in the lower species, and shorter chain length and increased saturation were noted also in the lower phyla. However, the workers call attention to the difficulty in controlling age in selecting such groups for study, and this may have a bearing on the types of lipids found. Akino (1969) examined the base and fatty acid composition of pig brain sphingolipids (ceramide, cerebroside, sulfatide, sphingomyelin, and ganglioside). Each sphingosine sphingolipid showed a characteristic base pattern, having C_{18}-sphingosine and C_{18}-dihydrosphingosine as the predominant bases, but there were considerable quantitative differences among the sphingolipids studied. Considerable C_{20}-sphingosine was found in ganglioside, and

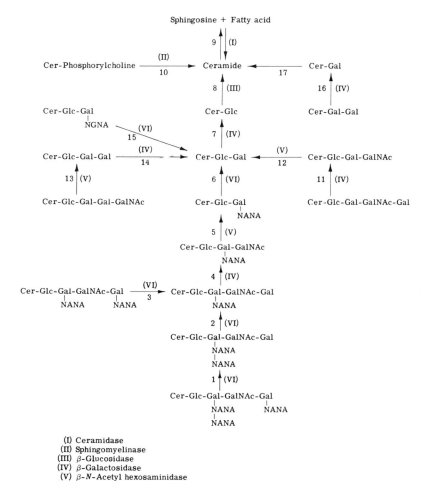

(I) Ceramidase
(II) Sphingomyelinase
(III) β-Glucosidase
(IV) β-Galactosidase
(V) β-*N*-Acetyl hexosaminidase
(VI) Sialidase

Fig. 3. Reactions involved in the hydrolysis of the sphingolipids. The arabic numbers are serial numbers of the reactions in the scheme; the roman numerals identify the enzymes. Abbreviations: Cer, ceramide; Glc, glucose; Gal, galactose; GalNAc, *N*-acetyl-glactosamine; NANA, *N*-acetyl neuraminic acid; NGNA, *N*-glycolyl-neuraminic acid. Enzymes: I, ceramidase; II, sphingomyelinase; III, β-glucosidase; IV, β-galactosidase; V, β-*N*-acetylhexosaminidase; VI, neuraminidase (or sialidase). Taken from Gatt (1970a).

small quantities in ceramide and sphingomyelin, but none was detected in cerebroside and sulfatide.

Attention is called to the comprehensive review on the chemistry and occurrence of sphingolipid long-chain bases by Karlsson (1970), although the review is not directed toward brain constituents.

C. Cerebrosides

(Galacto) cerebrosides are glycosylceramides in which a β-D-galacto-pyranosyl group is linked at the C-1 of sphingosine, and a fatty acid residue is linked to the C-2 amino group.

Two possible methods for the biosynthesis of cerebrosides, as indicated by *in vitro* experiments are: (1) addition of galactose to sphingosine at the 1-position of sphingosine to form galactopyschosine, followed by its N-acylation, and (2) N-acylation of sphingosine (forming ceramide), followed by the addition of galactose to the latter (for recent summaries of references to early work, see Basu *et al.*, 1971; Svennerholm, 1970a,b). Attempts to incorporate glucose or galactose directly into ceramide were largely unsuccessful until Basu *et al.* (1968) demonstrated that the reaction could be accomplished by two glycosyltransferases in particulate fractions of chicken brain. These transferases perform the following steps:

1. UDP-Glucose-^{14}C + ceramide $\rightarrow$ ceramide-glucose-^{14}C + UDP
2. UDP-Galactose^{14}C + ceramide-glucose $\rightarrow$ ceramide-glucose-galactose-^{14}C + UDP

Reaction 1 was subsequently shown to take place in rat brain subcellular preparations but with UDP-galactose and the formation, of course, of (largely) ceramide-galactose. The reaction also occurred to a lesser extent in rat liver and chicken liver and was accompanied by smaller amounts of other glycolipids (Fujino and Nakano, 1969).

Morell and Radin (1969) have described experiments in which crude microsomal fractions from young mice brains catalyze the reaction:

Hydroxy fatty acid-ceramide + UDP-galactose $\rightarrow$ hydroxy fatty acid-cerebroside
+ UDP

This system apparently does not work with nonhydroxylated fatty acid-ceramide.

Apparently cerebroside cannot pass the blood-brain barrier. When high specific activity tritium-labeled galactosyl ceramide was injected intravenously into monkeys, very little radioactivity appeared in brain after as much as 37 days (Burton and Sodd, 1969).

A detailed report of cerebroside biosynthesis and degradation has been made by Radin (1970). Attention was again called to the possibility that nonhydroxy fatty acid cerebroside may be synthesized by a route different from that of hydroxy fatty acid cerebroside. The properties of crude enzymes capable of degrading cerebroside were studied also. The principal products detected were ceramide, and (via conversion) sphingomyelin.

Basu *et al.* (1971) have recently shown that the reaction

$$\text{UDP-Galactose-}{}^{14}\text{C} + \text{ceramide} \rightarrow {}^{14}\text{C-galactocerebroside} + \text{UDP}$$

is catalyzed by an enzyme from chicken embryonic brain which is a galactosyltransferase different from the enzymes involved in the biosynthesis of gangliosides. The differences were based upon the centrifugation purification steps, which effectively separated the galactosyltransferase involved in ganglioside biosynthesis. As in the case of the report by Morell and Radin (1969) the transferase catalyzed the synthesis of cerebrosides containing α-hydroxy acids only.

Examination of the fatty acid composition, distribution, and general configuration of the cerebrosides has continued. Kishimoto *et al.* (1968) have isolated two glycolipids from pig brain. These were shown to be fatty acid esters of kerasin and cerebron in which the fatty acid moiety is attached to the 6-position of the galactose. The ester-linked fatty acids were primarily 16:0, 18:0, and 18:1. The amide-linked fatty acids showed the varied assortment of chain lengths characteristic of brain cerebrosides. The galactose in the cerebron ester was shown to exist in the β-pyranose form. On the basis of some prior observations by Klenk and Löhr (1967), Tamai (1968; see, for references to other low polarity glycolipids) has examined white matter of bovine brain for four "faster running glycolipids." All were characterized as ceramide monogalactosides containing fatty acid ester linkages. The long-chain base consisted principally of sphingosine (C_{18}). By special methylation procedures it was concluded that fatty acid esterification was present at carbons 3 and/or 6 of galactose. Further study to more precisely locate the fatty acid ester position was indicated. The kerasin and nervone fractions of human brain have been examined by Klenk and Schorsch (1968). The kerasin cerebroside yielded tetracosanoic acid as the principal fatty acid. Two minor kerasins containing tricosanoic acid and pentacosanoic acid were detected. The nervone cerebroside yielded a major constituent containing tetracosenoic acid and two minor cerebrosides containing pentacosenoic and hexacosenoic acid. The 2-hydroxy acids from bovine brain cerebrosides, as determined by GLC of the (-) methylformate esters, were determined to have the D-configuration (Hammarström, 1969). In a later investigation Hammarström and Samuelsson (1970) prepared 2-hydroxy acid ceramides labeled with deuterium in both the sphingosine and fatty acid moieties. On incubation with mouse brain microsomes it was found that both sphingosine and 2-hydroxy acid from the ceramide were incorporated into cerebroside. In a study of the subcellular fatty acid composition of mouse brain cerebrosides, Blass (1970) found that 2-hydroxy fatty acids constituted 80% of the fatty acids in myelin cerebrosides and about 55% of the fatty acids in both light and heavy microsomes. In myelin, the fatty acids consisted largely of those

C_{20} or longer, while in microsomes shorter chain fatty acids (C_{16} to C_{20}) predominated.

Attention must be called to a review on the chemistry and biochemistry of glycosphingolipids, which unfortunately was not available to us at the time this chapter was written (Gielen, 1971).

D. SULFATIDES

The sulfate donor or "active sulfate" in the biosynthesis of the brain sulfatides (cerebroside sulfate) and brain sulfated mucopolysaccharides (glycosaminoglycans) is 3'-phosphoadenosine-5-phosphosulfate (PAPS) and the reactions leading to its formation are believed to be according to the following steps (as summarized by Balasubramanian and Bachhawat, 1970):

$$\text{ATP} + \text{SO}_4{}^{2-} \xrightleftharpoons{\text{ATP-sulfurylase}} \text{APS} + \text{PP}_i$$

$$\text{APS} + \text{ATP} \xrightarrow{\text{APS-kinase}} \text{PAPS} + \text{ADP}$$

$$\overline{2\,\text{ATP} + \text{SO}_4{}^{2-} \xrightarrow{\hspace{2cm}} \text{PAPS} + \text{ADP} + \text{PP}_i}$$

The importance of sulfatides to the central nervous system has not yet been completely assessed. This is perhaps not unparalleled for relatively minor components of nervous tissues. Cumar et al. (1968) have shown that enzymes distributed in all brain particulate organelles examined, as well as the cytosol, contain enzymes that catalyze the transfer of sulfate-^{35}S from 3'-phosphoadenosine-5'-phosphosulfate-[35]S (PAP[35]S) to galactose-containing glycosphingolipids and to galactose and water-soluble galactosides. Special hydrolytic (acidic) and chromatographic methods established that the sulfate was in position 3 of the galactose moiety of the galactose-containing glycosphingolipids. The enzyme catalyzing the transfer of sulfate to the glycosphingolipids was shown to be different from that catalyzing the transfer to water-soluble compounds (e.g., galactose sulfate).

The review of Balasubramanian and Bachhawat cited above summarizes the recent literature prior to 1968 and stresses the significance of sulfatide as a myelin lipid and the changes occurring in content, and possible significance, in certain metabolic diseases. An additional review (Levitina, 1970) was not available to us in translation. A manuscript describing the sulfatide nature of a so-called "X-lipid" has been studied by Kreps et al. (1969b). The substance apparently occurs in the brains of all animals with a developed nervous system.

Table I: Gangliosides of Brain

		Notations		
Trivial name	Structure	Svenner-holm	Korey and Gonata	Kuhn and Wiegandt
Monosialosylgalac-tosyl ceramide	NANA$(2\rightarrow 3)$Gal$(1\rightarrow 1)$Cer	—	—	G_{gal}
Monosialosyllac-tosyl ceramide	NANA$(2\rightarrow 3)$Gal$(1\rightarrow 4)$Glc$(1\rightarrow 1)$Cer	G_{M3}	G_6	G_{lac}^1
Disialosyllactosyl ceramide	NANA$(2\rightarrow 8)$NANA$(2\rightarrow 3)$Gal$(1\rightarrow 4)$Glc$(1\rightarrow 1)$Cer	G_{D3}	G_{3A}	G_{lac}^2
N-acetylgalacto-saminyl-(sialo-syl)lactosyl ceramide	GalNHAc$(1\rightarrow 4)$Gal$(1\rightarrow 4)$Glc$(1\rightarrow 1)$Cer $\quad\quad\quad\quad 3 \atop \quad\quad\quad\quad \uparrow \atop \quad\quad\quad\quad 2$ NANA	G_{M2}	G_5	G_{CNTr11}^1
N-acetylgalacto-saminyl-(disialo-syl)lactosyl ceramide	GalNHAc$(1\rightarrow 4)$Gal$(1\rightarrow 4)$Glc$(1\rightarrow 1)$Cer $\quad\quad\quad\quad 3 \atop \quad\quad\quad\quad \uparrow \atop \quad\quad\quad\quad 2$ NANA$(2\rightarrow 8)$NANA	G_{D2}	G_{2A}	G_{GNTr11}^2
Galactosyl-N-ace-tylgalacto-saminyl-(sialo-syl)lactosyl ceramide	Gal$(1\rightarrow 3)$GalNHAc$(1\rightarrow 4)$Gal$(1\rightarrow 4)$Glc$(1\rightarrow 1)$Cer $\quad\quad\quad\quad 3 \atop \quad\quad\quad\quad \uparrow \atop \quad\quad\quad\quad 2$ NANA	G_{M1}	G_4	G_{GNT}^1
Sialosylgalactosyl-N-acetylgalacto-saminyl(sialo-syl)lactosyl ceramide	NANA$(2\rightarrow 3)$Gal$(1\rightarrow 3)$GalNHAc$(1\rightarrow 4)$Gal$(1\rightarrow 4)$Glc$(1\rightarrow 1)$Cer $\quad\quad\quad\quad 3 \atop \quad\quad\quad\quad \uparrow \atop \quad\quad\quad\quad 2$ NANA	G_{D1a}	G_3	G_{GNT}^{2a}
Galactosyl-N-ace-tylgalacto-saminyl-(disialo-syl)lactosyl ceramide	Gal$(1\rightarrow 3)$GalNHAc$(1\rightarrow 4)$Gal$(1\rightarrow 4)$Glc$(1\rightarrow 1)$Cer $\quad\quad\quad\quad 3 \atop \quad\quad\quad\quad \uparrow \atop \quad\quad\quad\quad 2$ NANA$(2\rightarrow 8)$NANA	G_{D1b}	G_2	G_{GNT}^{2b}
Disialosylgalacto-syl-N-acetyl-galactosaminyl-(sialosyl)lactosyl ceramide	NANA$(2\rightarrow 8)$NANA$(2\rightarrow 3)$Gal$(1\rightarrow 3)$GalNHAc$(1\rightarrow 4)$Gal$(1\rightarrow 4)$Glc$(1\rightarrow 1)$Cer $\quad\quad\quad\quad 3 \atop \quad\quad\quad\quad \uparrow \atop \quad\quad\quad\quad 2$ NANA	G_{T1a}	—	—
Sialosylgalactosyl-N-acetylgalacto-saminyl-(disialo-syl)lactosyl ceramide	NANA$(2\rightarrow 3)$Gal$(1\rightarrow 3)$GalNHAc$(1\rightarrow 4)$Gal$(1\rightarrow 4)$Glc$(1\rightarrow 1)$Cer $\quad\quad\quad\quad 3 \atop \quad\quad\quad\quad \uparrow \atop \quad\quad\quad\quad 2$ NANA$(2\rightarrow 8)$NANA	G_{T1b}	G_1	G_{GNT}^{3a}
Disialosylgalacto-syl-N-acetyl-galactosaminyl-(disialosyl)-lactosyl	NANA$(2\rightarrow 8)$NANA$(2\rightarrow 3)$Gal$(1\rightarrow 3)$GalNHAc$(1\rightarrow 4)$Gal$(1\rightarrow 4)$Glc$(1\rightarrow 1)$Cer $\quad\quad\quad\quad 3 \atop \quad\quad\quad\quad \uparrow \atop \quad\quad\quad\quad 2$ NANA$(2\rightarrow 8)$NANA	G_{Q1}	—	G_{GNT}^9

E. Gangliosides

While ganglioside isolation and structural determination has been an area of study for a number of years, only recently has the examination of the mode of biosynthesis and degradation of gangliosides been delineated. Excellent reviews on gangliosides have been published by Svennerholm (1970a,b). An effort will be made therefore to cover only the basic concepts and pathways involved in ganglioside metabolism and information added to the literature since the latest review. The ganglioside nomenclature of Svennerholm will be used primarily. The structures and nomenclature utilized by three different groups investigating the major brain gangliosides are shown in Table I.

1. *Distribution*

The original work of Klenk and Langerbeins (1941) demonstrated that gangliosides were present only in the gray matter of brain. More recent work has established that indeed the bulk of CNS gangliosides are concentrated in this tissue. Careful investigation has established that there is also a small cerebral ganglioside fraction associated with myelin (Suzuki *et al.*, 1967, 1968; Kamoshita *et al.*, 1969; Suzuki, 1970).

That the general rate of ganglioside accumulation in whole rat brain occurs over a relatively long time span is evident (Fig. 4) from the work

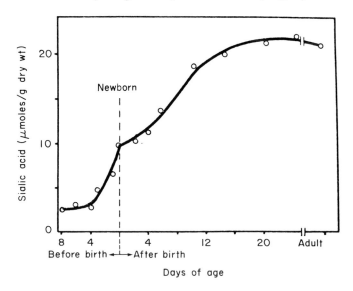

Fig. 4. Changes in total gangliosides of rat brain during development. Taken from Tettamanti (1971).

Table II
Ganglioside Distribution in Human Brain Tissue

Tissue	Total NANA (μg/gm wet wt)	Percentage distribution of NANA								Reference
		G_{M3}	G_{M2}	G_{M1}	G_{DIa}	G_{DIb}	G_{D2}	G_{T1}	G_{Q1}	
Cerebral cortex										
Newborn	400	1.0	3.6	14.6	71.6	1.8	1.1	7.3	—	Svennerholm (1964)
8 years	797	—	3.6	17.4	39.4	19.8	—	15.9	2.9	Suzuki (1965)
73 years	796	—	1.7	12.8	22.8	25.5	—	31.2	5.1	Suzuki (1965)
White matter										
Newborn	400	1.0	6.9	19.1	57.8	2.1	1.4	3.4	—	Svennerholm (1964)
8 years	73	—	1.7	20.4	42.9	12.5	—	16.0	5.9	Suzuki (1965)
73 years	191	—	1.9	12.6	18.4	30.4	—	27.9	7.9	Suzuki (1965)

of Tettamanti (1971). The types and amounts of individual gangliosides present also change with the age of the animal. This is partially evident from the data on humans in Table II. There are potential pitfalls when one makes a comparison of data from several different sources. A comprehensive study on rat and human brain has been recently published by Vanier *et al.* (1971). Figure 5 clearly shows that in the developmental period in both rat and human, after initially high levels of G_{M1} and G_{T1}, G_{D1a} quickly becomes the dominant ganglioside in percentage composi-

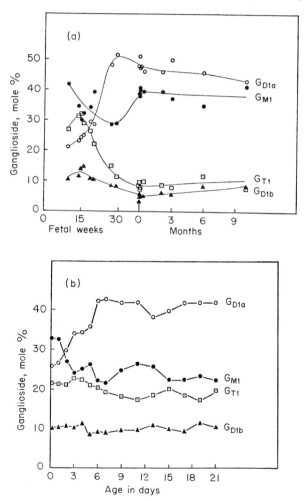

Fig. 5. (a) The ganglioside pattern in human frontal brain cortex during prenatal and early postnatal development. (b) The ganglioside pattern in rat cerebrum during postnatal development. Taken from Vanier *et al.* (1971).

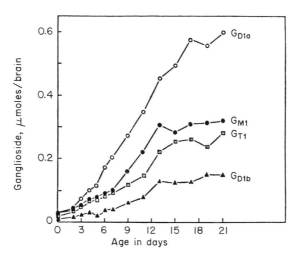

Fɪɢ. 6. Content of individual gangliosides in rat cerebrum during postnatal development. Taken from Vanier *et al.* (1971).

tion. This early dominance becomes even more evident when the actual quantities of gangliosides in rat cerebrum are plotted versus age of the animal (Fig. 6). With the approach of neuronal maturation in the human, the ganglioside distribution seems to be stabilized, with G_{D1a} becoming the predominant ganglioside (Fig. 7).

2. Biosynthesis

The elucidation of the biosynthetic pathways, both major and minor, of ganglioside formation is still incomplete. A general scheme of established pathways and several proposed pathways is shown in Fig. 8. A number of individual steps have been investigated and several of the enzymes partially localized (Table III). Most of the work thus far has indicated that the synaptosomal fraction of brain contains the bulk of the biosynthetic activity.

Since the bulk of the pathway studied has been conducted under *in vitro* conditions, some criticism has been leveled at the conclusions drawn, particularly with regard to what relationship, if any, exists between the pools of potential precursors available *in vitro* as opposed to *in vivo* conditions. Arce *et al.* (1971) have expressed the belief that, with regard to the N-acetylneuraminic acid (NANA) addition to gangliosides at least, there are rigid relationships between the enzymes capable of adding NANA to the substrate and the substrates that are available for NANA addition. There appear to be no general pools of say G_{M1} to the precursor of G_{D1b}, or G_{D1b} to the precursor for G_{T1b}, but a number of

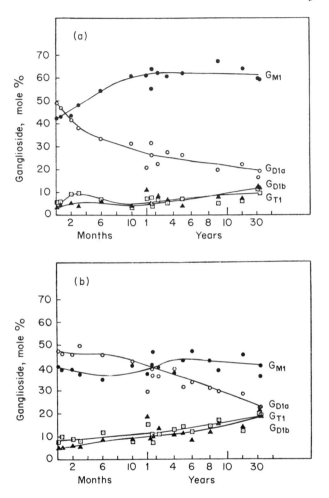

Fig. 7. (a) Developmental changes in the ganglioside pattern of human frontal white matter. (b) Developmental changes in the ganglioside pattern of human frontal brain cortex. Taken from Vanier *et al.* (1971).

small pools, some precursors for more complex gangliosides and some not. It would seem that *in vivo* membrane localization may play an important role in the manner in which products of gangliosides are formed and the type of compound synthesized. Only further investigation will answer this question.

3. Degradation

Several years ago it was determined that the half-life of gangliosides in developing brain was from 20 to 25 days (Burton, 1967; Suzuki, 1967).

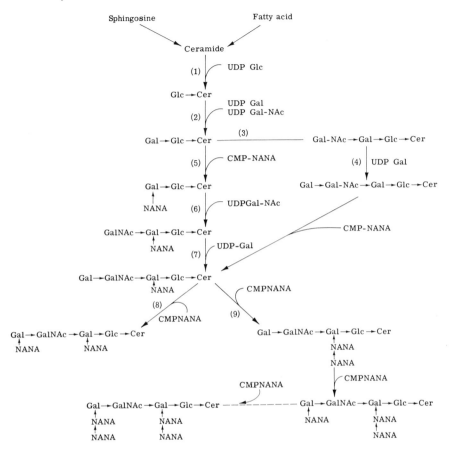

Fɪɢ. 8. Major pathways of ganglioside biosynthesis.

It was also found that as the animal matured, ganglioside turnover decreased (Suzuki, 1967). Much of the effort with regard to the individual enzymes involved in ganglioside degradation has been carried out in relation to certain genetic lipidoses in which several of these enzymes are partially or completely absent. The lipidoses will, however, be discussed in a later section of this chapter.

As is apparent in Fig. 9, the initial steps of ganglioside degradation involve the removal of several N-acetylneuraminic acid residues. The enzyme involved, neuraminidase (or sialidase), was originally thought to be ganglioside-specific (Leibovitz and Gatt, 1968). Examination by Tettamanti and Zambotti (1968) and Ohman *et al.* (1970) of pig and bovine neuraminidase respectively, has indicated that one enzyme was hydrolyzing the NANA residues from the gangliosides as well as from

Table III

Specific Enzymes Involved in Ganglioside Biosynthesis

Reaction number	Enzyme	Subcellular localization	Reference
1.	UDP-Glucose-ceramide glucosyltransferase	Particulate	Basu (1968)
2.	UDP-Galactose-glucosylceramide galactosyltransferase	Synaptosomes, microsomes, mitochondria	Hildebrand et al. (1970)
3.	UDP-N-Acetylgalactosamine:galactosylglucosylceramide N-Acetylgalactosaminyltransferase	Particulate	Handa and Burton (1969)
4.	UDP-Galactose:N-acetylgalactosaminylgalactosyl-glucosylceramide galactosyl transferase		
5.	CMP-N-Acetylneuraminic acid: galactosylglucosyl-ceramide N-acetylneuraminyl transferase	Particulate	Kaufman et al. (1967)
6.	UDP-N-Acetylgalactosamine: (N-acetylneuraminyl)-galactosylglucosylceramide N-acetylgalactosaminyl transferase	Microsomes, synaptic membranes	Dicesare and Dain (1971)
7.	UDP-Galactose:N-acetylgalactosaminyl-(N-acetyl-neuraminyl) galactosylglucosylceramide galactosyl transferase	Microsomes, crude mitochondria	Yip and Dain (1970)
8.	CMP-N-Acetylneuraminic acid: galactosyl-N-acetyl-galactosaminyl-(N-acetylneuraminyl) galactosyl-glucosylceramide N-Acetylneuraminyl transferase	Microsomes, crude mitochondria	Kaufman et al. (1968)
9.	CMP-N-Acetylneuraminic acid: N-acetylneuraminyl (galactosyl-N-acelylgalactosaminyl) galactosylglucosyl-ceramide CMP-N-acetylneuraminyl transferase	Microsomes, crude mitochondria	Kaufman et al. (1968)

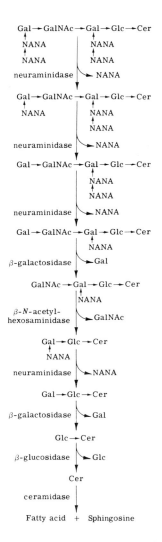

Fig. 9. Major pathways of ganglioside degradation.

other nonganglioside substrates. Ohman *et al.* (1970) have shown that of the ganglioside substrates examined, G_{D1b} was consistently hydrolyzed more slowly than the other natural gangliosides. This suggests that a NANA with a $2 \to 8$ glycosidic linkage was more resistant to attack than was the NANA having a $2 \to 3$ glycosidic linkage, as would be present in the other disialyl-ganglioside, G_{D1a}. Neuraminidase has been shown, by two research groups (Schengrund and Rosenberg, 1970; Ohman, 1971a), to be localized in the synaptosomal fractions. Ohman has questioned whether the enzyme is really synaptosomal or lysosomal in nature. He suggests that lysosomal material could be associated with the synaptosomal fraction either by being trapped naturally in the nerve endings or by the means of isolation used. Schengrund and Rosenberg have indicated that the enzymatic activity is associated with the synaptosomal membrane.

Definite differences in neuraminidase activity have been found with regard to various regions or age of the brain. Ohman (1971b) found that the enzyme activity of cerebral cortex was 10–25 times higher than in white matter. The cerebellar cortex had higher neuraminidase activity than did cerebral cortex. The hydrolysis of NANA from gangliosides seems to be also quite age dependent. Ohman and Svennerholm (1971) have indicated that neuraminidase activity is not present in human brain until a fetal age of 15–20 weeks. As the fetus developed, enzymatic activity continued to increase with greatest activity being found in the adult brain. A similar pattern has been described in the chick by Schengrund and Rosenberg (1971) with the exception that the chick brain had neuraminidase activity, of some sort, at all ages examined. Neuraminidase activity has also been found to increase with age in the rat (Roukema et al., 1970).

While it appears that only one neuraminidase enzyme is necessary to cleave the various NANA residues from gangliosides, it is equally evident that several glycosidases are involved in the removal of the other carbohydrate moieties. It had been assumed until the work of Gatt et al. (Gatt and Rapport, 1966; Gatt, 1967) that one glycosidase was responsible for the hydrolysis of both glucose and galactose. Gatt's successful separation of a β-glycosidase fraction and a β-galactosidase fraction indicates that at least two separate enzymes are involved in the cleavage of these two carbohydrates from gangliosides. Since there is present both an internal and an external galactosyl moiety, the possibility of at least two separate galactosidases is quite possible.

In contrast to the neuraminidase enzyme which was mainly in the synaptosomes, the β-galactosidase, β-glucosidase, and β-N-acetylhexosaminidase were found to be localized in the lysosomal subcellular fraction (Ohman, 1971a). The contrast does not end there, however, for when enzyme activity versus age of animal for the neuraminidase was compared to the glycosidases, two different profiles were apparent. The neuraminidase increased during development and was maximal in the adult. The glycosidases were of about the same enzymatic activity at all ages of animals examined (Ohman and Svennerholm, 1971). These differences in developing brain have also been demonstrated by Schengrund and Rosenberg (1971). It has been suggested by Ohman and Svennerholm (1971) that the low level of neuraminidase may be a way for the cell in the developing tissue to favor biosynthetic activities, since without neuraminidase splitting off NANA from the gangliosides, the ganglioside cannot be further degraded by the glycosidases.

The final step in ganglioside degradation, ceramide → sphingosine + fatty acid, is catalyzed by the enzyme ceramidase. Examination by several groups (Bowen and Radin, 1969a; Radin *et al.*, 1969) has established that ceramidase activity increases with development of the animal, as was the case with the neuraminidase. The subcellular localization of this enzyme has not as yet been determined.

4. Function

Gangliosides are localized in two fractions of the brain. A minor amount of ganglioside appears to serve a structural role in the myelin matrix (Suzuki, 1970). The bulk of the ganglioside in brain is found in the outer membrane of the nerve endings. What physiological role these gangliosides perform is still in question. Wiegant (1968) has suggested that they are involved in nerve impulse conduction. It has been demonstrated that the distribution of gangliosides resembles that of γ-aminobutyric acid (Lowden and Wolfe, 1964). Deul *et al.* (1968) have indicated that the binding of serotonin to synaptic vesicles may be mediated by gangliosides. Irwin (Irwin, 1969; Irwin and Samson, 1971) has also indicated that certain types of behavioral stimulation seem to be accompanied by alteration of ganglioside metabolism, compared to corresponding control animals. Whatever the specific role or roles of gangliosides in brain, it is clearly evident by now that they serve an active rather than a passive function.

VI. Cholesterol, Methyl Sterols, Trace Isoprenoids, and Other Trace Lipids

Considerable progress has been made during the past 4 years in elucidating the ability of CNS tissue to synthesize cholesterol (for reviews, see Paoletti *et al.*, 1969; Davison, 1970a,b,c). Recent work has been directed toward refining some of the individual steps in the biosynthetic process, the subcellular and cellular localization of the biosynthetic process, and perhaps more significantly, investigation of factors controlling the regulation of cholesterol biosynthesis within CNS tissue.

A. CHEMISTRY AND DISTRIBUTION

While cholesterol has been shown by many early investigators to be the major sterol of CNS tissue, recent precise physicochemical analytical

Table IV

STEROLS DETECTED IN CENTRAL NERVOUS SYSTEM TISSUE

Sterol	Found in adult brain	Reference	Found in developing brain	Reference
5α-Cholestanol	+	Fieser (1953); Weiss et al. (1968)	+	Weiss et al. (1968)
Desmosterol	+	Galli et al. (1968); Weiss et al. (1968); D'Hollander and Chevallier (1969); Ramsey et al. (1971f)	+	Stokes et al. (1956); Kritchevsky and Holmes (1962); Fumagalli and Paoletti (1963); Fumagalli et al. (1964); Weiss et al. (1968)
Lathosterol	+	Fieser (1953)	–	
5α-Cholesta-7,24-dien-3β-ol	+	Weiss et al. (1968); Ramsey et al. (1971a)	+	Kritchevsky et al. (1965); Weiss et al. (1968); Ramsey et al. (1971e)
5α-Cholesta-8-en-3β-ol	+	Weiss et al. (1968); Galli et al. (1968)	+	Weiss et al. (1968)
5α-Cholest-14-en-3β-ol	+	G. Galli et al. (1968, 1970)	–	
4α-Methyl-5α-cholest-7-en-3β-ol	+	Ramsey et al. (1971a)	+	Ramsey et al. (1971e)
4α-Methyl-5α-cholesta-7,24-dien-3β-ol	+	Ramsey et al. (1971a)	+	Ramsey et al. (1971e)
4α-Methyl-5α-cholest-8-en-3β-ol	+	Weiss et al. (1968); Galli et al. (1968)	+	Weiss et al. (1968); Galli et al. (1968); Ramsey et al. (1971e)
4α-Methyl-5α-cholesta-8,24-dien-3β-ol	+	Weiss et al. (1968); Galli et al. (1968)	+	Weiss et al. (1968); Galli et al. (1968); Ramsey et al. (1971e)
4α,4α-Dimethyl-5α-cholest-7-en-3β-ol	+	Ramsey et al. (1971a)	–	—
4,4-Dimethyl-5α-cholest-8-en-3β-ol	+	Weiss et al. (1968); Galli et al. (1968)	+	Weiss et al. (1968); Galli et al. (1968); Ramsey et al. (1971e)
4,4-Dimethyl-5α-cholesta-8,24-dien-3β-ol	+	Weiss et al. (1968); Galli et al. (1968); Ramsey et al. (1971a)	+	Weiss et al. (1968); Galli et al. (1968); Ramsey et al. (1971e)
4,4,14α-Trimethyl-5α-cholest-7-en-3β-ol	+	Ramsey et al. (1971a)	–	—
Dihydrolanosterol	+	Galli et al. (1968); D'Hollander and Chevallier (1969)	–	—
Lanosterol	+	Galli et al. (1968); Ramsey et al. (1971a)	+	Ramsey et al. (1971e)

techniques have tended to indicate that many other sterols are present in this tissue in trace amounts, and that not all of them are artifacts resulting from autooxidation (Paoletti *et al.*, 1969). Table IV lists neutral sterols thus far identified in developing and adult brain (other than cholesterol, of course). The experiments of van Lier and Smith (1969) have been especially informative in determining that compounds such as 26-hydroxycholesterol are not autooxidation artifacts. Exactly how all of these compounds are involved in brain cholesterol metabolism may provide an exciting area for future study.

B. BIOSYNTHESIS: YOUNG VERSUS ADULT BRAIN

In the late forties and up until the early sixties it was almost a biochemical axiom that young CNS tissue actively synthesized cholesterol but that this synthetic capacity was lost in the adult organ. Since then it has been generally accepted that adult brain tissue can synthesize cholesterol to a limited but measurable extent (see Kabara, 1967), for review). There seem to have been few attempts made to determine why the adult brain should be deficient in this respect. It has been tacitly assumed that the period of active myelination is the only period during which cholesterol biosynthesis is necessary. That adult brain can synthesize cholesterol has again been recently demonstrated by the experiments of Gautheron *et al.* (1969), in which MVA-2-^{14}C was injected intravenously into adult rats. Experiments of the latter type raise the question: why does mature brain tissue perform so poorly *in vitro* but synthesize cholesterol to an appreciable extent *in vivo?*

A partial answer to this problem has been presented by the experiments of Ramsey *et al.* (1971a,b) in which, as previously suggested by the experiments of Kelley *et al.* (1969), a "metabolic block" in the conversion of squalene to cholesterol appears to be a characteristic consequence of disrupting central nervous tissue on removal from its natural habitat. This phenomenon, which may be due to the instability of enzymes required for the squalene-to-cholesterol stage or to inhibitors released on disruption of the tissue, seem to apply to newborn as well as mature brain (Ramsey *et al.*, 1971a,b). At our present stage of knowledge it appears that only experiments in which labeled cholesterol precursors are presented *intracerebrally* can accurately assess the capacity of central nervous tissue to synthesize cholesterol. It may be pertinent to note that cofactor requirements in brain cell-free preparations are rather critical with respect to the conversion of squalene to cholesterol (Kelley *et al.*, 1969).

C. Subcellular Biosynthesis

Despite many years of effort expended on studies of brain cholesterol biosynthesis, only recently has an attempt been made to determine precisely which subcellular organelle is responsible for sterol biosynthesis in brain tissue. Possibly it has been accepted (see below) on the basis of studies on liver cholesterol biosynthesis, that the biosynthetic site in both organs must be the same. The extraordinary cellular complexity of CNS tissue as compared to that of liver tissue should preclude any such simple comparison. Nevertheless, it now appears clear that, as in liver, both the microsomal component of the endoplasmic reticulum *and* some contribution from the cytosol fractions are essential for cholesterol biosynthesis (Ramsey *et al.*, 1971a). Myelin and mitochondria were clearly excluded as biosynthetic sites. Such preparations from young as well as mature CNS tissue also failed to carry the biosynthetic process, except to a limited degree, past the squalene stage. A possible inhibiting factor in microsomal preparations was suggested by the initial work (Ramsey *et al.*, 1971b). The observation that microsomes are the subcellular site of brain cholesterol biosynthesis has been substantiated by Paoletti (1971).

If brain microsomes are the site of cholesterol biosynthesis, how do the other central nervous system subcellular organelles receive their cholesterol? This question has been partially answered in a series of investigations by Ramsey *et al.* (1971c,d) who studied the distribution of cholesterol and some of its immediate precursors in both immature and adult rat brain following intracerebral injection of labeled acetate and mevalonate. The deposition of steroidal material in brain with respect to age had been determined in terms of myelin and nonmyelin fractions by Cuzner (1968) and Davison (1970c). In this connection Rawlins *et al.* (1970) had determined that cholesterol is reutilized in peripheral nerve. The experiments of Ramsey *et al.* (1971c,d) adequately indicate that in both immature and adult brain, factors controlling the distribution of cholesterol, and especially the immediate 4,4-dimethyl and 4α-methyl sterol cholesterol precursors, strongly influence the rate at which cholesterol itself is deposited within subcellular organelles of the CNS. A complete knowledge of controlling factors would greatly add to our knowledge of the role cholesterol plays in the central nervous system.

D. Steryl Esters in the CNS

It has been the consensus of opinion for many years that while measurable amounts of "cholesteryl" esters are present in developing brain (Mandel *et al.*, 1949; Adams and Davison, 1959; Clarenburg *et al.*, 1963; Grafnetter *et al.*, 1965), steryl esters are not present in adult brain tissue (Fumagalli and Paoletti, 1963). Experiments conducted during the period 1967 to 1971, however, have suggested that there is a small but significant steryl ester content in the adult CNS. For example, Tichy (1967) indicated that the small but measurable steryl ester content in the corpus callosum of human adult brain was composed mainly of saturated and monounsaturated fatty acid esters of cholesterol. Alling and Svennerholm (1969) found that the major fatty acids esterified to sterols in adult human brain are oleic, palmitic, palmitoleic, and arachidonic. Of these, arachidonic was in highest concentration. That cholesteryl esters can be synthesized *in situ* by adult brain, albeit in small amounts, has been indicated by Kelley *et al.* (1969) with brain cell-free preparations, and by Ramsey *et al.* (1971b) with subcellular preparations of adult rat brain.

As further indication that our knowledge of brain cholesterol biosynthesis is far from complete, Ramsey *et al.* (1971e) have indicated that the *in vivo* biosynthetic pathway in adult rat brain differs from that *in vitro*. Thus following intracerebral injection of 2-^{14}C-MVA high specific activity lanosterol, 4,4-dimethyl-5α-cholesta-8(9)-24-dien-3β-ol, 4α-methyl-5α-cholesta-7,24-dien-3β-ol and 5α-cholesta-7,24-dien-3β-ol were formed 1 hour after intracerebral injection of the ^{14}C-labeled precursor. Labeled to a lesser extent were 4,4,14α-trimethyl-5α-cholest-7-en-3β-ol, 4α-methyl-5α-cholest-7-en-3β-ol, desmosterol, and cholesterol. 4α,14α-Dimethyl-5α-cholest-7-en-3β-ol was detected by mass only. Incubation of 2-^{14}C-MVA with adult rat brain cell-free preparations yielded highly

Table V

DISTRIBUTION OF STEROLS IN THE STERYL ESTER FRACTION FROM
DEVELOPING RAT BRAIN[a]

Compound	Sterol/gm wet wt of brain (μg)	Distribution of sterols in steryl ester fraction (%)
Cholesterol	5.55	54.3
4α-Methyl-5α-cholest-8-en-3β-ol	1.21	11.8
4α-Methyl-5α-cholest-7-en-3β-ol	0.67	6.6
4α-Methyl-5α-cholesta-8,24-dien-3β-ol	0.31	3.0
4α-Methyl-5α-cholesta-7,24-dien-3β-ol	1.70	16.6
4,4-Dimethyl-5α-cholesta-8,24-dien-3β-ol	0.79	7.7

[a] Taken from Ramsey *et al.* (1972).

labeled 4,4-dimethyl-5α-cholesta-14(15), 24-dien-3β-ol and 4α-methyl-5α-cholesta-14(15)-24-dien-3β-ol. These experiments suggest that a partial disruption or alteration of the cholesterol biosynthetic pathway (at the latter stages) occurs when the brain tissue is macerated.

In a recent investigation of the endogenous sterol content of developing (15-day-old) rat brain (Ramsey et al., 1972), it was found that cholesterol constituted only about half of the steryl ester fraction, the other sterols consisting largely of 4α-methyl mono- and diunsaturated sterols (Table V). In the free sterol fraction cholesterol was the major sterol component (91%), while 4α- and 4,4-dimethyl sterols, both mono- and diunsaturated, constituted (as a whole) a relatively minor group of constituents (Table VI). The reason for this unusual distribution was not apparent, but is discussed by Ramsey et al. (1972) with respect to analogous esterification of sterols by liver and a possible role in regulating sterol metabolism in developing brain.

Ramsey et al. (1971a,b,c) have established that developing brain can synthesize steryl esters in situ. In fetal and developing human brain the major fatty acids of the steryl ester fraction were shown to be oleic, palmitic, palmitoleic, and arachidonic (Alling and Svennerholm, 1969). The latter investigators and Eto and Suzuki (1971a) have suggested that steryl esters in the CNS may play a role in the metabolism of phosphoglyceride fatty acids. Further investigation of the significance of steryl esters in the CNS is indicated.

Table VI

DISTRIBUTION OF STEROLS IN THE FREE STEROL FRACTION FROM DEVELOPING RAT BRAIN[a]

Compound	Sterol/gm wet wt of brain (μg)	Distribution of sterol in free sterol fraction (%)
Cholesterol	12,700	91.4
Desmosterol	1,120	8.1
4α-Methyl-5α-cholest-8-en-3β-ol	8.93	0.064
4α-Methyl-5α-cholest-7-en-3β-ol	0.75	0.005
4α-Methyl-5α-cholesta-8,24-dien-3β-ol	4.67	0.034
4α-Methyl-5α-cholesta-7,24-dien-3β-ol	1.35	0.010
4,4-Dimethyl-5α-cholest-8-en-3β-ol	4.48	0.032
4,4-Dimethyl-5α-cholesta-8,24-dien-3β-ol	26.7	0.19
Lanosterol	17.3	0.12

[a] Taken from Ramsey et al. (1972).

Table VII

GAS CHROMATOGRAPHIC RETENTION INDEXES OF UNKNOWN ISOPRENOID HYDROCARBONS[a]

Compound	TLC Region:	GLC Phase SE-30				GLC Phase SE-52				GLC Phase OV-17			
		1	2	3	4	1	2	3	4	1	2	3	4
I		2800		2731	2687	2835		2788	2692	2964		2926	2989
II			2801	2770	2818		2844	2830	2839		2968	2993	3031
III				2820	2848			2865	2870			3031	3061
IV				2875				2896	2957			3065	3095

[a] Taken from Ramsey (1971).

Table VIII

GAS CHROMATOGRAPHIC RETENTION INDEXES OF UNKNOWN BRAIN ISOPRENOID HYDROCARBONS AFTER HYDROGENATION[a]

Compound	TLC Region:	GLC Phase SE-30				GLC Phase SE-52				GLC Phase OV-17			
		1	2	3	4	1	2	3	4	1	2	3	4
I		2668	2667	2690	2733	2669	2650	2738	2788	2628	2685	2734	2939
II			2742	2726	2793		2727	2785	2870		2745	2793	2976
III				2759	2812			2826	2900			2884	3016
IV				2804	2886				2957				3050

[a] Taken from Ramsey (1971).

E. TRACE ISOPRENOID COMPOUNDS IN BRAIN

The biosynthesis by brain, of isoprene hydrocarbons, in addition to squalene, was first indicated by Kelley *et al.* (1969). These hydrocarbons formed *in vitro* on incubation of adult brain cell-free preparations with MVA-2-14C, were examined in more detail by Ramsey (1971) and were found to have longer retention times than squalene on several GLC phases (Table VII), and upon hydrogenation, longer retention times than squalane (Table VIII). They could not be detected in nonsaponifiable fractions from adult brain subcellular fractions or liver homogenates incubated with MVA-2-14C. Squalene-like hydrocarbons have also been detected in bovine brain. The retention times of these hydrocarbons and their reduction products (Pt + H_2) were shorter than those of squalene and squalane respectively (Ramsey *et al.*, 1971f). The opposite was found for the unidentified rat brain hydrocarbons. Mass spectra of the naturally occurring hydrocarbons from bovine brain and their reduction products are shown in Fig. 10. The only formula for the hydrocarbon(s) consistent with the data was a hydrocarbon similar but not identical to that obtained from the presqualene pyrophosphate of Rilling (1966). Edmond *et al.* (1971) have substantiated the structure originally proposed by Rilling. A cyclopropane ring in a squalene-like hydrocarbon containing 5 double bonds was strongly indicated. The specific structures of these squalene-like hydrocarbons in rat and bovine brain require more detailed investigation, since they may have a pertinent bearing on the biosynthetic pathway of sterol formation in the CNS.

F. POSSIBLE CHOLESTEROL DEGRADATION BY CNS TISSUE

The "bile" acid 3α-hydroxy-5β-cholanoic acid (lithocholic acid) has been detected in trace amounts in experimental allergic encephalomye-litis-(EAE)-afflicted guinea pig brain (Naqvi *et al.*, 1969) and in multiple sclerosis brain tissue (Naqvi *et al.*, 1970a). Several monohydroxy bile acids were found to be demyelinating agents after intracerebral injection (Naqvi *et al.*, 1970b). When the same investigators injected labeled lithocholic acid intracerebrally, most of the compound was rapidly expelled from the brain, yet a small quantity of more polar and less polar metabolites were retained for several days. Naqvi and Nicholas (1970) have demonstrated the reduction of 3-keto-5β-cholanoic acid to lithocholic acid by guinea pig brain *in vitro*, and Martin and Nicholas (1972) have shown that the reverse process, the oxidation of lithocholic acid to 3-keto-5β-cholanoic acid can be accomplished by adult rat brain *in vitro*, and in addition have demonstrated that the same preparations

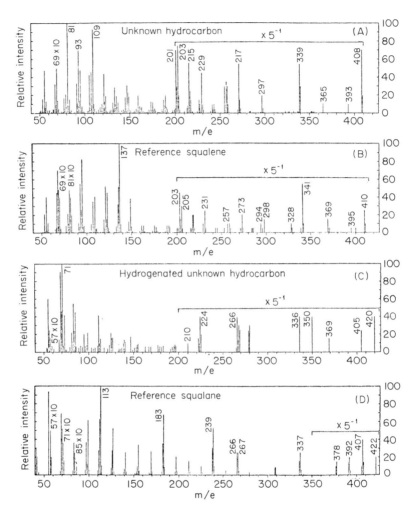

FIG. 10. Mass spectra of naturally occurring hydrocarbons from bovine brain and their reduction products. Mass spectra of (A) major unknown isoprenoid hydrocarbon a; (B) squalene standard; (C) hydrogenated unknown isoprenoid hydrocarbons, b; and (D) squalane standard. Spectra were obtained with an LKB model 9000 GLC-mass spectrograph with a 1% (w/w) SE-30 on Gas Chrom Q column at 200°C and at an ionizing voltage of 70 eV. Taken from Ramsey *et al.* (1971f).

can convert labeled lithocholic acid in 1–6% yield to the dihydroxysteroid 3α,6β-dihydroxy-5β-cholanoic acid.

Since cholesterol does undergo some degree of turnover in the brain (Davison, 1970a), and since Nicholas (1965) has suggested that acidic steroids might be produced in the brain by such turnover, the origin of the bile acids detected in EAE and multiple sclerosis brains raises the question as to the source of the acids. Since lithocholic acid is normally barely detectable in the bloodstream (Carey and Hanson, 1969) it seems highly possible that cholesterol degradation by brain may produce the acids, perhaps to a greater extent in the diseased organ, with consequent demyelination. Several investigations have produced evidence for the presence in brain of neutral cholesterol metabolites which could be precursors of such acidic compounds. For example, 24-hydroxycholesterol (cerebrosterol) has been detected in human brain (DiFrisco *et al.*, 1953; Ercoli and de Ruggieri, 1953; Ercoli *et al.*, 1953a; van Lier and Smith, 1969), and in horse brain (DiFrisco *et al.*, 1953; Ercoli *et al.*, 1953b; Fieser *et al.*, 1958) but was found to be absent from bovine brain (van Lier and Smith, 1971). On the other hand, 26-hydroxycholesterol has been identified in bovine brain (van Lier and Smith, 1971) but was found to be absent from human brain (van Lier and Smith, 1967). Both 7α- and 7β-hydroxycholesterol have been detected in human brain (van Lier and Smith, 1969). This observation [see van Lier and Smith (1969) for additional sources] is particularly interesting in view of the critical position of 7α-hydroxycholesterol in the biosynthesis of bile acids by liver. That brain microsomes can biosynthesize 24-hydroxycholesterol from cholesterol has been demonstrated by Dhar and Smith (1971) in about 0.5% yield.

All of these observations make it seem urgent that a thorough study of this aspect of brain cholesterol metabolism be given extensive investigation, both in the normal and in the diseased organ.

G. Other Trace Brain Lipids

Two different groups of investigators have indicated the presence of fluorescent lipids in brain. Geiger and Bampton (1966) have reported the presence of a fluorescent compound in the brains of rabbits killed with diisopropyl fluorophosphate. The structure of this compound as suggested by chemical synthesis and apparent identity with the brain compound is as shown in Fig. 10. The lipid thus appears to be a fatty acid ester of the *enol* form of acetopiperone. Lunt and Rowe (1969) have

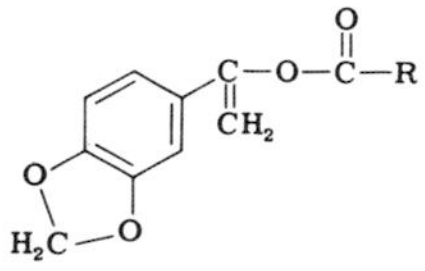

Fig. 11. Structure of diisopropyl fluorophosphate.

reported the presence of three fluorescent lipids in mouse brain slices incubated at 0°, and possibly something similar from ox brain stored at 0°. The compounds from the two different groups appeared to have a little in common from a structural standpoint. Vidrine *et al.* (1971) have not been able to verify the structure assigned to one fluorescent product described by Geiger and Bampton. Clearly these fluorescent materials should be subjected to more thorough investigation. Richter and Dannenberg (1969) have studied some neutral trace lipids in cattle and rabbit brain. A carotenoid, α-tocopherol, ubiquinone-10, lanosterol, dihydrolanosterol, several fatty acid and methyl esters, and dioctylphthalate (the latter, in our judgment, extremely puzzling) were detected. Several of these would appear to arise from the diet, but the need for further proof seems indicated.

VII. Myelin and Other Subcellular Fractions of the Brain

The lipid composition of myelin has recently been reviewed by Smith (1967) and Mokrasch (1969). Other brain subcellular fractions have also been discussed with reference to lipid composition by Dickerson (1968). We will therefore restrict this discussion to the *metabolism* of the lipids of brain subcellular fractions.

Several papers by Smith have demonstrated that the individual lipid components of myelin have different turnover rates. This phenomenon was demonstrated both *in vitro* (Smith, 1969a) and *in vivo* (Smith, 1968). In the intact brain the half-lives of phosphatidyl inositol and phosphatidyl choline were found to be much shorter than those of the other lipids (Table IX). In contrast, cerebroside and sulfatide in the myelin matrix had extremely long half-lives. As can be seen from Table IX the same general pattern of half-lives is also apparent in the crude mitochondrial fractions. These *in vivo* studies were conducted on adult animals, but the same type of lipid turnover was apparent in myelin of developing brains as well (Smith, 1969b). In a related study on myelin, Ansell and Spanner (1968c) showed that intracerebrally administered ^{14}C-ethanolamine yielded phosphatidyl ethanolamine undergoing significant turnover within a 9-week period. The turnover of the corresponding plasmologens was much slower.

In studying lecithin synthesis, Abdel-Latif, Smith, and Dasher (1970) utilized injected ^{14}C-choline and brief time periods to demonstrate an increase in specific activity of the lecithin in the synaptosomes. At the same time a decrease in the specific activity of microsomal lecithin was

Table IX

Estimated Half-Lives of Lipids and Proteins from Two
Subcellular Fractions[a]

Component	Myelin fraction (half-life)	Crude mito-chondrial fraction (half-life in days)
Total lipid	>6 months	17
Phosphatidyl inositol	18 days	11
Lecithin	41 days	12
Protein	35 days	21
Phosphatidyl serine	4 months	17
Ethanolamine phosphatide	>6 months	21
Sphingomyelin	>8 months	33
Cholesterol	>8 months	39
Cardiolipin	—	40
Cerebroside	>1 year	59
Sulfatide	>1 year	—

[a] Modified from Smith (1968).

observed. Interestingly enough, utilization of ^{14}C-choline, ^{14}C-glycerol, or ^{32}P-orthophosphate yielded three different half-lives for the lecithin labeled in both the microsomes and synaptosomes (Abdel-Latif and Smith, 1970). The half-lives determined were 11.7 days, 2.9 days, and 18.6 days, respectively. Although these different half-lives appear to be incongruous, such factors as endogenous pool size differences of the precursors and the ability of the precursors to pass through the blood-brain barrier may account for the different rates of turnover.

Lunt and Lapetina (1970a) have shown that isolated synaptosomes are also able to incorporate labeled choline and glycerol into phospholipids. It was interpreted that the labeling of these phospholipids did not necessarily represent *de novo* synthesis of phospholipids, but more likely an interchange of the moieties of the phospholipid molecule with the labeled material. The ability of synaptosomes to synthesize phospholipids (in part) is also reinforced by the finding that many of the enzymes related to phosphatidyl inositol biosynthesis can be found in synaptosomes (Harwood and Hawthorne, 1969).

A number of studies have now been reported on the lipid-synthesizing ability of brain microsomes. Aeberhard and Menkes (1968) have shown that microsomes as well as mitochondria are primarily responsible for fatty acid synthesis in brain; Ramsey *et al.* (1971a,b) have demonstrated that brain microsomes synthesize sterol; and several papers by Radin's group (Braun *et al.*, 1970; Morell and Radin, 1970; Morell *et al.*, 1970) have adequately shown the ability of brain microsomes to synthesize ceramide and cerebrosides.

Of considerable interest with respect to subcellular fractions and metabolism of the lipids therein, has been discovery of a myelin-like fraction (Banik and Davison, 1969). It has been suggested that this myelin-like fraction is a stage in the formation of compact myelin from glial plasma membrane (Agrawal *et al.*, 1970). This fraction is notably deficient in cerebroside when compared to mature myelin. These studies indicated that when the lipids of the myelin-like fraction were labeled with ^{14}C-acetate a precursor-product relationship could not be shown between the myelin-like and myelin fractions (Agrawal *et al.*, 1970). When these labeled lipids of the myelin and myelin-like fractions were further fractionated, the comparable lipid fractions in the two fractions contained similar amounts of label with the exception of the phosphatidyl choline fraction, which had a higher degree of labeling in the myelin-like fraction. What role this fraction plays in the construction of the myelin sheath has yet to be determined, but it definitely is a distinct entity present mainly during the period of most active myelin formation.

VIII. Effect of Undernutrition on Lipids of the Brain

It seems reasonably well established that, with some exceptions, the fully mature brain is refractive to marked changes in the diet, including malnutrition. The neonatal and developing brain, however, are now known to be highly susceptible to the nutrition of the mother and dietary restrictions during the period of active myelination. Dobbing, in three comprehensive reviews (Dobbing, 1968a,b,c) has summarized his own observations leading to the view that the brain "growth spurt" represents a vulnerable period in the development of both animals and humans. The reader is also referred to reviews by Davies (1969), Granoff and Howard (1969), and in *Nutrition Reviews* (1970). Two manuscripts of general interest were not available to us in translation (Krop and Winick, 1969; Winick and Rosso, 1969).

It is now amply substantiated that irreversible changes in brain lipids occur in animals deprived of proper nutrition neonatally or during the period of active myelination. Some recent observations are summarized in Table X. Other deficiencies, such as arrest of postnatal glial cell migration (Bass and Netsky, 1969), were also noted but cannot be evaluated here. It appears certain that the "earlier the malnutrition, the more severe the effect and the less the chance of recovery" (Bass *et al.*, 1970a). In general the effects appear to be irreversible, with some occasional con-

Table X

Changes in Brain Lipids in Nutritionally Deprived Animals

Nutritional deprivation	Age examined	Decreased lipid (Compared to normal)	Comments	Reference
Rats, neonatal	50 days	Cerebrosides, cholesterol, gangliosides	Histological observations	Bass and Netsky (1969)
Neonatal, hypothyroid	—	Total lipid, cerebrosides, cholesterol, gangliosides	Histological observations	Bass and Netsky (1969)
Rats, 21 days postnatal	Up to 50 days	Total lipids, gangliosides, sialic acid	Developing cerebrum only	Bass et al. (1970a)
Rats, neonatal, postweanling	4 weeks	Reduced ^{35}S into lipid, cerebrosides, cholesterol	—	Freedman (1970)
Rats, 5 to 60 days	—	Cholesterol, phospholipid, cerebroside	Cerebellum affected most severely	Culley and Lineberger (1968)
Mice, 2 to 16 days	Up to 9 months	Cholesterol (slightly)	—	Howard and Granoff (1968)
Rats, postnatal	Up to 9 weeks	Cholesterol (irreversibly depressed)	—	Guthrie and Brown (1968)
Rats, suckling	Adult	Reduced total lipid	—	Geison and Waisman (1970b)
Rats, postnatal	Up to 50 days	Total lipids, cerebrosides, cholesterol, proteolipid (of myelin)	Histological observations on cerebrum	Bass et al. (1970b)

tradictory reports (Chase *et al.*, 1971; Freedman, 1970). The relationship between the lipid deficiencies produced and the learning response is not as yet clear (Howard and Granoff, 1968; see also Freedman, 1970).

Bass *et al.* (1970b) have suggested that the severe abnormal accumulation of total cholesterol shown by their experiments (histological observations) in cortex and white matter of adult rats subjected to neonatal malnutrition "may result from inefficient deesterification, incomplete removal of sterol precursors, or decreased formation of free cholesterol." It would be of value to follow up these studies to pursue these suggestions further. Bass *et al.* postulate that this lipid abnormality and others are a consequence of decreased myelin formation resulting from damage to glial cell precursors which fail to undergo differentiation. Decreases in lipids of the cerebellum (as opposed to other gross sections of brain) in undernourished rats have been briefly reported by Dickerson and Jarvis (1970).

Considering the extent of malnutrition throughout the world, it appears to the authors of this chapter that if it is possible to relate to the human the above observations on malnutrition and brain development in the animal, one of the most significant developments in medical biochemistry of this century will have been accomplished. Some implications of this have been given in the reviews by Dobbing (1968a) and Davison (1968a) and more recently by Fishman *et al.* (1969) and Winick (1970a,b).

Dobbing *et al.* (1970) have also reported that the vulnerable period hypothesis (Dobbing, 1968b) also applies to susceptibility of this period to X-irradiation. Their data show that the growth of the brain is substantially and permanently affected by a simple exposure to such treatment. A large and disproportionate reduction in cerebellar weight was reminiscent of the same effect previously noticed in undernutrition (Culley and Lineberger, 1968; Chase *et al.*, 1969).

No clear-cut biochemical causative factors for mental deficiencies accompanying inborn errors of metabolism have as yet been defined. This applies especially to phenylketonuria. Geison and Waisman (1970a) have reported that after 3 weeks of age only moderate effects on accumulation of cerebral lipids are produced by excess dietary L-phenylalanine fed at almost toxic levels. However, Shah *et al.* (1968) have indicated that incorporation of mevalonic acid into cholesterol of brain homogenates from young rats treated with L-phenylalanine is inhibited, suggesting that earlier stages of cerebral maturation may be more susceptible to high levels of the amino acid with respect to effects on brain lipids. Subcutaneous injection of phenylalanine into newborn rats produced reduction of total brain cholesterol, cerebroside, and sulfatide (Chase and

O'Brien, 1970). Clearly the dietary relationship of L-phenylalanine to effects on brain lipids needs more evaluation. Vitamins and fatty acid deficiency effects on brain lipids have been subjected to investigation for the period covered in this chapter. Borgman and Haselden (1969) in subjecting rabbits to a vitamin E-deficient diet found that no significant alterations occurred in brain lipids providing the diet included 10% oleic acid. C. Galli *et al.* (1970) have reviewed the effects of dietary fatty acid deficiency on brain lipids and have presented data showing that an essential fatty acid deficient diet, when started early enough and prolonged, induces a decrease in brain total lipid and phospholipid concentration. An unexplained sex difference was noted, male rats reacting to the deficiency more than females.

Of interest to this general dietary problem are the data of Turchetto and Borri (1969), who fed weanling male rats a diet high in hydrogenated cocoanut oil (containing predominantly saturated fatty acids), olive oil (monounsaturated fatty acids), and peanut oil (polyunsaturated fatty acids), respectively. Apparently the rat brain requires a source of unsaturated fatty acids as the animal matures, since the hydrogenated cocoanut diet induced a progressive decrease in brain essential fatty acids (EFA), olive oil induced a significant fall in EFA up to 180 days, with recovery during the following period, while the olive oil diet induced no significant changes. On the other hand Hansen and Clausen (1969) fed young rats diets containing stearic, oleic, linoleic, and lauric acids respectively and found a direct relationship to the fat component of the diet only in the phosphatidylcholine fraction of the animals fed on stearic and oleic acids, respectively. The brain content on the whole of palmitic, stearic, and oleic acid showed a pattern related to age rather than diet. The slow response of brain to essential fatty acid dietary changes has been noted by Walker (1968).

An interesting effect of early dietary choline deficiency on brain growth of chicks has been noted by Jose *et al.* (1970). When newly hatched chicks were fed a choline-deficient diet for 8 to 10 days an inhibition of protein and an accumulation of proteolipid in the brains was found (previously observed in rats also). Since proteolipid reflects myelin content it was concluded that myelination was inhibited by the choline deficiency.

Finally, attention is called to the observations of Szepsenwol (1969), who in feeding mice on Purina mice chow supplemented with small amounts of various lipids (e.g., lecithin, cholesterol) found brain nerve cell tumor production in the frontal lobe, in reasonably high incidence. No good explanation for development of the tumors on this dietary regime were given.

IX. Lipids and the Developing Brain

Changes in the quantity and composition of brain lipids during maturation continue to draw interest, despite previous thorough studies (see Paoletti and Davison, 1971). Dalal and Einstein (1969) have studied the changes in various lipid classes of whole brain of rabbits varying in age from 1 to 170 days. The data obtained are shown in Table XI. Analogous data were obtained on myelin from ages to 170 days. These are shown in Table XII. The study also compares lipid protein of brain and cord myelin from several species of animals and gives information on central nervous system developmental changes that has not been presented elsewhere. This and the manuscripts by Horrocks (1968) and Eng and Noble (1968) again emphasize the difference between immature and mature myelin composition.

In addition, Barlow (1969) studied the development of sheep fetus myelin by morphological and histological methods. Differentiation of neurons and glia are responsible for the marked changes in lipid content that accompany early growth of the central nervous system. An attempt was made to describe how lipids are transported to the myelin sheath

Table XI

LIPIDS IN DEVELOPING RABBIT BRAIN[a]

	Percentage (on dry weight)						
Days after birth	Sph + IP[b]	SGP[c]	CGP[d]	EGP[e]	Cho-lesterol	Cerebro-sides	Total protein
1	2.47	3.67	15.37	8.49	0.51	0.90	56.37
5	2.50	3.40	15.03	8.02	1.05	2.30	56.43
7	3.30	3.30	15.00	8.40	2.00	2.77	55.56
9	3.50	3.42	15.48	8.50	5.90	8.40	56.31
12	3.40	3.30	14.00	7.30	5.60	7.66	55.37
14	3.46	3.36	14.38	7.00	7.20	9.00	51.37
18	3.70	3.20	14.00	6.90	8.40	9.60	48.44
30	4.05	3.06	12.50	6.49	11.80	11.80	42.25
60	4.00	2.95	12.00	6.78	12.84	13.40	43.44
90	4.40	3.00	11.80	7.10	15.80	15.60	33.69
120	4.55	2.80	10.70	6.55	14.80	14.17	40.56
170	4.80	2.60	8.80	6.40	15.56	15.17	43.62

[a] From Dalal and Einstein (1969).
[b] Sph + IP, sphingomyelin + inositol phosphatides.
[c] SGP, serine glycerophosphatide.
[d] CGP, choline glycerophosphatide.
[e] EGP, ethanolamine glycerophosphatide.

Table XII

COMPOSITION OF CORD MYELIN DURING DEVELOPMENT[a]

Days after birth	Total P-lipids	Sph + IP[b]	SGP[c]	CGP[d]	EGP[e]	Cho-lesterol	Cerebro-sides
			Molar percentage of total lipids				
5	57.14	6.19	3.65	27.60	19.70	3.90	1.07
8	56.15	6.29	3.70	26.56	19.60	8.00	3.06
9	60.84	6.62	3.87	30.30	20.05	11.60	6.93
14	55.14	6.51	3.73	25.97	18.93	20.00	7.31
170	42.23	10.60	6.20	13.10	12.33	32.90	24.00

[a] Taken from Dalal and Einstein (1969).
[b] Sph + IP, sphingomyelin + inositol phosphatides.
[c] SGP, serine glycerophosphatide.
[d] CGP, choline glycerophosphatide.
[e] EGP, ethanolamine glycerophosphatide.

during development of the latter. The embryonic development of beef brain, studied by Hooghwinkel and de Rooij (1968) has provided additional data showing lipid changes in developing brain.

Hauser (1968) has presented data for cerebroside sulfatide levels in rat brain from ages 8 days to adult (>250 days old). In animals less than 1 week old only very low levels of both lipids were detected. An unvarying ratio of the two lipids during growth was interpreted to indicate that the accumulation rate of sulfatides found in adult rat brain is very similar to that for the cerebrosides of myelin, although little or no sulfatide is found in myelin itself.

Changes in the fatty acid content of sphingolipids and the ratio of C_{18}-sphingosine and C_{18}-dihydrosphingosine were recently studied by Kawamura and Taketomi (1969) in developing rabbit brain. Dihydrosphingosine of cerebroside showed a predominant increase at ages 10 to 22 days, whereas in sphingomyelin and ganglioside the levels were lower at all ages. C_{20}-Sphingosine was present in ganglioside (in small amounts), and was already present in fetal brain, steadily increasing in amount with age. Other significant changes were noted. In short, the long-chain base compositions and fatty acids of all three sphingolipids differed from each other during growth. Sphingosine bases of cerebrosides, sulfatides, and sphingomyelin from selected areas of human brain ranging in age from premature infants to 59 years were examined by Isaacson and Moscatelli (1970). In immature sphingolipids as much as 10% of the total was 18:dihydrosphingosine; in adults 95% of the sphingosine was 18:sphingosine. 20:Sphingosine was tentatively identified in fetal, infant, and adult brain, decreasing in quantity in the older tissues. Thus there is general agreement between these observations and those presented by Kawamuri and Taketomi (1969).

Sheltawy and Dawson (1969) have presented a detailed study of changes in polyphosphoinositides during growth of the rat and guinea pig cerebral hemispheres. The maximum increase in concentration of both tri- and diphosphoinositide occurred during the period of myelination, but in the rat some of the compounds were present before significant myelination occurred. However, rapid turnover of triphosphoinositide in adult rat brains following treatment of the brains with ^{32}P indicated that the rapid turnover is independent of myelin deposition. Attention was called (again) to the rapid changes in polyphosphoinositides accompanying postmortem conditions.

Fatty acids in lecithin of developing rat, guinea pig, and rabbit brain subcellular fractions were studied by Skrbic and Cumings (1970). The lecithins were found to consist of at least two groups with dissimilar fatty acid profiles, with the acids from myelin showing little variation with age in any species examined. The data of Skrbic and Cumings indicate a progressively greater contribution of myelin lecithin to the total cerebral lecithins with increasing age (see also Svennerholm, 1968, for human brain analyses).

Using injected p-chlorophenyl alanine and phenylalanine to induce experimental phenylketonuria in rats, Foote and Tao (1968) studied changes in fatty acid content of cerebral lipids in developing rats (ages 12 to 31 days). Some variations in brain lipids were encountered, especially a lowered level of oleic acid. This retardation was compatible with the abnormally low 18:1/18:0 ratio of brains from phenylketonuric humans.

Radin et al. (1969) have studied changes in the activity of four enzymes (acid hydrolases) in brains from rats, ages 4 days to 320 days. The enzymes, lactosylceramide galactosidase, galactosylphenol galactosidase, glucosylceramide glucosidase, and sphingomyelin phosphocholine hydrolase are presumably lysosomal in origin. The activity of the first two enzymes rose with age until about 24 days, then declined somewhat. The other enzymes steadily declined in activity with increasing age. The authors attempt to interpret the data in terms of the hypothesis that lysosomal enzymes function in normal turnover of the lipids they influence. Roukema et al. (1970) have found that the activity of the enzymes sialidase, β-galactosidase, and β-galactosaminidase increase markedly in rat brain between the ages of 4 and 18 days. The biosynthetic enzyme, CMP-N-acetylneuraminic acid synthetase, however, increased rapidly to day 6, then declined gradually. Gangliosides and

Table XIII

Lipid or lipid class	Enzyme(s)	Reference
Phospholipids, general	α-Glycerophosphate dehydrogenase	Tipton and Dawson (1968)
	Diglyceride kinase	Lapetina and Hawthorne (1971)
	Phospholipase A	Webster (1970)
	Phospholipase A	Cooper and Webster (1970)
	Phospholipase A₁	Gatt (1968)
	Phosphatide acyl-hydrolase	Webster and Cooper (1968)
Digalactose diglyceride	α-Galactosidase	Rao and Pieringer (1970)
Plasmalogen	Plasmalogenase	Ansell and Spanner (1968a)
Sulfates	Arylsulfatase	Clendenon and Allen (1970)
Cerebrosides (see also sphingolipids, general)	Cerebroside galactosidase	Bowen and Radin (1969a,b)
	Cerebroside galactosidase	Bowen and Radin (1968a)
Phosphoinositides	CDP-Diglyceride inositol phosphatidate transferase	Salway *et al.* (1968)
	Phosphatidylinositol kinase	
	Diphosphoinositide kinase	
	Triphosphoinositide phosphomonoesterase	
	Diphosphoinositide kinase	
Ceramides (see also sphingolipids, general)	Ceramidase	Kai *et al.* (1968)
	Ceramidase	Gatt and Yavin (1969)
Sphingolipids, general	Neuraminidase	Yavin and Gatt (1969)
	β-N-Acetylhexosaminidase	Gatt (1970b)
	β-Galactosidase	Gatt (1970b)
	β-Glucosidase	Gatt (1970b)
	Ceramidase	Gatt (1970b)
	NADP-Dependent-3-oxosphanganine reductase	Stoffel *et al.* (1968)
	Ceramidase	Gatt (1969)
	Sphingomyelinase	Gatt (1969)
	β-Glucosidase	Gatt (1969)
	β-Galactosidase	Gatt (1969)
	β-N-Acetylhexosaminidase	Gatt (1969)
	Sialidase	Gatt (1969)
	Sphingomyelin synthetase	Michael (1971)
Gangliosides	Sialidase	Schengrund and Rosenberg (1970)

sialoglycoproteins increased in amounts markedly also, as for the three enzymes first mentioned.

Finally, in a manuscript not available in translation (Prokhorova *et al.*, 1970), the metabolism of phospholipids in immature and adult rats was studied, using ^{32}P and ^{14}C. A role of di- and triphosphoinositides in nerve impulse conduction was suggested. It is not possible to determine from the abstract how much activity in immature brain differs from that in adult brain.

X. Enzymes of Significance to Brain Lipids

Considerable effort has been given during the period covered by this chapter to investigation of the properties (and activity) of the many enzymes responsible for brain lipid biosynthesis and degradation. A detailed discussion or complete survey is beyond the scope of our review. In order to acquaint the reader with some of the progress made in this area, Table XIII has been prepared. Where it was felt particularly pertinent, reference to a specific enzyme has been included in other sections of this review. The investigations cited have been largely directed toward specific localization within the brain and subcellular localization.

XI. Proteolipids

Proteolipids are protein-lipid "combinations" which are unusual in that they are insoluble in water but are soluble in 2:1 chloroform-methanol. They occur in many tissues but all are particularly high in concentration in brain. The review of Eichberg *et al.* (1969) is particularly informative and has described most of the pertinent observations on these substances prior to 1968.

The following examples will illustrate recent work performed on these important constituents of the central nervous tissue. Soto *et al.* (1969) subjected total lipid extracts of cat brain gray and white matter to chromatography on Sephadex LH-20 to obtain what appeared to be two different proteolipids from the two types of tissue. One of these is apparently identical to a proteolipid present in nerve ending membranes and capable of binding ^{14}C-dimethyltubocurarine (De Robertis *et al.*, 1968). Both preparations contained lipid phosphorus in small amounts which were believed to be constituents of the proteolipid molecules themselves.

Manukyan (1969) studied the lipid components of brain proteolipids and found mono- and diphosphoinositide, sphingomyelin, lecithin, serine phosphatide, ethanolamine phosphatide, polyglycerophosphatides, and phosphatidic acid bound electrostatically to the protein moiety. Possibly these are the components indicated in the preparations of Soto *et al.*

Proteolipid protein having a molecular weight of approximately 200,000 was obtained in the studies of Komai *et al.* (1970) from bovine brain white matter. Possibly the same material was studied by Sherman and Folch-Pi (1970). The protein moiety could not be completely delipidated. Studies by optical rotatory dispersion and circular dichroism in various solvents indicated that the protein exhibited a helix content of 60–70% or 90% depending upon the solvent used for the determination. No random coil was observed in the studies.

XII. Lipids in Cell-Enriched Fractions of the Brain

The investigation of lipids in isolated neuronal and glial preparations is still at an infantile stage of development. Until very recently the major way of approaching the problem was to isolate individual cells or to investigate neuron-rich and glial-rich areas of the brain. A review, which includes in its text differences in lipid content of gray (neuron-rich) and white (glial-rich) matter, has recently appeared (Eichberg *et al.*, 1969).

The first bulk isolation of neuron-enriched and glial-enriched fractions from whole brain was reported by Rose (1965). Since then many reports of modified isolation techniques have been documented and undoubtedly more refined methods will be developed. It is not within the scope of this review to report on these isolation techniques.

The total lipids of glial cells have been reported to be considerably higher (5.6 times) than that of neuronal cells, even though the distribution of lipids within the two cells is remarkably similar (Freysz *et al.*, 1968; Norton and Poduslo, 1971). Using bovine white matter to isolate glial cells, Fewster and Mead found the major lipid components of the latter to be cholesterol, ethanolamine glycerophosphatides, cerebroside, and serine glycerophosphatides. Sphingomyelin, cerebroside sulfate, and inositol glycerophosphatides were present in lower proportions. No gangliosides were found in the glial cell preparations (Fewster and Mead, 1968). The presence of ganglioside in glial cells (astrocytes as identified by the authors) has been reported (Norton and Poduslo, 1971). These authors reported that this was due to the large proportions of cell membranes isolated in their glial cells when compared to their

Table XIV

Lipid Composition of Isolated Cell Types From Various Animals[a]

Lipid	Pig nerve cell perikarya[b]	Developing rat neuron[c]	Developing rat astrocyte[c]	Bovine glial cell[d]
Cholesterol	9.0	10.6	14.0	30.5
Total phospholipids	86.7	72.3	70.9	42.6
Phosphatidyl ethanolamine	28.3	18.2	20.1	17.0
Phosphatidyl serine	8.7	3.9	5.2	10.3
Phosphatidyl choline	46.7	39.9	36.3	14.0
Phosphatidyl inositol	—	4.9	3.5	1.3
Sphingomyelin	1.9	3.2	3.7	5.6
Plasmalogens	—	7.0	7.6	—
Galactolipid	—	2.1	1.8	—
Cerebroside	—	—	—	10.4
Cerebroside sulfate	—	—	—	4.3

[a] Expressed as weight percent of total lipid.
[b] Average of 3 preparations (Tamai et al., 1971).
[c] Average of 6 preparations (Norton and Poduslo, 1971).
[d] Average of 2 preparations (Fewster and Mead, 1968).

neuronal cells. These researchers found a completely different lipid distribution in the developing rat brain glial cells (Table XIV) from that reported by Fewster and Mead for bovine glial cells. In a report on neurons isolated from pig brain stems the chemical composition of neuronal cell perikarya is in agreement with the findings of Norton and Poduslo (Tamai et al., 1971; Norton and Poduslo, 1971). This report also contained the fatty acid composition of the phospholipids of the neuronal cell perikarya (Table XV).

The incorporation of labeled precursors into neuronal and glial cells has been examined for phospholipids and sterols (Freysz et al., 1969; Jones et al., 1971). Using $^{32}P_i$ incorporation in vivo Freysz et al. found that neuronal phospholipids exhibited a greater rate of turnover than glial phospholipids. In both cell types inositol and choline plasmalogen had the fastest rate of turnover, diphosphatidylglycerol had the lowest turnover, and phosphatidylcholine, phosphatidylethanolamine, and phosphatidylserine had intermediate turnover rates. Turnover in neuron sphingomyelin was higher than in glial cells (Freysz et al., 1969). Using 2-^{14}C-mevalonic acid as the lipid precursor, Jones et al. (1971) found that the glial-enriched fractions in vitro formed considerably more sterol than the neuronal-enriched fractions. Only when both fractions of cells were mixed, were sterol esters produced.

Table XV

FATTY ACID COMPOSITION OF THE TOTAL PHOSPHOLIPIDS AND OF INDIVIDUAL
PHOSPHOLIPID FRACTION OF NERVE CELL PERIKARYA[a]

Number of C atoms and double bonds	Fatty acids (wt %)			
		Nerve cell perikarya		
	Total	PE	PS	PC
16:0	22.9	8.9	3.2	38.2
16:1	0.9	0.3	0.6	0.7
18:0	26.1	40.5	53.1	16.6
18:1	25.4	8.6	6.7	31.4
18:2	1.0	0.3	0.4	0.5
20:1	2.8	1.6	0.3	4.6
20:4	7.8	10.9	24.8	3.3
22:4	2.0	4.7	1.6	0.7
22:6	9.5	22.9	7.4	2.6
Unidentified	1.6	1.3	1.9	1.4
Saturated	49.0 (53.1)[b]	49.4	56.3	54.8
Unsaturated	49.4 (45.4)[b]	49.3	41.8	43.8

[a] Table taken from Tamai *et al.* (1971).

[b] Values in parentheses indicate the calculated percentages of saturated or unsaturated fatty acid of the total phospholipid from those of the individual phospholipid fraction.

XIII. Metabolic Diseases of the Brain

Many excellent reviews on changes in brain lipid content in various diseases have appeared (Aronson and Volk, 1967; Schettler and Kahlke, 1967; Zeman, 1969; Raine, 1969; Brady, 1969; Kaufman *et al.*, 1969; O'Brien, 1969; Rapport, 1970; Davison, 1970b; Brady, 1970a,b,c,d; Jatzkewitz *et al.*, 1970; Saifer and Wishnow, 1970; Cumings, 1970; O'Brien *et al.*, 1971a; Bernsohn and Grossman, 1971; Yatsu, 1971; O'Brien, 1971). Obviously a complete review of all clinical and biochemical changes is beyond the scope of this review. Consequently many erudite reports on the disease states had to be omitted. For this section the main lipid and enzymatic defects are covered to illustrate the established biochemical work in this important area of biomedical research.

This section is divided into four main parts: Gangliosides, Neutral Lipids, Glycolipids, and Phospholipids. Each of these four main lipid classifications has then been divided into two sections consisting of

Table XVI

Major Lipid and Enzymatic Defects of the Central Nervous System

Disease	Lipid abnormality	Enzymatic defect	Reference
Generalized gangliosidosis and juvenile G_{M1} gangliosidosis	G_{M1}	β-Galactosidase	Ledeen et al. (1968); O'Brien et al. (1965)
Tay-Sachs	G_{M2}	Absence of hexosaminidase A	Klenk (1942); Svennerholm (1962); Okada and O'Brien (1968)
Sandhoff's	G_{M2}	Deficiency in both hexosaminidase A and B	Sandhoff et al. (1968); Sandhoff et al. (1968)
Juvenile G_{M2} gangliosidosis	G_{M2}	Hexosaminidase A partially deficient	K. Suzuki et al. (1969); Y. Suzuki et al. (1970)
G_{M3} Gangliosidosis	G_{M3}	None reported	Pilz et al. (1966)
Metachromatic leukodystrophy	Sulfatide	Sulfatide sulfatase	Jatzkewitz (1958) Mehl and Jatzkewitz (1965); Austin et al. (1965)
Globoid leukodystrophy	Cerebroside to sulfatide ratio elevated	Galactocerebroside β-galactosidase	Austin et al. (1961)
Gaucher's disease	Glucocerebroside	Glucocerebroside glucosidase	Suzuki and Suzuki (1970) Aghion (1934) Brady et al. (1965)
Fabry's disease	Ceramidetrihexoside, ceramidedihexoside	Ceramidetrihexoside galactosidase	Sweeley and Klionsky (1963)
Refsum's disease	Phytanic acid	α-Oxidation of phytanic acid	Brady et al. (1967) Klenk and Kahlke (1963) Mize et al. (1969)
Cerebrotendinous xanthomatosis	Cholestanol buildup	None reported	Menkes et al. (1968)
Wolman's disease	Triglyceride and cholesterol ester buildup	Lysosomal lipase	Crocker et al. (1965)
Niemann-Pick disease	Sphingomyelin	Sphingomyelin phosphocholine hydrolase	Patrick and Lake (1969) Klenk (1935) Brady et al. (1966)

changes in lipid patterns which show the major (Table XVI) and minor biochemical lipid abnormalities.

A. GANGLIOSIDES

Cerebral lipidoses in which the primary abnormality is in the disproportionate distribution of gangliosides are of three types. These involve the storage of gangliosides GM_1, GM_2, or GM_3.

GM_1 gangliosidosis can be subclassified into two groups (Derry *et al.*, 1968; O'Brien *et al.*, 1971b), generalized gangliosidosis and juvenile GM_1 gangliosidosis. Recently, Suzuki has listed three biochemical criteria for classifying the GM_1 gangliosidosis (Suzuki *et al.*, 1971a). These consist of GM_1 ganglioside storage in brain and visceral organs, visceral accumulation of keratin sulfate-like mucopolysaccharide, and β-galactosidase deficiency.

Generalized gangliosidosis was first recognized as a clinico-pathological entity in 1964 by Landing (Landing *et al.*, 1964). The onset of symptoms begins in early infancy before the age of 6 months with clinical and radiological skeletal changes, abnormal facies, and visceromegaly (Suzuki *et al.*, 1971a). The levels of GM_1 and GA_1 are ten times normal in the CNS in these patients (Suzuki *et al.*, 1969). The major enzyme deficiency has been reported by many to be the degradative enzyme β-galactosidase (Okada and O'Brien, 1968; MacBrinn *et al.*, 1969; Dacremont and Kint, 1968; Hooft *et al.*, 1969; Wolfe *et al.*, 1970; van Hoof and Hevs, 1968; Sloan *et al.*, 1969). One attempt to distinguish between general gangliosidosis and juvenile GM_1 gangliosidosis enzymatically has been to distinguish the three components of β-galactosidase: A, B, and C (O'Brien, 1969b). However, Suzuki reported some inconsistencies in attempting to distinguish between components A, B, C, and could attach no significance of the fast-moving component A in relation to clinical conditions (Suzuki *et al.*, 1971a).

Juvenile GM_1 gangliosidosis is distinguished from general gangliosidosis in that the onset of symptoms is in late infancy with normal facies, bones, and abdominal organ size (Suzuki *et al.*, 1971a). The magnitude of the cerebral storage of GM_1 and GA_1 is very close to that in generalized gangliosidosis (O'Brien *et al.*, 1971b), but GM_1 has not been found to accumulate in the visceral organs (Derry *et al.*, 1968; Suzuki *et al.*, 1969; Wolfe *et al.*, 1970; Hooft *et al.*, 1970) as in generalized gangliosidosis. The enzymatic defect is a deficiency in β-galactosidase.

GM_2 gangliosidosis can be subclassified into three groups as described by O'Brien (1969a): (1) Tay-Sachs disease, (2) Sandhoff's disease, and (3) Juvenile GM_2 gangliosidosis.

Tay-Sachs disease was demonstrated by Klenk in 1942 to be a ganglio-side storage disease (Klenk, 1942) and by Svennerholm in 1962 as a GM_2 ganglioside storage disease (Svennerholm, 1962). The levels of GM_2 in these pathological brains are 100–300 times as high as normal and the sialo-derivative (GA_2) levels are 20 times normal in Tay-Sachs disease (Sandhoff et al., 1968; Suzuki et al., 1969). There does not seem to be any storage of ganglioside in the visceral organs (Taketomi and Kawa-mura, 1969) but the pattern of the gangliosides in the visceral organs is altered (O'Brien et al., 1971b). Using cell cultures, Batzdorf et al. demonstrated that cultured cerebral tissue from Tay-Sachs disease stored GM_2 ganglioside (Batzdorf et al., 1969).

The enzymatic defect is in hexosaminidase, which can be separated into two components A and B. In Tay-Sachs disease hexosaminidase A is absent and hexosaminidase B is elevated (Okada and O'Brien, 1968). Kolodny et al. have demonstrated the inability to cleave the terminal N-acetylgalactosamine moiety from radioactively-labeled ganglioside GM_2 in muscle of Tay-Sachs disease (Kolodny et al., 1969). They used Tay-Sachs ganglioside which was labeled in the sialic acid moiety (Kolodny et al., 1970).

In Sandhoff's disease the CNS levels of GM_2 are 100 to 300 times normal as in Tay-Sachs disease but the levels of GA_2 are 100 times normal (Sandhoff et al., 1968; O'Brien et al., 1971b); Klibansky et al., 1970). The enzymatic defect is in both components of hexosaminidase which are deficient to about the same extent (Sandhoff et al., 1968; O'Brien et al., 1971; Suzuki et al., 1971b).

In juvenile GM_2 gangliosidosis the cerebral levels of GM_2 are 40 to 90 times as high as normal and the levels of GA_2 are 5 to 10 times normal (Suzuki et al., 1969). Hexosaminidase A is partially deficient in juvenile GM_2 gangliosidosis (O'Brien et al., 1971a; Suzuki et al., 1970).

GM_3 Gangliosidosis has been reported in one case by Pilz (Pilz et al., 1966). In this he found an accumulation of monosialo ceramide lactoside.

In many other diseases the patterns of gangliosides are altered. In these the main lipid defect is not in ganglioside storage as in the pre-ceding diseases but in another lipid as discussed below.

In Nieman-Pick disease GM_2 and GM_3 are in abnormal concentrations (Kamoshita et al., 1969; Philippart et al., 1969), but the disease affects only the relative concentrations of the gangliosides, not the composition of the gangliosides (Seiter and McCluer, 1970). That the composition of the ganglioside can change in the disease state has been shown in Kufs' disease where, along with regional differences, high levels of C_{18} dienoic fatty acid were found (Berra and Galli, 1971). In Alzheimer's disease the percentage of palmitic acid was higher than in controls in the ganglioside fatty acids (Cherayil, 1968).

In Alexander's disease there is a marked increase of GM_2 (Peiffer, 1968). Also in gargoylism the total lipid NANA is increased (Borri and Hooghwinkel, 1968) with an abnormal amount of a fast moving ganglioside on TLC being present (Abraham *et al.*, 1969). But in the "jimpy" mouse no quantitative or qualitative differences in the gangliosides could be found (Kostie *et al.*, 1969).

Subacute sclerosing leukoencephalitis CNS tissue has been examined with Norton, Poduslo, and Suzuki reporting ganglioside abnormality only in white matter with an increase in the minor gangliosides (G_{2A}, G_{3A}, G_4, and G_6 [Korey's nomenclature]) (Norton *et al.*, 1966). But others have found an abnormal pattern in both cortex and white matter (Ledeen *et al.*, 1968; Dayan and Cumings, 1969). Ledeen's group found an increase in G_5, G_6, G_{2A}, and G_{3A}, and G_6 [Korey's nomenclature] containing a large proportion of oleate and palmitate. Dayan and Cumings also found an increase in G_{M3} and G_{M4} in subacute sclerosing leukoencephalitis brain tissue.

Investigation of human intracranial tumors has shown that cerebellar and cerebral gliomas have a lower ganglioside content than normal brain tissue, Gliomas also have a relatively high quantity of the less polar gangliosides G_4 and G_3 with decreases in G_2 and G_1, and in meningiomas a higher percentage of G_{gal} was found (Fostic and Buchkeit, 1970). The enzymatic block of ganglioside biosynthesis in a DNA virus-transformed tumorigenic mouse cell line was found to be the enzyme catalyzing the transfer of N-acetylgalactosamine from UDP-N-acetylgalactosamine to hematosides (Cumar *et al.*, 1970).

B. Neutral Lipids

The diseases which affect the normal balance of neutral lipids in the central nervous system are few, if we exclude the general demyelinating diseases.

Three diseases which could be classified as neutral lipidoses are Refsum's disease, cerebrotendinous xanthomatosis, and Wolman's disease. Cerebrotendinous xanthomatosis is characterized by the storage of 5α-cholestan-3β-ol (cholestanol) (Menkes *et al.*, 1968; Schimschock *et al.*, 1968). In a study of the subcellular distribution of cholestanol in the diseased state, myelin was found to contain the largest amounts, with smaller amounts in all other subcellular fractions (Stahl *et al.*, 1971).

Refsum's disease is characterized by the accumulation of 3, 7, 11, 15-

tetramethylhexadecanoic acid (phytanic acid) of exogenous origin (Dereux *et al.*, 1968; Blass *et al.*, 1969; MacBrinn and O'Brien, 1968). Patients with Refsum's disease have a block in the α-oxidation of phytanic to pristanic acid (Menkes, 1971). Phytanic acid has been found in its highest proportions in choline glycerophosphatides but not in cholesteryl esters (MacBrinn and O'Brien, 1968). But cholesteryl esters of phytanic acid have been reported (Dereux *et al.*, 1968). In brain, phytanic acid seems to accumulate in myelin (MacBrinn and O'Brien, 1968; Blass *et al.*, 1969).

Wolman's disease is characterized by an elevated level of triglycerides and both free and esterified cholesterol in the CNS (Guazzi *et al.*, 1968; Kahana *et al.*, 1968; Marshall *et al.*, 1969; Menkes, 1971). An enzymatic defect of acid lipase in spleen and liver has been reported (Patrick and Lake, 1969).

The changes in neutral lipids which are not the primary lipid abnormalities in the CNS can be divided into two groups, sterol and fatty acid changes. The first of these involve sterol changes in the central nervous system. Desmosterol has been shown to be a constituent of glioblastomas and the presence of desmosterol accumulation has been postulated as an efficient method for the diagnosis of brain tumors (Grossi-Paoletti *et al.*, 1971).

A patient with Pelizaeus-Merzbacher disease was shown to have a 50% decrease in cholesterol when compared with control brains (Schneck *et al.*, 1971). This reduction along with reduction of other lipids was diagnosed as a congenital defect in myelinization. Also in marasmic children a reduction of CNS cholesterol has been found (Rosso *et al.*, 1970). In like manner a 50% reduction in cholesterol with a 27% increase in cholesterol esters was found in subacute sclerosing leukoencephalitis (Norton *et al.*, 1966). Steryl esters have been found in many pathological brain samples. In glioblastomas, Smith and White found an increase in triglyceride and steryl esters and in meningiomas a prominent hydrocarbon fraction (Smith and White, 1968). In brains from patients with Schilder's disease, G_{M1}-gangliosidosis, and Tay-Sachs disease cholesterol esters have been found and the source of the fatty acid moiety is most likely the β-linked fatty acids of lecithin (Eto and Suzuki, 1971b).

The second of these general lipid groups is fatty acids. In total lipids U-^{14}C-glucose uptake in the CNS has been shown to decrease in EAE (Smith, 1969b) and in hyperphenylalaninemia (Shah *et al.*, 1970). In multiple sclerosis brains deficiencies of 20:1 from ethanolamine glycerophosphatide and $C_{24:1}$ from cerebroside have been found (Gerstl *et al.*, 1970). Supporting the role that changes in the synthesis of $C_{20:1}$ influence the eventual predisposition of multiple sclerosis is the fact that fatty acid elongation reaches its maximum rate during myelination (Yatsu and Moss, 1970). Also in Alpers disease fatty acid synthesis in the mitochondrial fraction of gray matter is significantly reduced (Menkes and Grippo, 1969), while in globoid cell leukodystrophy nonmyelin fatty acids have an increased turnover and the turnover of fatty acids destined for incorporation into myelin is diminished (Menkes and Grippo, 1969).

Hagberg *et al.* (1968) have found a patient with a severe progressive encephalopathy with changes indicating marked disturbances in the metabolism of linolenic acid (Hagberg *et al.*, 1968). In the same light, rats bred and raised on a diet deficient in polyunsaturated fatty acids have been shown to have a higher susceptibility to allergic encephalomyelitis (Clausen and Moller, 1969). That deficiencies in essential fatty acid modify brain lipids has been shown recently in an extensive study by Paoletti's laboratory. Feeding a diet deficient in essential fatty acids, the ω6 family were elevated in the CNS. When control diets were substituted for the deficient diets the ω6 family rebounded above controls and ω9 family receded below control levels (White *et al.*, 1971; Galli *et al.*, 1970b).

C. GLYCOLIPIDS

The diseases which alter the glycolipid patterns of the central nervous system are four: (1) Gaucher's disease, (2) metachromatic leukodystrophy, (3) globoid leukodystrophy (Krabbe's disease), (4) Fabry's disease.

Gaucher's disease is a hereditary condition which involves the nervous system only in the acute, infantile form. An increase in glucocerebroside in nonneural tissues is the main course of this lipidosis (Schettler and Kahlke, 1967). This is due to a deficiency of glucocerebrosidase in the nonneural tissues (Brady *et al.*, 1965). The presence (Scaravilli and Tavolato, 1968) and absence (Freeman and Nevis, 1969) of lipid accumulation in the CNS have been recently reported.

Metachromatic leukodystrophy is a genetically determined neurological disease characterized by an elevation of sulfatide (Jatzkewitz, 1958; Pilz and Muller, 1969; Taori *et al.*, 1969; Muller and Pilz, 1968). Austin, Armstrong, and Sheaver (1965) found arylsulfatase A was markedly diminished in metachromatic leukodystrophy. Recently, Jatzkewitz and Mehl (1969) have shown that both arylsulfatase A and cerebroside-sulfatase activity are reduced in all metachromatic leukodystrophy cases examined.

Cultured fibroblasts derived from patients with metachromatic leukodystrophy have been shown to undergo enzyme replacement when grown on a medium containing arylsulfatase A (Porter *et al.*, 1971). Furthermore, inclusion granules of sulfatides in the cultured fibroblasts were cleared by addition of arylsulfatase A to the medium.

Krabbe's globoid cell leukodystrophy (GLD) is characterized by an almost total loss of myelin and oligodendroglia, severe astrocytic gliosis, and massive infiltration of the unique multinucleated globoid cells in white matter. Sulfatide is severely decreased in white matter but cerebroside in white matter is relatively preserved (Eto and Suzuki, 1971a; Eto *et al.*, 1970), even though others have found elevated cerebroside levels (Andrews and Cancilla, 1970; Andrews *et al.*, 1971). The ratio of cerebroside to sulfatide in myelin is seven to one (Cumings *et al.*, 1968b). But this is contrary to the findings of Eto, Suzuki, and Suzuki (1970) who isolated low levels of myelin in GLD patients with cerebroside and sulfatide in normal proportions. This led them to examine the sphingoglycolipids of patients with GLD. They identified gluco- and galactocerebrosides, lactosylceramide, digalactosylglucosyl-ceramide, two types of tetrahexosyl-ceramides and sulfatides (Eto and Suzuki, 1971a), Galactosylglucosylceramide had been previously identified (Evans and McCluer, 1969). Eto and Suzuki postulated that the visceral type of sphingoglycolipids may be constituents of globoid cells (Eto and Suzuki, 1971a).

The enzymatic defect is in the deficient activity of galactocerebroside β-galactosidase (K. Suzuki and Suzuki, 1970; Y. Suzuki and Suzuki, 1971; Suzuki *et al.*, 1970; Austin *et al.*, 1970).

Fabry's disease is an inborn error of glycolipid metabolism transmitted in an X-linked recessive manner. Two glycolipids accumulated in the visceral organs. One is trihexosyl ceramide, the other is dihexosyl ceramide. The latter glycolipid has recently been identified in cerebral tissues (Schibanoff *et al.*, 1969). The enzyme defect has been reported as a deficiency in a hydrolytic enzyme which cleaves the terminal galactose from trihexosyl ceramide (Brady *et al.*, 1967).

Other lipid changes in glycolipid patterns in the CNS have been examined. Two experimental mutants which have a defective myelination process are the "jimpy" and "quaking" mice. Deficiencies in cerebroside, sulfatide, and long-chain fatty acids especially C_{24} associated with these glycolipids have been reported (Reasor and Kanfer, 1969; Baumann *et al.*, 1968; Jacque *et al.*, 1969; Hogan and Joseph, 1970; Hogan *et al.*, 1970; Nussbaum *et al.*, 1969; Galli and Galli, 1968). The enzymatic defect has not as yet been fully determined (Nixon and Kanfer, 1971). Alterations in the activity of both synthetic enzymes (Neskovic *et al.*, 1969, 1970; Friedrich and Hauser, 1970) and degradative enzymes (Kurtz and Kanfer, 1970; Bowen and Radin, 1968a; Kurihara *et al.*,

1970) have been reported. Also in two other experimental diseases, experimental allergic encephalomyelitis (Vasan *et al.*, 1971) and leukodystrophy in minks (Anderson and Palludan, 1968) lower cerebroside and sulfatide levels have been reported.

In a case of increased ganglioside storage in the CNS an abnormality in cerebroside metabolism was reported (Haberland and Brunngraber, 1970). And in patients with generalized gangliosidosis, there is an increase in activity of cerebroside hydrolases (Brady *et al.*, 1970). In the same light, a case of an exceptional form of amaurotic idiocy associated with metachromatic leukodystrophy has been reported (Pilz and Jatzkewitz, 1968).

Cerebrosides and sulfatides are deficient in multiple sclerosis (Einstein *et al.*, 1970; Gerstl *et al.*, 1970) with no abnormality in the sphingosine bases (Moscatelli and Isaacson, 1969). Also in sclerosing leukoencephalitis (Haltia *et al.*, 1970; Norton *et al.*, 1966), in atypical leukodystrophy (Adachi *et al.*, 1970), in white matter tumors (Yanagihara and Cumings, 1968; Slagel *et al.*, 1967), and in phenylketonuria (Menkes and Aeberhard, 1969; Cumings *et al.*, 1968a; Barbato *et al.*, 1968) cerebrosides and sulfatides are deficient to some extent.

D. PHOSPHOLIPIDS

The only cerebral lipidosis which involves a phospholipid is Niemann-Pick disease.

Niemann-Pick disease is characterized by the accumulation of sphingomyelin and cholesterol in the CNS (Klenk, 1935; Philippart *et al.*, 1969). Niemann-Pick disease can be divided into four types as described by Crocker (Crocker, 1961). Types A and B have a low activity of sphingomyelinase while no deficiency of enzyme activity was detected in Niemann-Pick types C and D (Sloan, 1970). The lipid composition in brain of a Niemann-Pick patient was recently examined (Uda *et al.*, 1969). One possible experimental animal (a Siamese cat) has been reported with a sphingomyelin accumulation (Chrisp *et al.*, 1970).

In other diseases a lower phospholipid concentration in the CNS has been observed. This has been noted in marasmic children (Rosso *et al.*, 1970), in essential fatty acid deficiency conditions (C. Galli *et al.*, 1970), in tumor conditions (Slagel *et al.*, 1967), in "jimpy" mutant mice (Nussbaum *et al.*, 1969), in cases of subacute sclerosing leukoencephalitis (Norton *et al.*, 1966), and in victims of Refsum's disease (MacBrinn and O'Brien, 1968).

In the "quaking" mouse brain deficiencies in C_{24}-sphingomyelin have been reported (Reasor and Kanfer, 1969; Baumann *et al.*, 1968; Jacque *et al.*, 1969). Likewise, in a case of glycolipidosis C_{24}-sphingomyelin was diminished (Pilz and Jatzkewitz, 1968).

XIV. Summary and Conclusions

Obviously no comprehensive short summary can be given of a review encompassing so many aspects of lipid biochemistry, even though limited primarily to one organ or to one type of tissue. However, despite the exceptional diversity in structure of the substances discussed in this review, there is a common denominator for almost all of the compounds described: fatty acids, esterified in some manner to sterols, phospholipids, sphingolipids, etc. Why should long-chain fatty acids occupy such a prominent position in almost all of the lipids of the central nervous system? One facet now appears certain: fatty acids are inserted enzymatically in their respective positions in all of the brain lipids with a high degree of specificity. The concept of "random distribution," previously thought to be the norm for fatty acid distribution in triglycerides and phospholipids, for example, can no longer be accepted. Perhaps it is too early to develop a unified hypothesis for the function of fatty acids esterified in these various compounds. Nevertheless we take the liberty of recommending the following phases from selected published studies as suggestive of their overall function:

(1) "Phospholipids are generally considered to be 'membrane based.' Modification of brain lipid phospholipid species occurring in response to environmental temperature changes can be expected to regulate the operation of any or all the membranes in the nervous system. This increased expandibility of plasma membrane and myelin phospholipid species at low temperatures could assist in the maintenance of specific membrane 'fluidity' and permeability properties necessary to their efficient functioning. Modification of mitochondrial phospholipids may influence the kinetics of metabolic reactions. In this way *structural* and metabolic changes may be linked." [Roots (1968)]. It can be added that this "fluidity" is to a great extent influenced by the fatty acid content of the phospholipids.

(2) "In the liquid crystalline phase, the hydrocarbon chains are in a very mobile condition. . . .

"We can appreciate that, if the hydrocarbon chains of a particular phospholipid are flexing and twisting and are in a mobile condition in the solid state, they will be flexing and twisting *at least* as much as this in a monolayer at the same temperature." [Chapman (1966)].

ACKNOWLEDGMENT

We are indebted to John Paul Jones for help in assembling this manuscript.

References

Abdel-Latif, A. A., and Smith, J. P. (1970). *Biochim. Biophys. Acta* **218**, 134.

Abdel-Latif, A. A., Smith, J. P., and Dasher, C. A. (1970). *Proc. Soc. Exp. Biol. Med.* **134**, 850.

Abraham, J., Chakrapani, B., Singh, M., Kokrady, S., and Bachhawat, B. K. (1969). *Indian J. Med. Res.* **57**, 9.

Adachi, M., Schneck, L., Torii, J., and Volk, B. W. (1970). *J. Neuropathol. Exp. Neurol.* **29**, 601.

Adams, C. W. M., and Davison, A. N. (1959). *J. Neurochem.* **4**, 282.

Aeberhard, E., and Menkes, J. H. (1968). *J. Biol. Chem.* **243**, 3834.

Aeberhard, E., Grippo, J., and Menkes, J. H. (1969). *Pediat. Res.* **3**, 590.

Aghion, A. (1934). Thèse, Univ. de Paris, Paris.

Agranoff, B. W., Benjamin, J. A., and Hajra, A. K. (1969). *Ann. N. Y. Acad. Sci.* **165**, 755.

Agrawal, H. C., Banik, N. L., Bone, A. H., Davison, A. N., Mitchell, R. F., and Spohn, M. (1970). *Biochem. J.* **120**, 635.

Akino, T. (1969). *Tohoku J. Exp. Med.* **98**, 87.

Akulin, V. N., Chebotareva, M. A., and Kreps, E. M. (1969). *Zh. Evol. Biokhim. Fiziol.* **5**, 446. [*Chem. Abstr.* **72**, 52275z (1970).]

Alling, C., and Svennerholm, L. (1969). *J. Neurochem.* **16**, 751.

Anderson, H. A., and Palludan, B. (1968). *Acta Neuropathol.* **11**, 347.

Andrews, J. M., and Cancilla, P. A. (1970). *Arch. Pathol.* **89**, 53.

Andrews, J. M., Pasquale, A. C., Grippo, J., and Menkes, J. H. (1971). *Neurology* **21**, 337.

Ansell, G. B. (1968). *Sci. Basis Med.* p. 383.

Ansell, G. B. (1971). *In* "Chemistry and Brain Development," Proc. Advan. Study Inst. Chem. Brain Develop., Milan (R. Paoletti and A. N. Davison, eds.), Advan. Exp. Med. Biol., Vol. 13, p. 63. Plenum, New York.

Ansell, G. B., and Metcalfe, R. F. (1970). *Lipids* **5**, 734.

Ansell, G. B., and Spanner, S. (1967). *J. Neurochem.* **14**, 873.

Ansell, G. B., and Spanner, S. (1968a). *Biochem. J.* **108**, 207.

Ansell, G. B., and Spanner, S. (1968b). *Biochem. J.* **110**, 201.

Ansell, G. B., and Spanner, S. (1968c). *J. Neurochem.* **15**, 1371.

Ansell, G. B., and Spanner, S. (1970). *Biochem. J.* **117**, 11P.

Arce, A., Maccioni, H. J., and Caputto, R. (1971). *Biochem. J.* **121**, 483.

Aronson, S. M., and Volk, B. W., eds. (1967). *In* "Inborn Disorders of Sphingolipid Metabolism." Pergamon, New York.

Austin, J., Lehfeldt, D., and Maxwell, W. (1961). *J. Neuropathol. Exp. Neurol.* **20**, 284.

Austin, J., Armstrong, D., and Sheaver, L. (1965). *Arch. Neurol.* (*Chicago*) **13**, 593.

Austin, J., Suzuki, K., Armstrong, D., Brady, R. O., and Bachhawat, B. K., Schlenker, J., and Stumpf, D. (1970). *Arch. Neurol.* (*Chicago*) **23**, 502.

Balasubramanian, A. S., and Bachhawat, B. K. (1970). *Brain. Res.* **20**, 341.

Banik, N. L., and Davison, A. N. (1969). *Biochem. J.* 115, 1051.

Barbato, L., Barbato, I. W. M., and Hamanaka, A. (1968). *Brain Res.* 7, 399.

Barlow, R. M. (1969). *J. Comp. Neurol.* 135, 249.

Bass, N. H., and Netsky, M. G. (1969). *Trans. Amer. Neurol. Ass.* 94, 216.

Bass, N. H., Netsky, M. G., and Young, E. (1970a). *Arch. Neurol. (Chicago)* 23, 289.

Bass, N. H., Netsky, M. G., and Young, E. (1970b). *Arch. Neurol. (Chicago)* 23, 303.

Basu, S. (1968). *Fed. Proc. Fed. Amer. Soc. Exp. Biol.* 27, 346.

Basu, S., Kaufman, B., and Roseman, S. (1968). *J. Biol. Chem.* 243, 5802.

Basu, S., Schultz, A. M., Basu, M., and Roseman, S. (1971). *J. Biol. Chem.* 246, 4272.

Batzdorf, U., Sarlieve, L. L., Gold, V. A., and Menkes, J. H. (1969). *Arch. Neurol. (Chicago)* 20, 650.

Baumann, N. A., Jacque, C. M., Pollet, S. A., and Harpin, M. L. (1968). *Eur. J. Biochem.* 4, 340.

Bazan, N. G., Jr. (1970). *Biochim. Biophys. Acta* 218, 1.

Bazan, N. G., Jr., and Rakowski, H. (1970). *Life Sci.* 9, 501.

Behrens, N. H., Parodi, A. J., Leloir, L. F., and Krisman, C. R. (1971). *Arch. Biochem. Biophys.* 143, 375.

Bell, O. E., Jr., Blank, M. L., and Snyder, F. (1971). *Biochim. Biophys. Acta* 231, 579.

Bernsohn, J., and Grossman, H. J., eds. (1971). *In* "Lipid Storage Diseases." Academic Press, New York.

Bernsohn, J., and Stephanides, L. M. (1967). *Nature (London)* 215, 821.

Bernsohn, J., Stephanides, L. M., and Norgello, H. (1971). *Brain Res.* 28, 327.

Berra, B., and Galli, C. (1971). *Life Sci.* 10, 213.

Bickerstaffe, R., and Mead, J. F. (1968). *Lipids* 3, 317.

Bishop, H. H., and Strickland, K. P. (1970). *Can. J. Biochem.* 48, 269.

Blank, M. L., Wykle, R. L., Piantadosi, C., and Snyder, F. (1970). *Biochim. Biophys. Acta* 210, 442.

Blass, J. P. (1970). *J. Neurochem.* 17, 545.

Blass, J. P., Avigan, J., and Steinberg, D. (1969). *Biochim. Biophys. Acta* 187, 36.

Boone, S. C., and Wakil, S. J. (1970). *Biochemistry* 9, 1470.

Borgman, R. F., and Haselden, F. (1969). *S.C. Agr. Exp. Sta., Tech. Bull.* No. 1029.

Bornstein, M. B., and Crain, S. M. (1965). *Science* 148, 1242.

Borri, P. F., and Hooghwinkel, G. J. M. (1968). *Pathol. Eur.* 3, 416.

Bourre, J. M., Pollet, S. A., Dubois, G., and Baumann, N. A. (1970). *C. R. Acad. Sci., Ser. D* 271, 1221.

Bowen, D. M., and Radin, N. S. (1968a). *Biochim. Biophys. Acta* 152, 599.

Bowen, D. M., and Radin, N. S. (1968b). *Advan. Lipid Res.* 6, 255.

Bowen, D. M., and Radin, N. S. (1969a). *J. Neurochem.* 16, 457.

Bowen, D. M., and Radin, N. S. (1969b). *J. Neurochem.* 16, 501.

Brady, R. O. (1969). *New Engl. J. Med.* 281, 1243.

Brady, R. O. (1970a). *Clin. Chem.* 16, 811.

Brady, R. O. (1970b). *Biochem. J.* 117, 8P.

Brady, R. O. (1970c). *Annu. Rev. Med.* 21, 317.

Brady, R. O. (1970d). *Chem. Phys. Lipids* 5, 261.

Brady, R. O., Kanfer, J. N., and Shapiro, D. (1965). *Biochem. Biophys. Res. Commun.* **18**, 221.

Brady, R. O., Kanfer, J. N., Mock, M. B., and Fredrickson, D. S. (1966). *Proc. Nat. Acad. Sci. U. S.* **55**, 366.

Brady, R. O., Gal, A. E., Bradley, R. M., Martensson, E., Warshaw, H. C., and Laster, L. (1967). *New Engl. J. Med.* **276**, 1163.

Brady, R. O., O'Brien, J. S., Bradley, R. M., and Gal, A. E. (1970). *Biochim. Biophys. Acta* **210**, 193.

Braun, P. E., Morell, P., and Radin, N. S. (1970). *J. Biol. Chem.* **245**, 335.

Burton, R. M. (1967). *In* "Lipids and Lipidoses" (E. G. Schetter, ed.), p. 122. Springer-Verlag, Berlin and New York.

Burton, R. M., and Sodd, M. A. (1969). *Lipids* **4**, 496.

Capella, P., Galli, C., and Fumagalli, R. (1968). *Lipids* **3**, 431.

Carey, J. B., and Hansen, R. F. (1969). "Bile Acid Metabolism," p. 5. Thomas, Springfield, Illinois.

Chang, M., and Ballou, C. E. (1967). *Biochem. Biophys. Res. Commun.* **26**, 199.

Chapman, D. (1966). *Ann. N. Y. Acad. Sci.* **137**, 745.

Chase, H. P., and O'Brien, D. (1970). *Pediat. Res.* **4**, 96.

Chase, H. P., Lindsley, W. F. B., and O'Brien, D. (1969). *Nature (London)* **221**, 554.

Chase, H. P., Dabiere, C. S., Welch, N., and O'Brien, D. (1971). *Pediatrics* **47**, 491.

Cherayil, G. D. (1968). *J. Lipid Res.* **9**, 207.

Chetverikov, D. A., Gasteva, S. V., Dvorkin, V. Y., Shmelev, A. A., and Bobkov, V. A. (1970). *Vses. Konf. Neirokhim. Nerv. Sist., Dokl., 5th, 1969* p. 274. [*Chem. Abstr.* **75**, 2783e (1971).]

Chrisp, C. E., Ringler, D. H., Abrams, G. D., Radin, N. S., and Brekert, A. (1970). *J. Amer. Vet. Med. Ass.* **156**, 616.

Clarenburg, R., Chaikoff, I. L., and Morris, M. D. (1963). *J. Neurochem.* **10**, 135.

Clarke, D. W., and Gittens, B. (1968). *Can. J. Physiol. Pharmacol.* **46**, 507.

Clausen, J., and Moller, J. (1969). *Int. Arch. Allergy Appl. Immunol.* **36**, 224.

Clendenon, N. R., and Allen, N. (1970). *J. Neurochem.* **17**, 865.

Cooper, M. F., and Webster, G. R. (1970). *J. Neurochem.* **17**, 1543.

Crocker, A. C. (1961). *J. Neurochem.* **7**, 69.

Crocker, A. C., Vawter, G. F., Neuhauser, E. B. D., and Rosowsky, A. (1965). *Pediatrics* **35**, 627.

Culley, W. J., and Lineberger, R. O. (1968). *J. Nutr.* **96**, 375.

Cumar, F. A., Barra, H. S., Maccioni, H. J., and Caputto, R. (1968). *J. Biol. Chem.* **243**, 3807.

Cumar, F. A., Brady, R. O., Kolodny, E. H., McFarland, V. W., and Mora, P. T. (1970). *Proc. Nat. Acad. Sci. U. S.* **67**, 757.

Cumings, J. N. (1970). *Handb. Clin. Neurol.* **10**, 325.

Cumings, J. N., Grundt, I. K., and Yanagihara, T. (1968a). *J. Neurol., Neurosurg. Psychiat.* **31**, 334.

Cumings, J. N., Thompson, E. J., and Goodwin, H. (1968b). *J. Neurochem.* **15**, 243.

Cuzner, M. L. (1968). Ph.D. Thesis, Univ. of London, London.

Dacremont, G., and Kint, J. A. (1968). *Clin. Chim. Acta* **21**, 421.

D'Adamo, A. F., Jr. (1970). *In* "Handbook of Neurochemistry" (A. Lajtha, ed.), Vol. 3, p. 525. Plenum, New York.

Dahl, D. R. (1968). *J. Neurochem.* **15**, 815.

Dalal, K. B., and Einstein, E. R. (1969). *Brain Res.* **16**, 441.

Davidson, J. B., and Stanacev, N. Z. (1970). *Can. J. Biochem.* **48**, 633.
Davies, P. A. (1969). *Proc. Nutr. Soc.* **28**, 66.
Davison, A. N. (1968a). *Proc. Nutr. Soc.* **27**, 83.
Davison, A. N. (1968b). "Applied Neurochemistry, Contemporary Neurology Series," Ch. 4, p. 178. Davis, Philadelphia, Pennsylvania.
Davison, A. N. (1970a). In "Lipid Metabolism" (M. Florkin and E. H. Stotz, ed.), Comprehensive Biochemistry, Vol. 18, p. 293. Elsevier, Amsterdam.
Davison, A. N. (1970b). In "Handbook of Neurochemistry" (A. Lajtha, ed.), Vol. 3, p. 547. Plenum, New York.
Davison, A. N. (1970c). In "Myelination" (A. N. Davison and A. Peters, eds.), p. 80. Thomas, Springfield, Illinois.
Dawson, R. M. C. (1969). *Ann. N. Y. Acad. Sci.* **165**, 774.
Dayan, A. D., and Cumings, J. N. (1969). *Arch. Dis. Childhood* **44**, 187.
Debuch, H., Friedemann, H., and Müller, J. (1970). *Hoppe-Seylers Z. Physiol. Chem.* **351**, 613.
De Jimenez, E. S., and Cleland, W. W. (1969). *Biochim. Biophys. Acta* **176**, 685.
Dereux, J., Lowenthal, A., Mardens, Y., and Karcher, D. (1968). *Pathol. Eur.* **3**, 468.
De Robertis, E., Fiszer, S., Pasquini, J. M., and Soto, E. F. (1969). *J. Neurobiol.* **1**, 41.
Derry D. M., Fawcett, J. S., Andermann, F., and Wolfe, L. S. (1968). *Neurology* **18**, 340.
Deul, D. H., Haisma, J. A., and Van Breeman, J. F. L. (1968). *Progr. Brain Res.* **29**, 125.
Dhar, A. K., and Smith, L. L. (1971). *Fed. Proc. Fed. Amer. Soc. Exp. Biol.* **30**, 1140. Abstr.
D'Hollander, F., and Chevallier, F. (1969). *Biochim. Biophys. Acta* **176**, 146.
Dhopeshwarkar, G. A., and Mead, J. F. (1970). *Biochim. Biophys. Acta* **210**, 250.
Dhopeshwarkar, G. A., Maier, R., and Mead, J. F. (1969). *Biochim. Biophys. Acta* **187**, 6.
Dhopeshwarkar, G. A., Subramanian, C., and Mead, J. F. (1971). *Biochim. Biophys. Acta* **231**, 8.
Diamond, I. (1971). *Arch. Neurol. (Chicago)* **24**, 333.
Dicesare, J. L., and Dain, J. A. (1971). *Biochim. Biophys. Acta* **231**, 385.
Dickerson, J. W. T. (1968). In "Applied Neuochemistry" (A. N. Davison and J. Dobbing, eds.), p. 48. Davis, Philadelphia, Pennsylvania.
Dickerson, J. W. T., and Jarvis, J. (1970). *Proc. Nutr. Soc.* **29**, Suppl. 4A/5A, 29.
DiFrisco, S., de Ruggieri, P., and Ercoli, A. (1953). *Bull. Soc. Ital. Biol. Sper.* **29**, 1351.
Dobbing, J. (1968a). In "Psychopharmacology, Dimensions and Perspectives" (C. R. B. Joyce, ed.), p. 345. Lippincott, Philadelphia, Pennsylvania.
Dobbing, J. (1968b). *Proc. Nutr. Soc.* **27**, 83.
Dobbing, J. (1968c). In "Applied Neurochemistry" (A. N. Davison and J. Dobbing, eds.), Vols. 4 and 5, p. 287. Davis, Philadelphia, Pennsylvania.
Dobbing, J., Hopewell, J. W., Lynch, A., and Sands, J. (1970). *Exp. Neurol.* **28**, 442.
Durell, J., and Garland, J. T. (1969). *Ann. N. Y. Acad. Sci.* **165**, 743.
Dvorkin, V. Y. (1969). *Tr. Vses. Konf. Biokhim. Nerv. Sist., 4th, 1966* p. 396. [*Chem. Abstr.* **74**, 11373c (1971).]
Dvorkin, V. Y., and Kiselev, G. V. (1969). *Biokhimiya* **34**, 1245. [*Chem. Abstr.* **72**, 86432p (1970).]

Edmond, J., Popják, G., Wong, S., and Williams, V. P. (1971). *J. Biol. Chem.* **246**, 6254.

Eichberg, J., Hauser, G., and Karnovsky, M. L. (1969). In "The Structure and Function of Nervous Tissue" (G. H. Bourne, ed.), Vol. 3, p. 185. Academic Press, New York.

Einstein, E. R., Dalal, K. B., and Csejtey, J. (1970). *J. Neurol. Sci.* **11**, 109.

Eng, L. F., and Noble, E. P. (1968). *Lipids* **3**, 157.

Ercoli, A., and de Ruggieri, P. (1953). *J. Amer. Chem. Soc.* **75**, 3284.

Ercoli, A., Di Frisco, S., and de Ruggieri, P. (1953a). *Gazz. Chim. Ital.* **83**, 78.

Ercoli, A., Di Frisco, S., and de Ruggieri, P. (1953b). *Bull. Soc. Ital. Biol. Sper.* **29**, 494.

Eto, Y., and Suzuki, K. (1971a). *J. Neurochem.* **18**, 1007.

Eto, Y., and Suzuki, K. (1971b). *J. Neurochem.* **18**, 503.

Eto, Y., Suzuki, K., and Suzuki, K. (1970). *J. Lipid Res.* **11**, 473.

Etzrodt, A., and Debuch, H. (1970). *Hoppe-Seylers Z. Physiol. Chem.* **351**, 603.

Evans, J. E., and McCluer, R. H. (1969). *J. Neurochem.* **16**, 1393.

Fewster, M. E., and Mead, J. F. (1968). *J. Neurochem.* **15**, 1041.

Fieser, L. F. (1953). *J. Amer. Chem. Soc.* **75**, 4395.

Fieser, L. F., Yuang, W. Y., and Bhattacharyya, B. K. (1958). *J. Org. Chem.* **23**, 459.

Fishman, M. A., Prensky, A. L., and Dodge, P. R. (1969). *Nature (London)* **221**, 552.

Foote, J. L., and Tao, R. V. (1968). *Life Sci.* **7**, 1187.

Formby, B. (1968). *Mol. Pharmacol.* **4**, 288.

Fostic, D., and Buchkeit, F. (1970). *Life Sci.* **9**, 589.

Freedman, L. S. (1970). *Diss. Abstr. B* **31**(3), 1367.

Freeman, F. R., and Nevis, A. H. (1969). *Neurology* **19**, 87.

Freysz, L., Bieth, R., Judes, C., Sensenbrenner, M., Jacob, M., and Mandel, P. (1968). *J. Neurochem.* **15**, 307.

Freysz, L., Bieth, R., and Mandel, P. (1969). *J. Neurochem.* **16**, 1417.

Friedrich, V. L., and Hauser, G. (1970). *Fed. Proc. Fed. Amer. Soc. Exp. Biol.* **29**, 410.

Fujino, Y., and Nakano, M. (1969). *Biochem. J.* **113**, 573.

Fujino, Y., and Negishi, T. (1968). *Biochim. Biophys. Acta* **152**, 428.

Fumagalli, R., and Paoletti, R. (1963). *Life Sci.* **5**, 291.

Fumagalli, R., Grossi, E., Paoletti, P., and Paoletti, R. (1964). *J. Neurochem.* **11**, 561.

Galli, C., and Galli, D. (1968). *Nature (London)* **220**, 165.

Galli, C., White, H. B., Jr., and Paoletti, R. (1970). *J. Neurochem.* **17**, 347.

Galli, C., White, H. B., Jr., and Paoletti, R. (1971). In "Chemistry and Brain Development" Proc. Advan. Study Inst. Chem. Brain Develop., Milan (R. Paoletti and D. Kritchevsky, eds.), Advan. Exp. Med. Biol., Vol. 13, p. 425. Plenum, New York.

Galli, G., Paoletti, E. G., and Weiss, J. F. (1968). *Science* **162**, 1495.

Galli, G., Kienle, M., Caltabeni, F., Fiecchi, A. Paoletti, E. G., and Paoletti, R. (1970). *Advan. Enzyme Regul.* **8**, 311.

Gasteva, S. V., and Raize, T. E. (1970). *Byull. Eksp. Biol. Med.* **70**, 31. [*Chem. Abstr.* **74**, 135a (1971).]

Gatt, S. (1967). *Inborn Disord. Sphingolipid Metab., Proc. Int. Symp. Cereb. Sphingolipidoses, 3rd, Brooklyn, N. Y., 1965* p. 261.

Gatt, S. (1968). *Biochim. Biophys. Acta* **159**, 304.

Gatt, S. (1969). *In* "Lipids" (J. M. Lowenstein, ed.), Methods in Enzymology, Vol. 14, p. 134. Academic Press, New York.

Gatt, S. (1970a). *Chem. Phys. Lipids* **5**, 235.

Gatt, S. (1970b). *Biochem. J.* **117**, 4P.

Gatt, S., and Rapport, M. M. (1966). *Biochim. Biophys. Acta* **113**, 567.

Gatt, S., and Yavin, E. (1969). *In* "Lipids" (J. M. Lowenstein, ed.), Methods in Enzymology, Vol. 14, p. 139. Academic Press, New York.

Gautheron, C., Petit, L., and Chevallier, F. (1969). *Exp. Neurol.* **25**, 18.

Geiger, W. B., and Bampton, A. E. (1966). *Nature (London)* **212**, 510.

Geison, R. L., and Waisman, H. A. (1970a). *J. Neurochem.* **17**, 469.

Geison, R. L., and Waisman, H. A. (1970b). *J. Nutr.* **100**, 315.

Gerstl, B., Eng, L. F., Tavaststjerna, M., Smith, J. K., and Kruse, S. L. (1970). *J. Neurochem.* **17**, 677.

Gielen, W. (1971). *Chimia* **25**, 81.

Gilliland, K. M., and Moscatelli, E. A. (1969). *Biochim. Biophys. Acta* **187**, 221.

Grafnetter, D., Grossi, E., and Marganti, P. (1965). *J. Neurochem.* **12**, 145.

Granoff, D. M., and Howard, E. (1969). *J. Pediat.* **75**, 732.

Grossi-Paoletti, E., Paoletti, P., and Fumagalli, R. (1971). *J. Neurosurg.* **34**, 454.

Guazzi, G. C., Martin, J. J., Philippart, M., Roels, H., van der Eecken, H., Vrints, L., Delbeke, M. J., and Hooft, E. (1968). *Eur. Neurol.* **1**, 334.

Guthrie, H. A., and Brown, M. L. (1968). *J. Nutr.* **94**, 419.

Haberland, C., and Brunngraber, E. G. (1970). *Arch. Neurol. (Chicago)* **23**, 481.

Hagberg, B., Sourander, P., and Svennerholm, L. (1968). *Acta Paediat. Scand.* **57**, 495.

Haltia, M., Sourander, P., and Svennerholm, L. (1970). *Acta Neuropathol.* **14**, 284.

Hammarström, S. (1969). *FEBS (Fed. Eur. Biochem. Soc.), Lett.* **5**, 192.

Hammarström, S., and Samuelsson, B. (1970). *Biochem. Biophys. Res. Commun.* **41**, 1027.

Handa, S., and Burton, R. M. (1969). *Lipids* **4**, 589.

Hansen, I. B., and Clausen, J. (1968). *Lab. Invest.* **22**, 231.

Hansen, I. B., and Clausen, J. (1969). *Z. Ernaehrungswiss.* **9**, 278.

Harwood, J. L., and Hawthorne, J. N. (1969). *J. Neurochem.* **16**, 1377.

Hauser, G. (1968). *J. Neurochem.* **15**, 1237.

Haverkate, F., and van Deenen, L. L. M. (1965). *Biochim. Biophys. Acta* **106**, 78.

Hawthorne, J. N., and Kai, M. (1970). *In* "Handbook of Neurochemistry" (A. Lajtha, ed.), Vol. 3, Ch. 17, p. 491. Plenum, New York.

Heitzman, R. J., and Skipworth, S. (1969). *J. Neurochem.* **16**, 121.

Henning, R., and Stoffel, W. (1969). *Hoppe-Seyler's Z. Physiol. Chem.* **350**, 827.

Hildebrand, J., Stoffyn, P., and Hanser, G. (1970). *J. Neurochem.* **17**, 403.

Himwich, W. A. (1970). *In* "Physiology of the Perinatal Period" (U. Stave, ed.), Vol. 2, p. 717. Appleton, New York.

Hinzen, D. H., Isselhard, W., Fuesgen, I., and Mueller, V. (1970). *Pfluegers Arch.* **318**, 117.

Hogan, E. L., and Joseph, K. C. (1970). *J. Neurochem.* **17**, 1209.

Hogan, E. L., Joseph, K. C., and Schmidt, G. (1970). *J. Neurochem.* **17**, 75.

Holub, B. J., Kuksis, A., and Thompson, W. (1970). *J. Lipid Res.* **11**, 558.

Hooft, C., Senesael, L., Delbeke, M. J., Kint, J. A., and Dacremont, G. (1969). *Eur. Neurol.* **2**, 225.

Hooft, C., Vlietinck, R. F., Dacremont, G., and Kint, J. A. (1970). *Eur. Neurol.* **4**, 1.

Hooghwinkel, G. J. M., and De Rooij, R. E. (1968). *Chromatogr. Electrophor., Symp. Int., 4th, 1966* p. 298.

Horrocks, L. A. (1968). *J. Neurochem.* **15**, 483.

Howard, E., and Granoff, D. M. (1968). *J. Nutr.* **95**, 111.

Irwin, L. N. (1969). *Brain Res.* **15**, 518.

Irwin, L. N., and Samson, F. E., Jr. (1971). *J. Neurochem.* **18**, 203.

Isaacson, E., and Moscatelli, E. A. (1070). *J. Neurochem.* **17**, 365.

Ivanova, T. N., Rubel, L. N., and Semenova, N. A. (1969). *Tr. Vses. Konf. Biokhim. Nerv. Sist., 4th, 1966* p. 386. [*Chem. Abstr.* **74**, 40169w (1971).]

Jacque, C. M., Harpin, M. L., and Baumann, N. A. (1969). *Eur. J. Biochem.* **11**, 218.

Jatzkewitz, H. (1958). *Hoppe-Seyler's Z. Physiol. Chem.* **311**, 297.

Jatzkewitz, H., and Mehl, E. (1969). *J. Neurochem.* **16**, 19.

Jatzkewitz, H., Mehl, E., and Sandhoff, K. (1970). *Biochem. J.* **117**, 6P.

Joffe, S. (1969). *J. Neurochem.* **16**, 715.

Jones, J. P., Ramsey, R. B., and Nicholas, H. J. (1971). *Life Sci.* **10**, 997.

Jose, J. M., Seifter, E., Rettura, G., Cefaloni, A., and Levenson, S. M. (1970). *Poultry Sci.* **49**, 649.

Kabara, J. J. (1967). *Advan. Lipid Res.* **5**, 279.

Kahana, D., Berant, M., and Wolman, M. (1968). *Pediatrics* **42**, 70.

Kai, M., and Hawthorne, J. N. (1969). *Ann. N. Y. Acad. Sci.* **165**, 761.

Kai, M., Salway, J. G., and Hawthorne, J. N. (1968). *Biochem. J.* **106**, 791.

Kamoshita, S., Aron, A. M., Suzuki, K., and Suzuki, K. (1969). *Amer. J. Dis. Child.* **117**, 379.

Kanfer, J. N. (1970). *Chem. Phys. Lipids* **5**, 159.

Kanfer, J. N., and Bates, S. (1970). *Lipids* **5**, 718.

Karlsson, K. (1970). *Chem. Phys. Lipids* **5**, 6.

Kaufman, B., Basu, S., and Roseman, S. (1967). *Inborn Disord. Sphingolipid Metab., Proc. Int. Symp. Cereb. Sphingolipidoses, 3rd, Brooklyn, N. Y., 1965* p. 193.

Kaufman, B., Basu, S., and Roseman, S. (1968). *J. Biol. Chem.* **243**, 5804.

Kaufman, M. A., Roizin, L., and Gold, G. (1969). *Progr. Neurol. Psychiat.* **24**, 104.

Kawamura, N., and Taketomi, T. (1969). *Jap. J. Exp. Med.* **39**, 383.

Kelley, M. T., Aexel, R. T., Herndon, B. L., and Nicholas, H. J. (1969). *J. Lipid Res.* **10**, 166.

Kishimoto, Y., Wajda, M., and Radin, N. S. (1968). *J. Lipid Res.* **9**, 27.

Kishimoto, Y., Agranoff, B. W., Radin, N. S., and Burton, R. M. (1969). *J. Neurochem.* **16**, 397.

Kiyasu, J. Y., Pieringer, R. A., Paules, H., and Kennedy, E. P. (1963). *J. Biol. Chem.* **238**, 2293.

Klenk, E. (1935). *Hoppe-Seyler's Z. Physiol. Chem.* **235**, 24.

Klenk, E. (1942). *Ber. Deut. Chem. Ges. B* **75**, 1632.

Klenk, E., and Kahlke, W. (1963). *Hoppe-Seyler's Z. Physiol. Chem.* **333**, 133.

Klenk, E., and Langerbeins, H. (1941). *Hoppe-Seyler's Z. Physiol. Chem.* **270**, 185.

Klenk, E., and Löhr, J. P. (1967). *Hoppe-Seyler's Z. Physiol. Chem.* **348**, 1712.

Klenk, E., and Schorsch, E. U. (1968). *Hoppe-Seyler's Z. Physiol. Chem.* **349**, 653.

Klibansky, C., Saifer, A., Feldman, N. I., Schneck, L., and Volk, B. W. (1970). *J. Neurochem.* **17,** 339.

Kolodny, E. H., Brady, R. O., and Volk, B. W. (1969). *Biochem. Biophys. Res. Commun.* **37,** 526.

Kolodny, E. H., Brady, R. O., Quirk, J. M., and Kanfer, J. N. (1970). *J. Lipid Res.* **11,** 144.

Komai, Y., Hiraiwa, N., and Takahashi, Y. (1970). *Jap. J. Exp. Med.* **40,** 401.

Kostie, D., Nussbaum, J. L., and Mandel, P. (1969). *Life Sci.* **8,** 1135.

Kreps, E. M., Chebotareva, M. A., and Akulin, V. N. (1969a). *Comp. Biochem. Physiol.* **31,** 419.

Kreps, E. M., Patrikeeva, M. V., Smirnov, A. A., Chirkovskaya, E. V., and Vaver, V. A. (1969b). *Zh. Evol. Biokhim. Fiziol.* **5,** 360. [*Chem. Abstr.* **72,** 220h (1970).]

Kritchevsky, D., and Holmes, W. L. (1962). *Biochem. Biophys. Res. Commun.* **7,** 128.

Kritchevsky, D., Tepper, S. A., Di Tullio, N. W., and Holmes, W. L. (1965). *J. Amer. Oil Chem. Soc.* **42,** 1024.

Krop, T. M., and Winick, M. (1969). *Pediatria (Santiago)* **12,** 151.

Kurihara, T., Nussbaum, J. L., and Mandel, P. (1970). *J. Neurochem.* **17,** 993.

Kurtz, D., and Kanfer, J. N. (1970). *Science* **168,** 259.

Lajtha, A., ed. (1969–1970). "Handbook of Neurochemistry," Vols. 1, 2, and 3. Plenum, New York.

Landing, B. H., Silverman, F. N., Craig, J. M., Jacoby, M. D., Lahey, M. E., and Chadwick, D. L. (1964). *Amer. J. Dis. Child.* **108,** 503.

Lapetina, E. G., and Hawthorne, J. N. (1971). *Biochem. J.* **122,** 171.

Lapetina, E. G., and Rodriquez De Lores Arnaiz, G. (1969). *Biochim. Biophys. Acta* **176,** 643.

Lapetina, E. G., Soto, E. F., and De Robertis, E. (1968). *J. Neurochem.* **15,** 437.

Lapetina, E. G., Rodriquez De Lores Arnaiz, G., and De Robertis, E. (1969). *J. Neurochem.* **16,** 101.

Lapetina, E. G., Lunt, G. G., and De Robertis, E. (1970). *J. Neurobiol.* **1,** 295.

Larrabee, M. G. (1968). *J. Neurochem.* **15,** 803.

Ledeen, R., Salsman, K., and Cabrera, M. (1968). *J. Lipid Res.* **9,** 129.

Lee, J. W., and Barnes, M. M. (1969). *Brit. J. Nutr.* **23,** 289.

Leibovitz, Z., and Gatt, S. (1968). *Biochim. Biophys. Acta* **152,** 136.

Lesch, P., and Bernhard, K. (1968). *Helv. Chim. Acta* **51,** 652.

Levitina, V. M. (1970). *Usp. Sovrem. Biol.* **69,** 113. [*Chem. Abstr.* **73,** 21247h (1970).]

Lippel, K., and Mead, J. F. (1968). *Biochim. Biophys. Acta* **152,** 669.

Little, J. R., Hori, S., and Spitzer, J. J. (1969). *Amer. J. Physiol.* **217,** 919.

Lowden, J. A., and Wolfe, L. S. (1964). *Can. J. Biochem.* **42,** 1587.

Lunt, G. G., and Lapetina, E. G. (1970a). *Brain Res.* **17,** 164.

Lunt, G. G., and Lapetina, E. G. (1970b). *Brain Res.* **18,** 451.

Lunt, G. G., and Rowe, C. E. (1968). *Biochim. Biophys. Acta* **152,** 681.

Lunt, G. G., and Rowe, C. E. (1969). *Life Sci.* **8,** 885.

Lunt, G. G., Canessa, O. M., and De Robertis, E. (1971). *Nature (London) New Biol.* **230,** 187.

Lynen, F. (1954). *Nature (London)* **174,** 962.

MacBrinn, M. C., and O'Brien, J. S. (1968). *J. Lipid Res.* **9,** 552.

MacBrinn, M. C., Okada, S., Ho, M. W., Hu, C. C., and O'Brien, J. S. (1969). *Science* 163, 946.

Mandel, P., Bieth, R., and Stoll, R. (1949). *C. R. Soc. Biol.* 143, 1224.

Manukyan, K. G. (1969). *Tr. Vses. Konf. Biokhim. Nerv. Sist., 4th, 1966* p. 375. [*Chem. Abstr.* 74, 29755p (1971).]

Marshall, W. C., Ockenden, B. G., Fosbrooke, A. S., and Cumings, J. N. (1969). *Arch. Dis. Childhood* 44, 331.

Martensson, E., and Kanfer, J. (1968). *J. Biol. Chem.* 243, 497.

Martin, C. W., and Nicholas, H. J. (1972). *Steroids* 19, 549.

Martin, D. L. (1970). *REACTS, Proc. Reg. Educ. Annu. Chem. Teach. Symp. 1st*, 159 (H. Heikkinen, ed.). [*Chem. Abstr.* 75, 184(2216x) (1971).]

Mehl, E., and Jatzkewitz, H. (1965). *Biochem. Biophys. Res. Commun.* 19, 407.

Menkes, J. H. (1971). *Trans. Amer. Soc. Neurochem.* 2, 52.

Menkes, J. H., and Aeberhard, E. (1969). *J. Pediat.* 74, 924.

Menkes, J. H., and Grippo, J. (1969). *Trans. Amer. Neurol. Ass.* 94, 301.

Menkes, J. H., Schimschock, J. R., and Swanson, P. D. (1968). *Arch. Neurol. (Chicago)* 19, 47.

Michael, S. (1971). *Can. J. Biochem.* 49, 306.

Michell, R. H., Hawthorne, J. N., Coleman, R., and Karnovsky, M. L. (1970). *Biochim. Biophys. Acta* 210, 86.

Mize, C. E., Herndon, J. H., Jr., Blass, J. P., Milne, G. W. A., Follansbee, C., Laudat, P. and Steinberg, D. (1969). *J. Clin. Invest.* 48, 1033.

Mokrasch, L. C. (1969). *In* "Handbook of Neurochemistry" (A. Lajtha, ed.), Vol. 2, p. 171. Plenum, New York.

Morell, P., and Radin, N. S. (1969). *Biochemistry* 8, 506.

Morell, P., and Radin, N. S. (1970). *J. Biol. Chem.* 245, 342.

Morell, P., Costantino-Ceccarini, E., and Radin, N. S. (1970). *Arch. Biochem. Biophys.* 141, 738.

Moscatelli, E. A., and Isaacson, E. (1969). *Lipids* 4, 550.

Muller, D., and Pilz, H. (1968). *Pathol. Eur.* 3, 294.

Naqvi, S. H. M., and Nicholas, H. J. (1970). *Steroids* 16, 297.

Naqvi, S. H. M., Herndon, B. L., Kelley, M. T., Bleisch, V., Aexel, R. T., and Nicholas, H. J. (1969). *J. Lipid Res.* 10, 115.

Naqvi, S. H. M., Ramsey, R. B., and Nicholas, H. J. (1970a). *Lipids* 5, 578.

Naqvi, S. H. M., Herndon, B. L., Del Rosario, L., and Nicholas, H. J. (1970b). *Lipids* 5, 964.

Neskovic, N., Nussbaum, J. L., and Mandel, P. (1969). *FEBS (Fed. Eur. Biochem. Soc.), Lett.* 3, 199.

Neskovic, N., Nussbaum, J. L., and Mandel, P. (1970). *Brain Res.* 21, 39.

Nicholas, H. J. (1965). *J. Amer. Oil Chem. Soc.* 42, 40.

Nicholas, H. J., and Thomas, B. E. (1961). *Brain* 84, 320.

Nixon, R., and Kanfer, J. N. (1971). *Life Sci.* 10, 71.

Norton, W. T., and Brotz, M. (1963). *Biochem. Biophys. Res. Commun.* 12, 198.

Norton, W. T., and Poduslo, S. E. (1971). *J. Lipid Res.* 12, 84.

Norton, W. T., Poduslo, S. E., and Suzuki, K. (1966). *J. Neuropathol. Exp. Neurol.* 25, 582.

Nussbaum, J. L., Neskovic, N., and Mandel, P. (1969). *J. Neurochem.* 16, 927.

Nutr. Rev. (1970). 28, 110.

O'Brien, J. S. (1969a). *Lancet* ii, 805.

O'Brien, J. S. (1969b). *J. Pediat.* **75**, 167.

O'Brien, J. S. (1971). *New Engl. J. Med.* **284**, 893.

O'Brien, J. S., Stern, M. B., Landing, B. M., O'Brien, J. K., and Donnell, G. N. (1965). *Amer. J. Dis. Child.* **109**, 338.

O'Brien, J. S., Okada, S., Ho, M. W., Fillerup, D. L., Veath, M. L., and Adams, K. (1971a). *Fed. Proc. Fed. Amer. Soc. Exp. Biol.* **30**, 956.

O'Brien, J. S., Okada, S., Ho, M. W., Fillerup, D. L., Veath, M. L., and Adams, K. (1971b). *In* "Lipid Storage Diseases" (J. Bernsohn and H. J. Grossman, eds.). Academic Press, New York.

Ohman, R. (1971a). *J. Neurochem.* **18**, 89.

Ohman, R. (1971b). *J. Neurochem.* **18**, 531.

Ohman, R., and Svennerholm, L. (1971). *J. Neurochem.* **18**, 79.

Ohman, R., Rosenberg, A., and Svennerholm, L. (1970). *Biochemistry* **9**, 3774.

Okada, S., and O'Brien, J. S. (1968). *Science* **160**, 1002.

Openshaw, H., and Bortz, W. M. (1968). *Diabetes* **17**, 80.

Ovsepyan, L. M., and Karagezyan, K. G. (1969). *Biol. Zh. Arm.* **22**, 49. [*Chem. Abstr.* **73**, 23105j (1970).]

Oyler, J. M., Jones, K. L., and Goetsch, D. D. (1970). *Amer. J. Vet. Res.* **31**, 1801.

Palmer, G. C., and Davenport, G. R. (1969). *Brain Res.* **13**, 394.

Pande, S. V., and Mead, J. F. (1968). *Biochim. Biophys. Acta* **152**, 636.

Paoletti, E. G. (1971). *Advan. Exp. Med. Biol.* **13**, 41.

Paoletti, R., and Davison, A. N., eds. (1971). "Chemistry and Brain Development," Proc. Advan. Study Inst. Chem. Brain Develop., Milan. Advan. Exp. Med. Biol., Vol. 13. Plenum, New York.

Paoletti, R., Paoletti, E. G., and Fumagalli, R. (1969). *In* "Handbook of Neurochemistry" (A. Lajtha, ed.), Vol. 1, p. 195. Plenum, New York.

Patrick, A. D., and Lake, B. D. (1969). *Nature* (*London*) **222**, 1067.

Peiffer, J. (1968). *Pathol. Eur.* **3**, 305.

Pfeifer, P. M., and Barnes, M. M. (1969). *Biochem. J.* **114**, 68P.

Philippart, M., Martin, L., Martin, J. J., and Menkes, J. H. (1969). *Arch. Neurol.* (*Chicago*) **20**, 227.

Piantadosi, C., and Snyder, F. (1970). *J. Pharm. Sci.* **59**, 283.

Pilz, A., and Jatzkewitz, A. (1968). *Pathol. Eur.* **3**, 409.

Pilz, H., and Muller, D. (1969). *J. Neurol. Sci.* **9**, 585.

Pilz, H., Sandhoff, K., and Jatzkewitz, H. (1966). *J. Neurochem.* **13**, 1273.

Pomazanskaya, L. F., Pravdina, N. I., and Zabelinskii, S. A. (1967). *Zh. Evol. Biokhim. Fiziol.* **3**, 3. [*Chem. Abstr.* **66**, 101937d (1967).]

Porcellati, G., Biasion, M. G., and Arienti, G. (1970a). *Lipids* **5**, 725.

Porcellati, G., Biasion, M. G., and Pirotta, M. (1970b). *Lipids* **5**, 734.

Porter, M. T., Fluharty, A. L., and Kihara, H. (1971). *Science* **172**, 1263.

Possmayer, F., Balakrishnan, G., and Strickland, K. P. (1968). *Biochim. Biophys. Acta* **164**, 79.

Pratt, J. H., Berry, J. F., Kaye, B., and Goetz, F. C. (1969). *Diabetes* **18**, 556.

Pravdina, N. I., and Chebotareva, M. A. (1971). *Zh. Evol. Biokhim. Fiziol.* **7**, 41. [*Chem. Abstr.* **74**, 107220b (1971).]

Prokhorova, M. I., Bespalova, M. A., Vinogradov, A. G., Zuber, V. L., Romanoff, L. J., Sokolova, G. P., Tumanova, Y. S., and Flerov, M. A. (1970). *Vses. Konf. Neirokhim. Nerv. Sist., Dokl., 5th, 1968* p. 259. [*Chem. Abstr.* **75**, 2276s (1971).]

Prottey, C., Salway, J. G., and Hawthorne, J. N. (1968). *Biochim. Biophys. Acta* **164**, 238.

Radin, N. S. (1970). *Chem. Phys. Lipids* **5**, 178.

Radin, N. S., Hof, L., Bradley, R. M., and Brady, R. O. (1969). *Brain Res.* **14**, 497.

Rahmann, H., and Korfsmeier, K. H. (1968). *Histochemie* **16**, 315.

Raine, D. N. (1969). *Lancet* **ii**, 959.

Ramsey, R. B. (1971). Ph.D Thesis, St. Louis Univ., St. Louis, Missouri.

Ramsey, R. B., Jones, J. P., Naqvi, S. H. M., and Nicholas, H. J. (1971a). *Lipids* **6**, 154.

Ramsey, R. B., Jones, J. P., Naqvi, S. H. M., and Nicholas, H. J. (1971b). *Lipids* **6**, 225.

Ramsey, R. B., Jones, J. P., and Nicholas, H. J. (1971c). *J. Neurochem.* **18**, 1485.

Ramsey, R. B., Jones, J. P., Rios, A., and Nicholas, H. J. (1971d). *J. Neurochem.* **19**, 101.

Ramsey, R. B., Aexel, R. T., and Nicholas, H. J. (1971e). *J. Biol. Chem.* **246**, 6393.

Ramsey, R. B., Aexel, R. T., and Nicholas, H. J. (1971f). *J. Neurochem.* **18**, 2245.

Ramsey, R. B., Aexel, R. T., Jones, J. P., and Nicholas, H. J. (1972). *J. Biol. Chem.* **247**, 3471.

Rao, K. S., and Pieringer, R. A. (1970). *J. Neurochem.* **17**, 483.

Rao, K. S., Wenger, D. A., and Pieringer, R. A. (1970). *J. Biol. Chem.* **245**, 2520.

Rapport, M. M. (1970). *In* "Handbook of Neurochemistry" (A. Lajtha, ed.), Vol. 3, p. 509. Plenum, New York.

Rawlins, F. A., Hedley-Whyte, E. T., Villegas, G., and Uzman, B. G. (1970). *Lab. Invest.* **22**, 237.

Reasor, M., and Kanfer, J. N. (1969). *Life Sci.* **8**, 1055.

Richter, R., and Dannenberg, H. (1969). *Hoppe-Seyler's Z. Physiol. Chem.* **350**, 1213.

Rilling, H. (1966). *J. Biol. Chem.* **241**, 3233.

Roots, B. I. (1968). *Comp. Biochem. Physiol.* **25**, 457.

Roozemond, R. C. (1970). *J. Neurochem.* **17**, 179.

Rose, S. P. R. (1965). *Nature (London)* **206**, 621.

Roseman, S. (1968). *In* "Cystic Fibrosis of the Pancreas," Proc. Int. Conf., 4th (E. Rossi and E. Stoll, eds.), Part II, p. 244. Karger, Basel.

Rosenberg, A. (1970). *In* "Handbook of Neurochemistry" (A. Lajtha, ed.), Vol. 3, p. 453. Plenum, New York.

Rossiter, R. J., and Strickland, K. P. (1970). *In* "Handbook of Neurochemistry" (A. Lajtha, ed.), Vol. 3, p. 467. Plenum, New York.

Rosso, P., Hormazabal, J., and Winick, M. (1970). *Amer. J. Clin. Nutr.* **23**, 1275.

Roukema, P. A., Van den Eijnden, D. H., Heijlman, D. H., and Van der Berg, G. (1970). *FEBS (Fed. Eur. Biochem. Soc.), Lett.* **9**, 267.

Rouser, G., Kritchevsky, G., Simon, G., and Nelson, G. J. (1967). *Lipids* **2**, 37.

Rouser, G., Yamamoto, A., and Kritchevsky, G. (1971). *In* "Chemistry and Brain Development," Proc. Advan. Study Inst. Chem. Brain Develop., Milan (R. Paoletti and A. N. Davison, eds.), Advan. Exp. Med. Biol., Vol. 13, p. 91. Plenum, New York.

Rumsby, M. G., and Rossiter, R. J. (1968). *J. Neurochem.* **15**, 1473.

Saifer, A., and Wishnow, D. E. (1970). *Handb. Clin. Neurol.* **10**, 265.

Salway, J. G., Harwood, J. L., Kai, M., White, G. L., and Hawthorne, J. N. (1968). *J. Neurochem.* **15**, 221.

Sanchez De Jimerez, E., and Cleland, W. W. (1969). *Biochim. Biophys. Acta* **76**, 685.

Sandhoff, K., Andreae, U., and Jatzkewitz, H. J. (1968). *Life Sci.* 7, 283.

Saxena, P. K. (1969). *Acta Anat.* 73, 569.

Scaravilli, F., and Tavolato, B. (1968). *Acta Neurol. Psychiat. Belg.* 68, 674.

Schengrund, C. L., and Rosenberg, A. (1970). *J. Biol. Chem.* 245, 6196.

Schengrund, C. L., and Rosenberg, A. (1971). *Biochemistry* 10, 2424.

Schettler, G., and Kahlke, W. (1967). *In* "Lipids and Lipidoses" (G. Schettler, ed.), p. 260. Springer-Verlag, Berlin and New York.

Schibanoff, J. M., Kamoshita, S., and O'Brien, J. S. (1969). *J. Lipid Res.* 10, 515.

Schimschock, J. R., Alvord, E. C., and Swanson, P. D. (1968). *Arch. Neurol. (Chicago)* 18, 688.

Schmid H. O., and Takahashi, T. (1970). *J. Lipid Res.* 11, 412.

Schneck, L., Adachi, M., and Volk, B. W. (1971). *Neurology* 21, 817.

Segal, W., and Wysocki, S. J. (1970). *Biochem. J.* 119, 43P.

Seiter, C. W., and McCluer, R. H. (1970). *J. Neurochem.* 17, 1525.

Shah, S. (1971). *J. Neurochem.* 18, 395.

Shah, S., Peterson, N. A., and McKean, C. M. (1968). *Biochim. Biophys. Acta* 164, 604.

Shah, S., Peterson, N. A., and McKean, C. M. (1970). *J. Neurochem.* 17, 279.

Sheltawy, A., and Dawson, R. M. C. (1969). *Biochem. J.* 111, 147.

Sherman, G., and Folch-Pi, J. (1970). *J. Neurochem.* 17, 597.

Skrbic, T. R., and Cumings, J. N. (1970). *J. Neurochem.* 17, 85.

Slagel, D. L., Dittmer, J. C., and Wilson, C. B. (1967). *J. Neurochem.* 14, 789.

Sloan, H. R. (1970). *Chem. Phys. Lipids* 5, 250.

Sloan, H. R., Uhlendorf, B. W., Jacobson, C. B., and Fredrickson, D. S. (1969). *Pediat. Res.* 3, 532.

Slotboom, A. J., and Bonsen, P. P. M. (1970). *Chem. Phys. Lipids* 5, 301.

Smirnov, A. A., and Chirkovskaya, E. V. (1969). *Tr. Vses. Konf. Biokhim. Nerv. Sist., 4th, 1966* p. 445. [*Chem. Abstr.* 74, 29904m (1971).]

Smith, M. E. (1967). *Advan. Lipid Res.* 5, 241.

Smith, M. E. (1968). *Biochim. Biophys. Acta* 164, 285.

Smith, M. E. (1969a). *J. Neurochem.* 16, 83.

Smith, M. E. (1969b). *J. Neurochem.* 16, 1099.

Smith, R. R., and White, H. B., Jr. (1968). *Arch. Neurol. (Chicago)* 19, 54.

Snyder, F., Rainey, W. T., Jr., Blank, M. L., and Christie, W. H. (1970a). *J. Biol. Chem.* 245, 5853.

Snyder, F., Malone, B., and Blank, M. L. (1970b). *J. Biol. Chem.* 245, 1790.

Snyder, F., Hibbs, M., and Malone, B. (1971). *Biochim. Biophys. Acta* 231, 409.

Soto, E. F., Pasquini, J. M., Placido, R., and LaTorre, J. L. (1969). *J. Chromatogr.* 41, 400.

Stahl, W. L., Sumi, S. M., and Swanson, P. D. (1971). *J. Neurochem.* 18, 403.

Stanacev, N. Z., Isaac, D. C., and Brookes, K. B. (1968). *Biochim. Biophys. Acta* 152, 806.

Stoffel, W. (1970). *Chem. Phys. Lipids* 5, 139.

Stoffel, W., and Lekim, D. (1971). *Hoppe-Seyler's Z. Physiol. Chem.* 352, 501.

Stoffel, W., Lekim, D., and Sticht, G. (1968). *Hoppe-Seyler's Z. Physiol. Chem.* 349, 1637.

Stoffel, W., Lekim, D., and Heyn, G. (1970). *Hoppe-Seyler's Z. Physiol. Chem.* 351, 875.

Stokes, W. M., Fish, W. A., and Hickey, F. C. (1956). *J. Biol. Chem.* 220, 415.

Sun, G. Y., and Horrocks, L. A. (1969a). *J. Neurochem.* 16, 181.

Sun, G. Y., and Horrocks, L. A. (1969b). *J. Lipid Res.* 10, 153.

Sun, G. Y., and Horrocks, L. A. (1970). *Lipids* **5**, 1006.

Suzuki, K. (1965). *J. Neurochem.* **12**, 969.

Suzuki, K. (1967). *J. Neurochem.* **14**, 917.

Suzuki, K. (1970). *J. Neurochem.* **17**, 209.

Suzuki, K., and Suzuki, Y. (1970). *Proc. Nat. Acad. Sci. U. S.* **66**, 302.

Suzuki, K., Poduslo, S. E., and Norton, W. T. (1967). *Biochim. Biophys. Acta* **144**, 375.

Suzuki, K., Poduslo, J. F., and Poduslo, S. E. (1968). *Biochim. Biophys. Acta* **152**, 576.

Suzuki, K., Suzuki, K., and Kamoshita, S. (1969). *J. Neuropathol. Exp. Neurol.* **28**, 25.

Suzuki, Y., and Suzuki, K. (1971). *Science* **171**, 73.

Suzuki, Y., Austin, J., Armstrong, D., Suzuki, K., Schlenker, J., and Fletcher, T. (1970). *Exp. Neurol.* **29**, 65.

Suzuki, Y., Crocker, A. C., and Suzuki, K. (1971a). *Arch. Neurol. (Chicago)* **24**, 58.

Suzuki, Y., Jacob, J. C., Suzuki, K., Kutty, K. M., and Suzuki, K. (1971b). *Neurology* **21**, 313.

Svennerholm, L. (1962). *Biochem. Biophys. Res. Commun.* **9**, 436.

Svennerholm, L. (1964). *J. Neurochem.* **11**, 839.

Svennerholm, L. (1968). *J. Lipid Res.* **9**, 570.

Svennerholm, L. (1970a). *In* "Lipid Metabolism" (M. Florkin and E. H. Stotz, eds.), Comprehensive Biochemistry, Vol. 18, p. 201. Elsevier, Amsterdam.

Svennerholm, L. (1970b). *In* "Handbook of Neurochemistry" (A. Lajtha, ed.), Vol. 3, p. 425. Plenum, New York.

Swartz, J. G., and Mitchell, J. E. (1970). *J. Lipid Res.* **11**, 544.

Sweeley, C. C., ed. (1970). "Chemistry and Metabolism of Sphingolipids" (Int. Symp.), A Collection of Papers, Dedicated to Dr. H. E. Carter, in Chemistry and Physics of Lipids, Vol. 5, No. 1.

Sweeley, C. C., and Klionsky, B. (1963). *J. Biol. Chem.* **238**, 3148.

Szepsenwol, J. (1969). *Pathol. Microbiol.* **34**, 1.

Tabakoff, B., and Erwin, V. G. (1970). *J. Biol. Chem.* **245**, 3263.

Taketomi, T., and Kawamura, N. (1969). *J. Biochem. (Tokyo)* **66**, 165.

Tamai, Y. (1968). *Jap. J. Exp. Med.* **38**, 65.

Tamai, Y., Matsukawa, S., and Satake, M. (1971). *Brain Res.* **26**, 149.

Taori, G. M., Mathew, N. T., Bhaktaviziam, A., and Bachhawat, B. K. (1969). *Indian J. Med. Res.* **57**, 5.

Tesoriero, G., Vento, R., and Cacioppo, F. (1970). *Ital. J. Biochem.* **19**, 155. [*Chem. Abstr.* **74**, 40056g (1971).]

Tettamanti, G. (1971). *Advan. Exp. Med. Biol.* **13**, 75.

Tettamanti, G., and Zambotti, V. (1968). *Enzymologia* **31**, 61.

Thompson, G. A., Jr. (1968). *Biochim. Biophys. Acta* **152**, 409.

Thompson, G. A., Jr. (1970). *In* "Lipid Biochemistry" (M. Florkin and E. H. Stotz, eds.), Comprehensive Biochemistry, Vol. 18, p. 157. Elsevier, Amsterdam.

Thompson, W. (1969). *Biochim. Biophys. Acta* **187**, 150.

Tichy, J. (1967). *J. Neurochem.* **14**, 555.

Tipton, K. F., and Dawson, A. P. (1968). *Biochem. J.* **168**, 95.

Turchetto, E., and Borri, P. F. (1969). *Nutr. Dieta* **11**, 34.

Uda, Y., Yanagawa, N., and Nakazawa, Y. (1969). *Bull. Tokyo Med. Dent. Univ.* **16**, 211.

van Hoof, F., and Hevs, H. G. (1968). *Eur. J. Biochem.* **7**, 34.

Vanier, M. T., Holm, M., Ohman, R., and Svennerholm, L. (1971). *J. Neurochem.* 18, 581.

van Lier, J. E., and Smith, L. L. (1967). *Biochemistry* 6, 3269.

van Lier, J. E., and Smith, L. L. (1969). *Tex. Rep. Biol. Med.* 27, 167.

van Lier, J. E., and Smith, L. L. (1971). *Lipids* 6, 85.

Vasan, N. S., Abraham, J., and Bachhawat, B. K. (1971). *J. Neurochem.* 18, 59.

Vidrine, W., Martin, C. M., and Nicholas, H. J. (1971). Unpublished observations.

Walker, B. L. (1968). *J. Nutr.* 94, 469.

Walker, C. O., McCandless, D. W., McGarry, J. D., and Schenker, S. (1970). *J. Lab. Clin. Med.* 76, 569.

Wang, J. H. (1970). *Proc. Nat. Acad. Sci. U. S.* 67, 916.

Warner, H. R., and Lands, W. E. M. (1963). *J. Amer. Chem. Soc.* 85, 60.

Webster, G. R. (1970). *Biochem. J.* 117, 10P.

Webster, G. R., and Cooper, M. F. (1968). *J. Neurochem.* 15, 795.

Weiss, J. F., Galli, G., and Grossi-Paoletti, E. (1968). *J. Neurochem.* 15, 563.

Wenger, D. A., Petitpas, J. W., and Pieringer, R. A. (1968). *Biochemistry* 7, 3700.

Wenger, D. A., Rao, K. S., Pieringer, R. A., and Petitpas, J. W. (1970). *J. Biol. Chem.* 245, 2513.

White, H. B., Jr., Galli, C., and Paoletti, R. (1971). *J. Neurochem.* 18, 869.

Weigandt, H. (1968). *Angew. Chem. Int. Ed.* 7, 87.

Winick, M. (1970a). *Amer. J. Dis. Child.* 120, 416.

Winick, M. (1970b). *Med. Clin. N. Amer.* 54, 1413.

Winick, M., and Rosso, P. (1969). *Pediatria (Santiago)* 12, 159.

Witting, L. A. (1967). *Lipids* 2, 109.

Witting, L. A., and Horwitt, M. K. (1967). *Lipids* 2, 89.

Wolfe, L. S., Callahan, S. J., Fawcett, J. S., Andermann, F., and Scriver, C. R. (1970). *Neurology* 20, 23.

Wood, R., and Healy, K. (1970). *J. Biol. Chem.* 245, 2640.

Wykle, R. L., and Snyder, F. (1970). *J. Biol. Chem.* 245, 3047.

Wykle, R. L., Blank, M. L., and Snyder, F. (1970). *FEBS (Fed. Eur. Biochem. Soc.), Lett.* 12, 57.

Yanagihara, Y., Salway, J. G., and Hawthorne, J. N. (1969). *J. Neurochem.* 16, 1133.

Yagihara, T., and Cumings, J. N. (1968). *Trans. Amer. Neurol. Ass.* 93, 51.

Yatsu, F. M. (1971). *Calif. Med.* 114, 1.

Yatsu, F. M., and Moss, S. (1970). *Nature (London)* 227, 1132.

Yavin, E., and Gatt, S. (1969). *Biochemistry* 8, 1692.

Yip, G. B., and Dain, J. A. (1970). *Biochim. Biophys. Acta* 206, 252.

Zahler, W. L., and Cleland, W. W. (1969). *Biochim. Biophys. Acta* 176, 699.

Zeman, W. (1969). *Lipids* 4, 76.

Enzymatic Systems That Synthesize and Degrade Glycerolipids Possessing Ether Bonds[1]

FRED SNYDER

Medical Division, Oak Ridge Associated Universities,
Oak Ridge, Tennessee

I. Introduction

Ether bonds in glycerolipids were first detected in biological materials during the first quarter of this century. The O-alkyl linkage ($R'OCH_2CH_2R$, where R' represents glycerol) was initially found in marine organisms, whereas the O-alk-1-enyl linkage[2] ($R'OCH=CHR$, where R' represents glycerol) was first detected in mammalian cells.

[1] Supported in part by the U. S. Atomic Energy Commission, Grant E-596B from the American Cancer Society, and Grant CA 11949.02 from the National Institutes of Health.

[2] Lipids containing this type of ether linkage are called plasmalogens.

Section II discusses the nomenclature and illustrates the structures of known O-alkyl and O-alk-1-enyl lipid classes that are of biological interest. Much of the earlier research on ether lipids was devoted to investigating the chemical structure of the O-alkyl and O-alk-1-enyl moieties and determining their occurrence as specific lipid classes in biological materials. The chemical structure of the two basic types of ether linkages is now firmly established and their distribution in nature is known to be widespread since they exist to some extent in most cells of the animal and plant kingdom. Review articles have covered the subject of ether-linked lipids from a number of viewpoints (Bodman and Maisin, 1958; Rapport and Norton, 1962; Klenk and Debuch, 1963; Mangold and Baumann, 1967; Hartree, 1964; Goldfine, 1968; Snyder, 1969, 1971; Thompson and Kapoulas, 1969; Piantadosi and Snyder, 1970); and a recent book (edited by Snyder, 1972a) entitled *Ether Lipids: Chemistry and Biology* provides a detailed account of the literature on the history, chemistry, analyses, metabolism, and biology of these compounds through 1970.

Tsujimoto and Toyama (1922) are generally given credit for the discovery of O-alkyl lipids; however, as pointed out by Debuch (1972), it appears that the substance ("astrol") isolated from starfish by Dorée (1909) and Kossel and Edlbacher (1915) was an alkylglycerol. The O-alkyl moiety is at the 1-position (Davies *et al.*, 1933) of glycerol in both "neutral lipids" and phospholipids; alkyl diol lipids (dialkoxypentane) also occur naturally (Varanasi and Malins, 1969).

Feulgen and Voit's (1924) histological studies were the first account of plasmalogens that appeared in the literature. After many years of research by numerous investigators, Rapport and co-workers (Rapport *et al.*, 1957; Rapport and Franzl, 1957) proved that the unique properties of plasmalogens were due to an O-alk-1-enyl moiety. The O-alk-1-enyl moiety is located at position 1 of the glycerol portion of the molecule (Klenk and Debuch, 1954; Marinetti and Erbland, 1957; Marinetti *et al.*, 1959; Debuch, 1959a,b), and the double bond has a *cis* configuration in both the polar (Norton *et al.*, 1962; Warner and Lands, 1961; Cymerman Craig *et al.*, 1966) and nonpolar plasmalogens (Schmid *et al.*, 1967a,b). In most tissues, plasmalogens exist mainly as alk-1-enylacylglycero-3-phosphorylethanolamine; however, other phospholipid classes and neutral lipids ("neutral plasmalogens") are known to contain the O-alk-1-enyl moiety (see review by Snyder, 1969). Alk-1-enyl ethylene-glycol lipids and related diols have also been detected in nature (see review by Bergelson, 1969).

In this chapter, I have attempted to summarize conclusions drawn from enzyme studies on the biosynthesis and degradation of alkyl and alk-1-enyl bonds in glycerolipids and their precursors; *in vivo* results and chemical syntheses are discussed only where they have provided new insights on possible reaction mechanisms. At the present time, the function of the ether-linked lipids in biological systems is unknown, although their structural role in membranes, especially surface membranes, has become apparent in a number of investigations (Pfleger *et al.*, 1968; Cotman *et al.*, 1969; Nozawa and Thompson, 1971; Kleinig *et al.*, 1971).

II. Nomenclature and Structural Formulas

A. GENERAL

Chromatographic isolation procedures and subsequent identifications in biochemical investigations, as well as chemical syntheses, have led to the discovery of a large number of distinct ether-linked lipid classes. Those lipid classes that contain ether bonds are generally structural analogs of the well-established acylated lipid classes. The terms alkyl and alk-1-enyl specify the nature of the ether linkage with respect to carbon atoms 1 (α) and 2 (β) of the aliphatic moiety attached to glycerol or glycol. These terms are not intended to reflect any other characteristic of the aliphatic moiety such as unsaturation or substituted groupings. Ether lipids that contain only a single alkyl or alk-1-enyl moiety have it located at the *sn*-1 position of glycerolipids. Dialkyl glycerolipids have been found in extremely halophilic microorganisms (Kates, 1972), whereas trialkylglycerols have only been synthesized in the organic laboratory (Baumann, 1972). No one has described di- or tri-alk-1-enyl glycerolipids from any source. Although 2-alkylglycerols have not been found in nature, they do serve as useful models in assessing the acylglycerol (monoglyceride) pathway that leads to the synthesis of triacylglycerols. S-Alkyl glycerolipids have been isolated from bovine heart tissue (Ferrell and Radloff, 1970) and their metabolism has been investigated in rats (Snyder *et al.*, 1969c); however, nothing is yet known about the mechanisms responsible for the biosynthesis or breakdown of the S-alkyl lipids.

The nomenclature of lipids as proposed by the Commission on Biochemical Nomenclature, sponsored by the International Union of Pure and Applied Chemistry and the International Union of Biochemistry (IUPAC-IUB, 1967), suggests rules for the naming of ether-linked glycerolipids. The general names used throughout this chapter reflect the recommended usage, except that for simplicity stereospecific (*sn*) numbering has not been used; in this article, unless otherwise stated, the prefixes represent the order of substituents at the three different positions of glycerol, i.e., the first prefix indicates the substituent at carbon position 1, the second prefix indicates the substituent at carbon position 2, and the third prefix indicates the substituent at carbon position 3. For example, alkylacylglycerylphosphorylcholine specifically indicates 1-alkyl-2-acyl-*sn*-glycero-3-phosphorylcholine. As proposed in the IUPAC-IUB rules, the prefix "*O*" has been omitted when the ether moiety is clearly on glycerol. Therefore, in this chapter, the *O* has only been retained to specify oxygen ether linkages for terms such as *O*-alkyl lipids or *O*-alk-1-enyl lipids where a term such as lipid does not necessarily imply glycerolipid. The structural formulas of ether-lipids illustrated in this section (Parts B, C, and D) introduce the reader to the various types of *O*-alkyl and *O*-alk-1-enyl lipid classes encountered in the field of biology.

B. Major Ether-Linked Lipids Isolated from Biological Materials

$$H_2C-OCH_2CH_2R$$
$$\underset{\displaystyle RCOCH}{\overset{\displaystyle O}{\underset{\|}{}}} |$$
$$\underset{H_2COCR}{\overset{O}{\underset{\|}{}}} |$$

Alkyldiacylglycerol

(1)

$$H_2C-OCH=CHR$$
$$\underset{\displaystyle RCOCH}{\overset{\displaystyle O}{\underset{\|}{}}} |$$
$$\underset{H_2COCR}{\overset{O}{\underset{\|}{}}} |$$

Alk-1-enyldiacylglycerol

(2)

$$H_2C-OCH_2CH_2R$$
$$\underset{\displaystyle RCOCH}{\overset{\displaystyle O}{\underset{\|}{}}} |$$
$$H_2CO-\underset{OH}{\overset{O}{\underset{|}{\overset{\|}{P}}}}-O\text{-base}$$

(base = choline, ethanolamine, or serine)

Alkylacylglycero-
phosphorylcholine

Alkylacylglycero-
phosphorylethanolamine

Alkylacylglycero-
phosphorylserine

(3)

$$H_2C-OCH=CHR$$
$$\underset{\displaystyle RCOCH}{\overset{\displaystyle O}{\underset{\|}{}}} |$$
$$H_2CO-\underset{OH}{\overset{O}{\underset{|}{\overset{\|}{P}}}}-O\text{-base}$$

(base = choline, ethanolamine, or serine)

Alk-1-enylacylglycero-
phosphorylcholine

Alk-1-enylacylglycero-
phosphorylethanolamine

Alk-1-enylacylglycero-
phosphorylserine

(4)

Chemical and chromatographic analysis of the complex lipids requires that the ester groupings be removed and this can be effectively done by

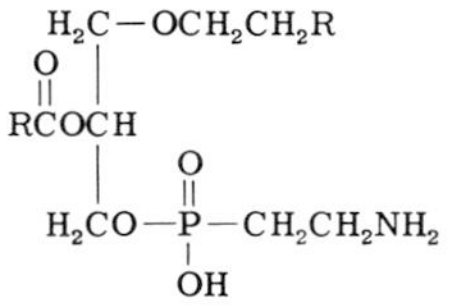

H₂C—OCH₂CH₂R
$$\underset{\text{O}}{\underset{\|}{\text{RCOCH}}}$$
| O
| ||
H₂CO—P—CH₂CH₂NH₂
|
OH

Alkylacylglycero-
phosphonoethanolamine

(5)

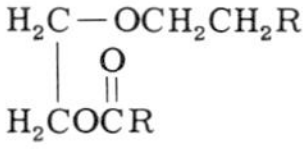

H₂C—OCH₂CH₂R
| O
| ||
H₂COCR

Alkylacyl-
ethyleneglycol

(6)

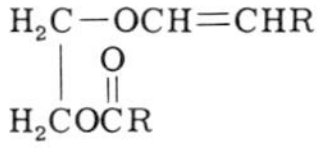

H₂C—OCH=CHR
| O
| ||
H₂COCR

Alk-1-enylacyl-
ethyleneglycol

(7)

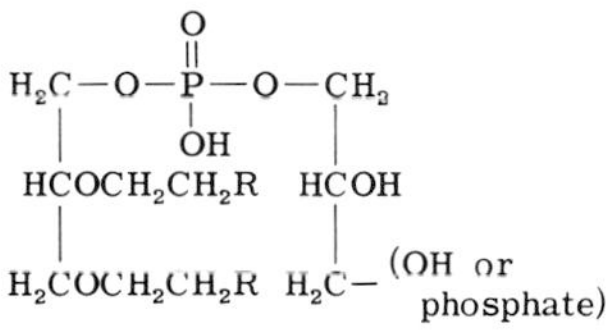

O
||
H₂C—O—P—O—CH₂
| | |
| OH |
HCOCH₂CH₂R HCOH
| |
| (OH or
H₂COCH₂CH₂R H₂C— phosphate)

Dialkylglycerophosphoryl-
glycerophosphate

Dialkylglycerophosphorylglycerol

(8)

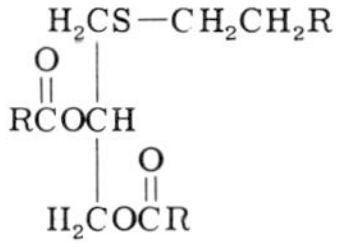

H₂CS—CH₂CH₂R
$$\underset{\text{O}}{\underset{\|}{\text{RCOCH}}}$$
| O
| ||
H₂COCR

S-Alkyldiacylglycerol

(9)

using reducing agents such as LiAlH₄ or NaAlH₂(OCH₂CH₂OCH₃)₂, which do not affect the ether linkages or the unsaturation in the ether-linked aliphatic moiety. The acyl moieties are converted to fatty alcohols, and the phosphorylbase esters are freed by the reducing agents. For example, reduction of lipids with formulas (1–5) yields alkylglycerols (10) and alk-1-enylglycerols (11). The common names for the alkylglycerols (formula 10) are based on the source of fish oils from which they were isolated and are mainly of historical importance, al-

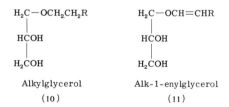

H₂C—OCH₂CH₂R
|
HCOH
|
H₂COH

Alkylglycerol

(10)

H₂C—OCH=CHR
|
HCOH
|
H₂COH

Alk-1-enylglycerol

(11)

though they are often still used by many investigators in this field: Chimyl alcohol possesses a 16:0 *O*-alkyl moiety, batyl alcohol possesses an 18:0 *O*-alkyl moiety, and selachyl alcohol possesses an 18:1 *O*-alkyl moiety. Although the free alkylglycerols are derived from more complex naturally occurring lipids, it will be seen later that these compounds can also be formed *in vitro* under certain conditions.

C. Ether-Linked Intermediates Isolated from Enzymatic Systems

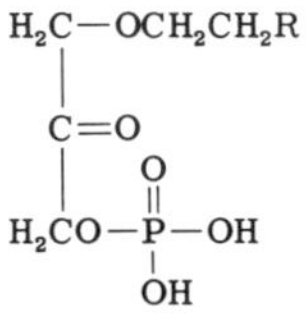

$H_2C-OCH_2CH_2R$
|
$C=O$
| O
| ‖
$H_2CO-P-OH$
|
OH

Alkyldihydroxy-
acetone-P

(12)

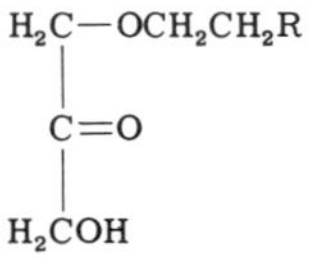

$H_2C-OCH_2CH_2R$
|
$C=O$
|
H_2COH

Alkyldihydroxy-
acetone

(13)

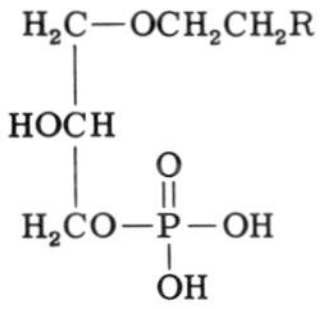

$H_2C-OCH_2CH_2R$
|
$HOCH$
| O
| ‖
$H_2CO-P-OH$
|
OH

Alkylglycerophosphate

(14)

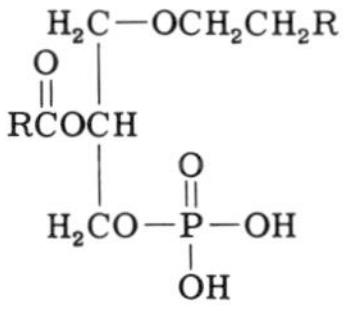

$H_2C-OCH_2CH_2R$
O |
‖
$RCOCH$
| O
| ‖
$H_2CO-P-OH$
|
OH

Alkylacyl-
glycerophosphate

(15)

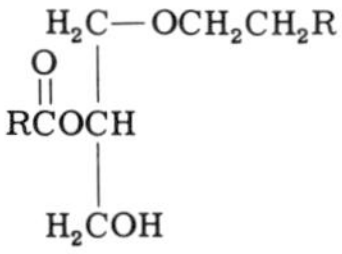

$H_2C-OCH_2CH_2R$
O |
‖
$RCOCH$
|
H_2COH

Alkylacylglycerol

(16)

D. Miscellaneous Ether-Linked Lipids

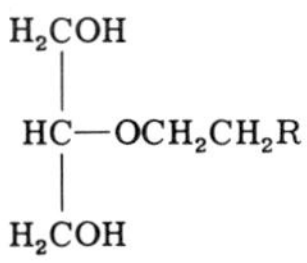

H_2COH
|
$HC-OCH_2CH_2R$
|
H_2COH

2-Alkylglycerol

(17)

$H_2C-OCH=CHR$
O |
‖
$RCOCH$
|
H_2COH

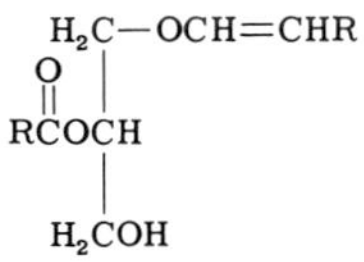

Alk-1-enylacyl-
glycerol

(18)

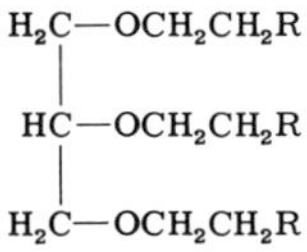

$H_2C-OCH_2CH_2R$
|
$HC-OCH_2CH_2R$
|
$H_2C-OCH_2CH_2R$

Trialkylglycerol

(19)

$H_2C-OCH_2CH_2R$
|
$HC-OCH_2CH_2R$
|
H_2COH

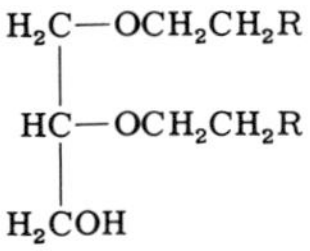

Dialkylglycerol

(20)

The *O*-alk-1-enyl analogs of formulas (**20–22**) are also of potential bio-logical significance; however, neither the *O*-alkyl nor *O*-alk-1-enyl glyc-erolipids of this type have been documented in living cells.

H₂C—OCH₂CH₂R

C=O
$$\underset{OH}{H_2CO-\overset{\overset{\displaystyle O}{\|}}{P}-O\text{-base}}$$
(base = choline, ethanolamine, or serine)

1-*O*-Alkyl-3-*O*-phosphoryl-choline-2-propanone

1-*O*-Alkyl-3-*O*-phosphoryl-ethanolamine-2-propanone

1-*O*-Alkyl-3-*O*-phosphoryl-serine-2-propanone

(21)

H₂C—OCH₂CH₂R

HCOH
$$\underset{OH}{H_2CO-\overset{\overset{\displaystyle O}{\|}}{P}-O\text{-base}}$$
(base = choline, ethanolamine, or serine)

Alkylglycerophosphoryl-choline (alkyl-GPC)

Alkylglycerophosphoryl-ethanolamine (alkyl-GPE)

Alkylglycerophosphoryl-serine (alkyl-GPS)

(22)

III. Methods of Analysis

Abbreviated flow diagrams of methods that our laboratory has successfully used to identify alkyl glycerolipids (Fig. 1) and alk-1-enyl glycerolipids (Fig. 2) illustrate some of the important chemical reactions available for the analyses of minute quantities of labeled products formed in metabolic studies. More extensive treatment of this subject can be

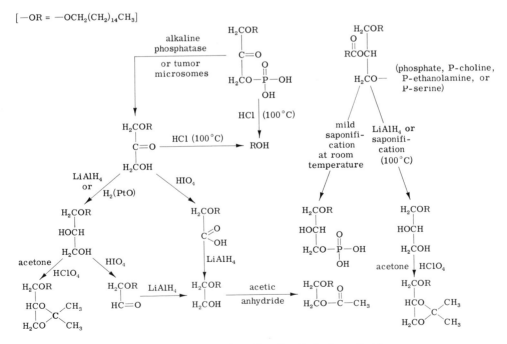

FIG. 1. Reactions used to identify alkyl glycerolipids.

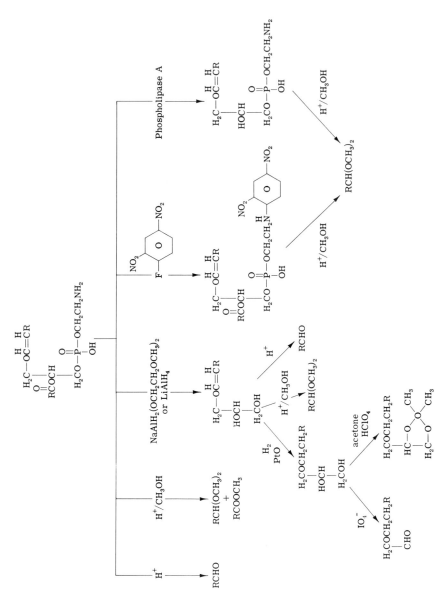

Fig. 2. Reactions used to identify plasmalogens (alk-1-enyl glycerolipids).

found in a number of articles that specifically review chemical, physical, and chromatographic methods applicable to the analysis of ether-linked lipids (Thompson and Kapoulas, 1969; Snyder, 1971; Piantadosi and Snyder, 1970; Hanahan, 1972; Horrocks, 1972). Several investigators have also reviewed the literature on the chemical syntheses of ether-linked lipids (Piantadosi and Snyder, 1970; Baumann, 1972; Gigg, 1972; Kates, 1972; Piantadosi, 1972a,b).

IV. Biosynthesis

A. FORMATION OF ETHER-LINKED PRECURSORS

1. *Formation of Fatty Alcohols*

Fatty alcohols are synthesized by enzymes that reduce fatty acids and fatty aldehydes. Reductases of this type have been detected in normal rat liver (Tietz *et al.*, 1964; Pfleger *et al.*, 1967; Stoffel *et al.*, 1970), in tumors (Snyder and Malone, 1970), in brain (Tabakoff and Erwin, 1970), in *Euglena gracilis* (Kolattukudy, 1970), and in *Clostridium butyricum* (Day *et al.*, 1970); the reductases have been reported to occur in the soluble and particulate fractions of cells. Interconversions of the aliphatic moieties can be depicted according to the following overall reaction:

$$RCOSCoA \leftrightarrow RCHO \leftrightarrow ROH$$

Formation of the acyl-CoA complex appears to be the only activation step required.

The specificity for NADPH (see footnote 3) or NADH and their oxidized forms in these reactions and the subcellular localization of the reductases vary according to the enzyme source. In *Euglena* and bacteria, specificity for NADH was reported, although NADPH appeared to partially substitute for NADH in the reduction of the aldehyde to alcohol in *Euglena*. In mammalian systems, NADPH was specifically required for the reductases associated with the conversion of the aldehyde to alcohol in brain and with the conversion of acid to alcohol in tumors; however, a slight synergistic effect of NADPH plus NADH was observed in the tumor preparation. Stoffel *et al.* (1970) reported that the aldehyde reductase from rat liver could utilize either NADH or NADPH. The

[3] Abbreviations used in this chapter: CoA, coenzyme A; ATP, adenosine-5′-triphosphate; NADP+, nicotinamide adenine dinucleotide phosphate; NADPH, reduced nicotinamide adenine dinucleotide phosphate; NAD+, nicotinamide adenine dinucleotide; NADH, reduced nicotinamide adenine dinucleotide; CDP, cytidine diphosphate.

specificity of nucleotides for the oxidative steps has not been studied to the same extent as for the reductive steps, but at least in preputial gland tumors (Snyder and Malone, 1970) and Ehrlich ascites cells (Snyder et al., 1971a) the oxidative reactions appear to be strictly NAD-linked.

2. Dihydroxyacetone Phosphate and Acyldihydroxyacetone Phosphate

The glycerol portion of ether-linked lipids is derived from dihydroxy-acetone-P, which is formed via the normal glycolytic pathway. The reader is referred to any good biochemistry text for an appropriate discussion of these pathways and their significance. The triose phosphate isomerase that catalyzes the reaction between dihydroxyacetone-P and glyceraldehyde-3-P can be difficult to deal with in studies designed to ascertain precursors of the "glycerol" moiety of lipid molecules. For example, equilibrium favors dihydroxyacetone-P by 96 to 4, yet higher concentrations of glyceraldehyde-3-P than of dihydroxyacetone-P occur in Ehrlich ascites cells (Garfinkel and Hess, 1964). Potent inhibitors [1-hydroxy-3-chloro-2-propanone synthesized by Hartman (1968, 1970) and glycidol phosphate synthesized by Rose and O'Connell (1969)] of the triose-P isomerase that have been used in investigations of the active site of triose-P isomerase can also be important tools in studies of "glycerol" sources in lipid metabolism (Wykle and Snyder, 1969, 1970; Snyder et al., 1970a); 1-hydroxy-3-chloro-2-propanone completely inhibits the isomerase without any effect on the enzymes that are responsible for synthesis of the ether bond in glycerolipids.

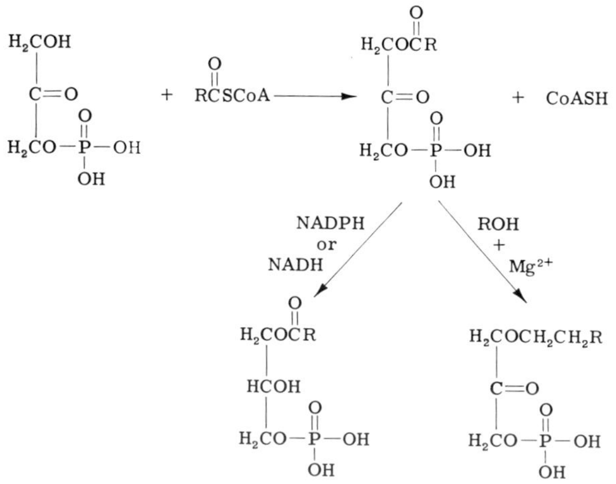

FIG. 3. Biosynthesis of acyldihydroxyacetone-P and alkyldihydroxyacetone-P.

Subsequent results by Hajra (1970) demonstrated that acyldihydroxy-acetone-P served as an immediate precursor of alkyldihydroxyacetone-P, a reaction that will be discussed in the following Part B of this section. Acyldihydroxyacetone-P can be formed by acylation of dihydroxyace-tone-P (Hajra and Agranoff, 1968a) as depicted in Fig. 3.

Hajra and Agranoff (1968b) have reported that reduction of the ke-tone group of acyldihydroxyacetone-P in liver mitochondria from guinea pigs is catalyzed by an NADPH specific-linked reductase, whereas Rao *et al.* (1970), Wykle *et al.* (1972b), and Grigor and Snyder (1971) have found that in other tissue preparations both NADH and NADPH can serve as hydrogen donors; however, the reductase requires higher levels of NADH.

B. FORMATION OF ETHER BONDS

1. *Alkyl Bonds*

In 1968, our laboratory discovered a cell-free system in which the *O*-alkyl bonds were derived from hexadecanol (Snyder *et al.*, 1969a); in this system CoA, ATP, and Mg^{++} were required as cofactors. A subse-quent study with subcellular fractions demonstrated that glyceraldehyde-3-P could serve as the precursor of the glycerol portion of *O*-alkyl lipids when the microsomal fraction was the sole source of the enzyme (Snyder *et al.*, 1969d). However, we later found that even extensively washed microsomes contained triose-P isomerase (Snyder *et al.*, 1970e), and that glyceraldehyde-3-P or dihydroxyacetone-P served equally well as precursors of alkyl glycerolipids. The problem was finally resolved by using a triose-P isomerase inhibitor (Wykle and Snyder, 1969, 1970; Snyder *et al.*, 1970a), kinetic studies (Hajra, 1969), and glycerophos-phate dehydrogenase (Hajra, 1969); these investigations clearly demon-strated that only dihydroxyacetone-P could serve as the triose phosphate precursor.

Hajra (1970) was able to explain the dihydroxyacetone-P, CoA, ATP, and Mg^{++} requirements by demonstrating that acyldihydroxyacetone-P could substitute for these components. This observation indicated that the alkyl ether bond is formed by exchange of the acyl group of acyldi-hydroxyacetone-P and free long-chain fatty alcohols (Hajra, 1970; Wykle *et al.*, 1972b). The exchange reaction depicted in Fig. 3 indicates that Mg^{++} ions are required, but it is not well documented. The first detect-able product in this reaction (alkyldihydroxyacetone-P) can be dephos-phorylated to alkyldihydroxyacetone (see Section V,B,2), and the ketone group of both *O*-alkyl lipids can be reduced by a microsomal reductase (see Section IV,C).

In experiments using double labeling techniques, Wykle and Snyder (1970) demonstrated that [14]C- or ^{3}H-labeled fatty alcohols and [14]C- or ^{32}P-labeled dihydroxyacetone-P were incorporated into alkyldihydroxy-acetone-P in a 1:1 molar ratio; similar studies have been done with 2-^{3}H-dihydroxyacetone-P as a substrate (Wykle, 1970) (Fig. 4). Both the oxygen (Snyder *et al.*, 1970c) and the hydrogen (Wykle and Snyder, 1970) atoms on carbon atom number 1 of 1-^{14}C-1-^{3}H-hexadecanol or ^{18}O-hexadecanol are retained in the O-alkyl moiety formed.

Identification of the ketone-containing alkyl glycerolipids has been documented by chemical and chromatographic techniques of identification (Snyder *et al.*, 1970a,b; Wykle and Snyder, 1970) as summarized in Fig. 1 or by the chemical synthesis (Piantadosi *et al.*, 1970, 1971) that is depicted in Fig. 5. O-Alkyl ketone analogs of choline and ethanolamine phospholipids have not yet been detected in biological systems, but they have been synthesized in the organic laboratory (Piantadosi *et al.*, 1972).

Although the exchange mechanism for formation of the O-alkyl linkage in glycerolipids is not fully understood, it should be noted that Murooka *et al.* (1970) have described a similar type reaction in an investigation of the mechanism responsible for alkylation of homoserine in *Corynebacterium acetophilum* as illustrated in the reaction:

$$HOCH_2CH_2CHNH_2COOH + CH_3COSCoA \rightarrow CH_3\overset{\overset{\displaystyle O}{\|}}{C}OCH_2CH_2CHNH_2COOH \xrightarrow{CH_3OH}$$
$$CH_3OCH_2CH_2CHNH_2COOH$$

Enzymatic systems that synthesize the O-alkyl bond in glycerolipids via the fatty alcohol-acyldihydroxyacetone-P system have been detected in preputial gland tumors (Snyder *et al.*, 1969a,d, 1970a,b,c,d), in Ehrlich ascites cells (Wykle and Snyder, 1970), in brain (Hajra, 1969, 1970; Snyder *et al.*, 1971b), in liver (Hajra, 1969, 1970; Snyder *et al.*, 1971b), in human leukemic cells (Snyder *et al.*, 1971c), in L-M fibroblasts grown

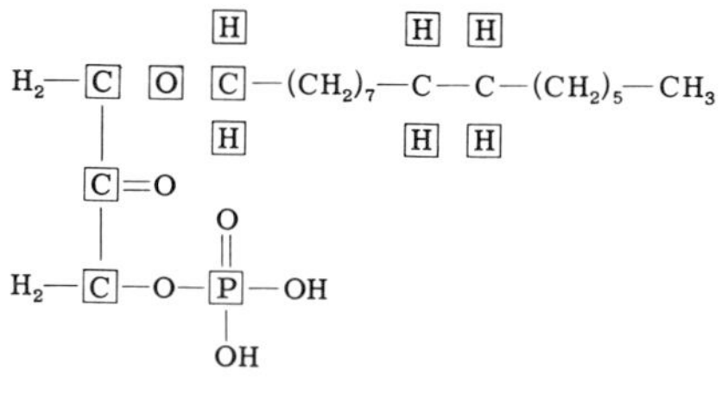

FIG. 4. Labeling of alkyldihydroxyacetone-P by [14]C- and ^{32}P-labeled dihydroxy-acetone-P and 1-[14]C-, 1-[3]H-, 9,10-^{3}H, and ^{18}O-hexadecanol. The atoms in boxes show the location of label in the product synthesized by microsomes from tumor cells.

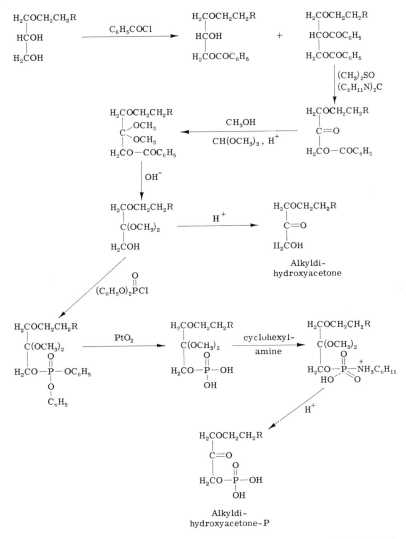

FIG. 5. The chemical synthesis of alkyldihydroxyacetone and alkyldihydroxy-acetone-P. (See Piantadosi *et al.*, 1971, for details.)

as suspension cultures (Snyder *et al.*, 1970e), in starfish (Snyder *et al.*, 1969b), in *Tetrahymena* (Kapoulas and Thompson, 1969), and in dog-fish liver (Malins and Sargent, 1971). At the present time, the most active enzymatic preparations have been derived from neoplastic cells and starfish, both also rich sources of alkyl glycerolipids.

2. Alk-1-enyl Bonds

A number of *in vivo* investigations [see chapter by Snyder (1972b) for references] have provided strong evidence for Thompson's (1968) concept that an O-alkyl moiety can be transformed to an O-alk-1-enyl moiety in glycerolipids. Recently, our laboratory described an enzyme system that can catalyze such a conversion. The key to the exploration of substrates and cofactors required for plasmalogen biosynthesis was provided when we were able to prepare a cell-free system from Ehrlich ascites cells that synthesized O-alk-1-enyl bonds in glycerolipids (Wykle *et al.*, 1970; Snyder *et al.*, 1971a). The system contained the same substrates (fatty alcohols and dihydroxyacetone-P) and cofactors (CoA, ATP, and Mg^{++}) as required for the synthesis of O-alkyl bonds, but in addition required $NADP^+$ or NAD^+. The only other difference in the two systems was that microsomes alone were needed for the biosynthesis of alkyl glycerolipids, whereas both microsomal and soluble fractions were needed for the biosynthesis of alk-1-enyl glycerolipids. More recent data have demonstrated that the NADP (or NAD) is reduced by enzymes in the soluble fraction (Wykle *et al.*, 1972a). Similar results were obtained when homogenates of preputial gland tumors were used.

U-^{14}C-Labeled dihydroxyacetone-P and 9,10-^{3}H-hexadecanol were incorporated into the alkylglycerols and the alk-1-enylglycerols isolated from the enzymatic products after $LiAlH_4$ reduction; the molar ratios of $^3H/^{14}C$ in both classes of ether-linked glycerolipids were identical, indicating that they were synthesized from the same precursors. In addition, fatty acids and fatty aldehydes did not serve as substrates for the synthesis of ethanolamine plasmalogens (Snyder *et al.*, 1971a).

In subsequent experiments, we prepared alkylacylglycerol-P as a substrate containing ^{3}H in the 9,10-position of the O-alkyl moiety and U-^{14}C- in the glycerol portion. This doubly labeled substrate was incorporated, in the absence of CoA, into alk-1-enylacylglycerylphosphorylethanolamine without any alteration in the $^3H/^{14}C$ ratio. These data represent the first enzymatic evidence for a direct conversion of an O-alkyl group to an O-alk-1-enyl group on a glycerolipid molecule. Other results that showed ethanolamine plasmalogen biosynthesis was stimulated by CDP-ethanolamine (Wykle *et al.*, 1971) suggest that the transformation of an O-alkyl linkage to an O-alk-1-enyl linkage occurs directly on alkylacylglycerylphosphorylethanolamine.

Recent investigations have indicated that a mixed-function oxidase is responsible for the biosynthesis of plasmalogens in tumor (Wykle *et al.*, 1972a; Snyder *et al.*, 1972), brain (Blank *et al.*, 1972), and intestinal (Paltauf, 1972) preparations, and that 1-alkyl-2-acyl-*sn*-glycero-3-

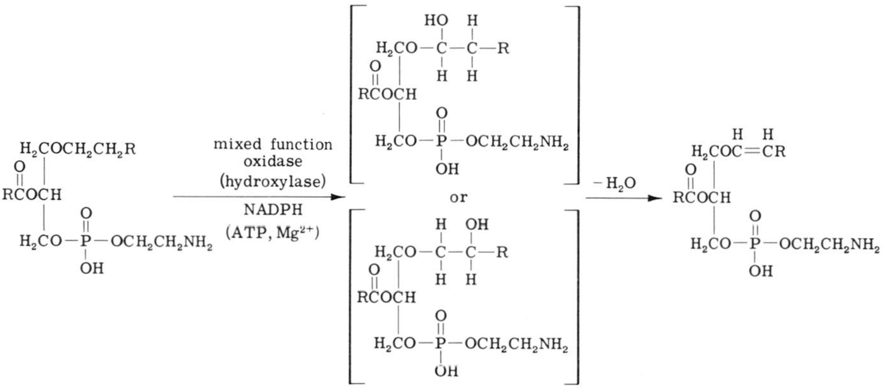

FIG. 6. Proposed pathway for the biosynthesis of ethanolamine plasmalogens. Other substituents instead of the hydroxyl moieties depicted could also participate in this type of reaction.

phosphorylethanolamine is the substrate; both ATP and Mg^{++} stimulate plasmalogen synthesis in this system. The overall reaction is illustrated in Fig. 6. Since cyanide inhibits this reaction and carbon monoxide does not, it seems that the microsomal electron transport system requiring cytochrome b_5, rather than P-450, is involved. The desaturation mechanism thus appears to be similar to that responsible for the synthesis of monoenoic acids.

Although the actual mechanism for plasmalogen biosynthesis remains unknown, data based on an unidentified component isolated in both *in vivo* and *in vitro* studies suggest that a substitution reaction(s) could occur on the *O*-alkyl moiety with the subsequent net elimination of two hydrogens on the 1- and 2-carbon atoms of the ether-linked aliphatic moiety (Blank *et al.*, 1970). Stoffel and LeKim (1971) have determined the stereospecificity of the hydrogen loss that occurs when the *O*-alk-1-enyl moiety is formed *in vivo*. In this important contribution, they used stereospecifically labeled species of hexadecanol labeled with tritium at the 1- and 2-positions; tritium was lost only from the hexadecanol having a 1S,2S configuration to give the *cis*-configuration of the *O*-alk-1-enyl linkage. An experiment of this type has not yet been done in a cell-free system.

C. Reduction of the Ketone Group in Alkyl Glycerolipids

There are two ketone-containing *O*-alkyl glycerolipids that have been carefully characterized in cell-free systems: alkyldihydroxyacetone-P and alkyldihydroxyacetone (Snyder *et al.*, 1970b; Wykle and Snyder, 1970).

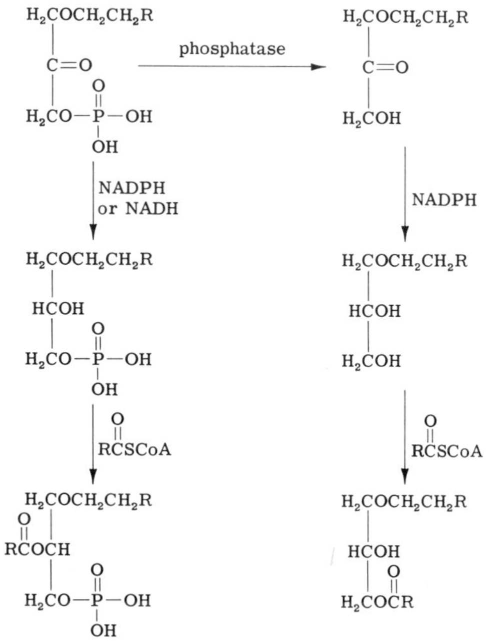

FIG. 7. Reactions involved in the biosynthesis of alkylacylglycerol-P and 1-alkyl-3-acylglycerols from alkyldihydroxyacetone-P.

In addition, both classes of compounds have been prepared by chemical synthesis (Piantadosi *et al.*, 1970, 1971). The alkyldihydroxyacetone-P can be dephosphorylated by phosphatases in the microsomal and soluble fractions of cells (Fig. 7). Microsomal reductases that utilize the two *O*-alkyl ketone substrates differ in their specificity for the reduced nucleotide (Fig. 7). Either NADPH or NADH will serve as hydrogen donors for the reduction of alkyldihydroxyacetone-P, whereas NADPH is much more effective than NADH for the reduction of alkyldihydroxyacetone (Wykle *et al.*, 1972b; Grigor and Snyder, 1971). Since the extent of phosphatase activity in the enzyme systems can mask the nucleotide specificity for alkyldihydroxyacetone-P, one must use caution in assessing nucleotide specificities for these lipid classes.

D. FORMATION OF ESTER BONDS

After the reduction of alkyldihydroxyacetone-P by the NADPH- or NADH-linked reductase, acylation of the hydroxyl group occurs at the 2-position of the glycerol moiety. In the presence of CoA, ATP, and Mg^{++}, the endogenous fatty acids of the microsomes serve as precursors of the acyl moieties (Wykle and Snyder, 1970; Hajra, 1970). However, the phosphate group at the 3-position of the glycerol moiety is mandatory for acylation to occur at the 2-position, since 1-alkylglycerols are only acylated at the 3-position and the 1-alkyl-3-acylglycerols do not serve as substrates for acyl transferases in the mammalian systems tested thus far (Snyder *et al.*, 1970f).

The alkylacylglycerol-P synthesized mimics the role of diacylglycerol-P in the biosynthesis of more complex lipids (Wykle and Snyder, 1970). After the phosphate group is removed by an Mg⁺⁺-dependent phosphatase in the microsomal or soluble fractions, the product, 1-alkyl-2-acylglycerol, can then react with acyl-CoA's (Snyder *et al.*, 1970b), CDP-phosphorylethanolamine (Snyder *et al.*, 1970d) or CDP-phosphorylcholine (Snyder *et al.*, 1970d). Figure 8 depicts how alkylacylglycerol-P participates in the formation of the complex lipids that contain *O*-alkyl bonds.

Phosphorylbase-alk-1-enylacylglycerol transferase systems that synthesize the *O*-alk-1-enyl analogs of ethanolamine and choline phosphoglycerides have been documented in rat liver (Kiyasu and Kennedy, 1960), rat brain (McMurray, 1964; Ansell and Metcalfe, 1971), and ox heart (Poulos *et al.*, 1968). These transferases are strongly inhibited by calcium ions (Kennedy and Weiss, 1956).

The transferases that utilize alkylacylglycerols and alk-1-enylacylglycerols appear to be identical to those that catalyze the same type of reactions in the biosynthesis of triacylglycerols and diacylphosphoglycerides from diacylglycerols (Kennedy, 1957). However, the reactions in-

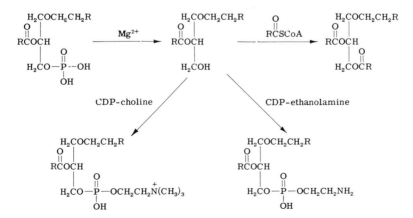

FIG. 8. Reactions involved in the biosynthesis of complex alkyl glycerolipids from alkylacylglycerol-P.

volving the ether-linked substrates are generally slower than those involving the ester-linked substrates.

V. Degradation

A. CLEAVAGE OF ETHER BONDS

1. O-Alkyl Cleavage Enzymes

In 1964 Tietz *et al.* demonstrated that rat liver microsomes contained a tetrahydropteridine-hydroxylase that could split the ether bond present in alkylglycerols. The hydroxylation requirements in the O-alkyl cleavage reaction are identical to those required for the hydroxylation of phenyl-alanine (Kaufman, 1959). An NADPH-linked reductase associated with the soluble fraction regenerates the tetrahydropteridine from the dihy-dropteridine produced during the hydroxylation step. Tietz *et al.* (1964) proposed a mechanism whereby the α-carbon of the O-alkyl moiety was hydroxylated to yield the unstable hemiacetal structure illustrated in Fig. 9. The hemiacetal spontaneously breaks down to produce the first detectable products: glycerol and long-chain fatty aldehydes. Depending on the incubation conditions, the fatty aldehyde can be oxidized to the acid or reduced to the alcohol. At neutral pH, and in the presence of added NAD⁺, only fatty acids are produced (Tietz *et al.*, 1964; Pfleger *et al.*, 1967), whereas in the absence of NAD⁺, fatty aldehydes (Tietz *et al.*, 1964; Pfleger *et al.*, 1967) and fatty alcohols (Pfleger *et al.*, 1967) also accumulate.

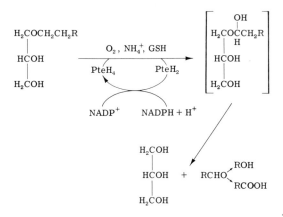

FIG. 9. Proposed reaction for the biocleavage of alkylglycerols by a microsomal enzyme system from rat liver.

Pfleger and colleagues (1967) further investigated the O-alkyl cleavage enzyme in a number of species (rats, dogs, guinea pigs, gerbils, mice, hamsters, rabbits, and slugs) and in various tissues (liver, intestine, perirenal fat, and brain). Only the liver and intestine exhibited significant ether cleavage activities, and the activities in livers of different species varied considerably. Liver preparations from male rats possessed greater cleavage activities than similar preparations from female rats.

Mitochondrial supernatants from cells rich in ether-linked lipids exhibited low or no ether cleavage activity. More extensive data verified this conclusion, since the cleavage enzyme was absent or depressed in mitochondrial supernatants from a variety of cancer cells (Soodsma *et al.*, 1970) and brain (Snyder *et al.*, 1971b).

Tietz *et al.* (1964) found that the bulk of the O-alkyl cleavage activity was associated with the microsomes of rat liver. Although Pfleger *et al.* (1967), using zonal centrifugation procedures, found a significant amount of the cleavage activity in the soluble fraction of rat liver, they did not carry out recovery studies to determine what proportion of the total activity had been solubilized.

Soodsma and co-workers (1972) reinvestigated the O-alkyl cleavage system with the purpose of determining product formation and subcellular localization of the enzyme under optimal conditions. This work revealed that the bulk of the cleavage activity in rat liver resides in the microsomes and that ammonium ions and sulfhydryl groups are required for maximum activity which occurs at approximately pH 9.0. The cofactor requirements and other properties of the O-alkyl cleavage reaction agreed in principle with those of the earlier investigations (Tietz *et al.*, 1964; Pfleger *et al.*, 1967).

Kapoulas *et al.* (1969) described an enzymatic system in *Tetrahymena pyriformis* that cleaves the ether linkage in alkylglycerols that appears to differ from that found in rat liver. For example, a tetrahydropteridine requirement could not be demonstrated in the *Tetrahymena* system, even by using tetrahydropteridine inhibitors. Furthermore, the *Tetrahymena* system formed an alcohol-like product which, on the basis of $^3H/^{14}C$ ratios, could not be a primary fatty alcohol. These data indicate that the cleavage of the O-alkyl moiety of alkylglycerols is accomplished by completely different enzymes in mammals and protozoa.

2. O-Alk-1-enyl Cleavage Enzymes

Bergmann *et al.* (1957) discovered that extracts from *Escherichia coli* and *Bacillus subtilis* cleaved the O-alk-1-enyl moiety of plasmalogens, whereas identically prepared extracts from other bacteria and yeast did not exhibit such activity. Thiele (1959) reported similar cleavage activities for a number of acetone extracts of fresh organs that were incubated at 37° with plasmalogens. The lipid product formed was a long-chain fatty aldehyde. Since chelating agents added to the system inhibited the cleavage of the O-alk-1-enyl moiety, Thiele (1959) concluded that a stable metal-complex probably catalyzed the reaction.

More detailed investigations of the formation of fatty aldehydes derived from the O-alk-1-enyl chain of plasmalogens have been described for enzyme systems prepared from livers (Warner and Lands, 1961) and brains (Ansell and Spanner, 1965) of rats. Although the overall reaction catalyzed is similar for both tissues, the systems exhibit marked differences in their substrate and cofactor specificities.

Warner and Lands (1961) found that the ether grouping in 1-alk-1-enylglycerylphosphorylcholine can be readily hydrolyzed by rat liver microsomes in the absence of any added cofactors (Fig. 10). The liver enzyme is specific for only this molecular species of O-alk-1-enyl-linked phospholipid, i.e., cleavage does not occur if the hydroxyl group is replaced with an acyl moiety at the 2-position of the glycerol portion or if choline is replaced with ethanolamine at the 3-position of the glycerol portion. The O-alk-1-enyl cleavage enzyme from rat liver is labile if subjected to heat, acid, alkali, or chymotrypsin, whereas lyophilization,

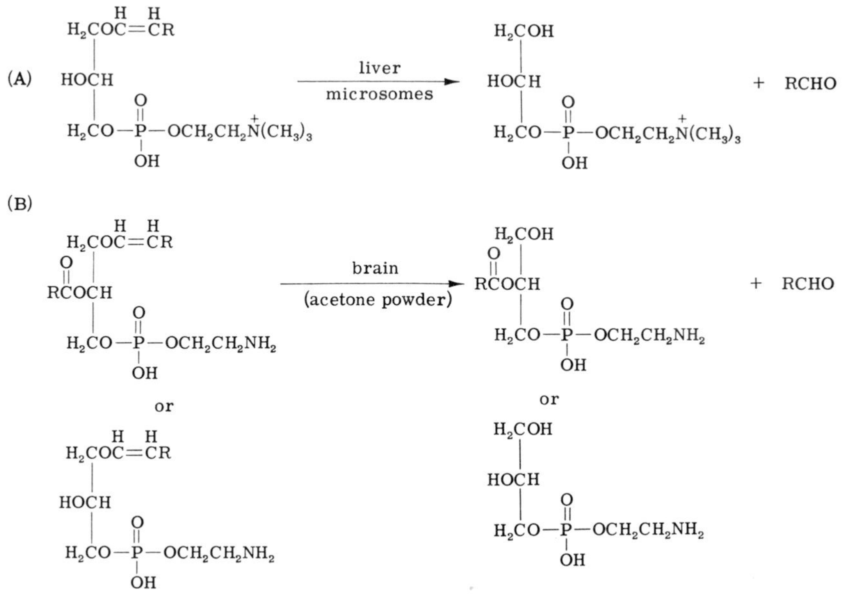

Fig. 10. Proposed reactions for the biocleavage of alk-1-enyl phospholipids by enzymes from livers (A) and brains (B) of rats.

Mg^{++}, Ca^{++}, or chelating agents had no effect on hydrolysis of the substrate. Inactivation of the enzyme caused by exposing the microsomes to phospholipases A or C, freezing and thawing, or imidazole (and derivatives) could be reversed by the addition of exogenous diacyl phosphoglycerides (Ellingson and Lands, 1968). Acyl moieties at both the 1- and 2-positions of the glycerol moiety of the phospholipids were required for reactivation.

Several years after the O-alk-1-enyl hydrolase in liver was discovered, Ansell and Spanner (1965) described an O-alk-1-enyl cleavage preparation (an acetone powder) from brain that exhibited requirements different from those reported for the liver system. The O-alk-1-enyl hydrolase from brain preferentially hydrolyzes 1-alk-1-enyl-2-acylglycerylphosphorylethanolamine, but it can also hydrolyze 1-alk-1-enylglycerylphosphorylethanolamine to some extent (Fig. 10). Furthermore, the enzyme from brain requires magnesium ions for optimal activity.

B. Cleavage of Ester Bonds

1. *Lipases*

Pancreatic lipase (Snyder and Piantadosi, 1968; Slotboom *et al.*, 1967; Gigg and Gigg, 1967), plasma or adipose tissue triacylglycerol lipase (Greten *et al.*, 1970), and plasma or adipose tissue monoacylglycerol lipase (Greten *et al.*, 1970) act primarily on nonpolar glycerolipid substrates that possess ether bonds (Fig. 11), but they have no effect on either the O-alkyl or O-alk-1-enyl moieties per se.

Specificity of pancreatic lipase for the 1- and 3-acyl moieties of glycerolipids is borne out by results obtained from investigations where alkyldiacylglycerols (Snyder and Piantadosi, 1968) and alk-1-enyldiacylglycerols (Gigg and Gigg, 1967; Slotboom *et al.*, 1967) were tested as substrates. Products formed from the alkyldiacylglycerols are alkylacylglycerols, free fatty acids, and to some extent free alkylglycerols (Snyder and Piantadosi, 1968) whereas products formed from alk-1-enyldiacylglycerols are alk-1-enylacylglycerols, free fatty acids, and alk-1-enylglycerols (Gigg and Gigg, 1967; Slotboom *et al.*, 1967). The 2-acyl moiety in both the O-alkyl and O-alk-1-enyl products can migrate to the 3-position where deacylation will occur to form the free forms of the glyceryl ethers.

The mono- and triacyl-glycerol lipases isolated from postheparin plasma of humans or NH$_4$OH extracts of adipose tissue and hearts of rats hydrolyze the acyl moieties in either 1,2-dioctadecyl-3-oleylglycerol or 1,3-dioctadecyl-2-oleylglycerol. Therefore, unlike pancreatic lipase,

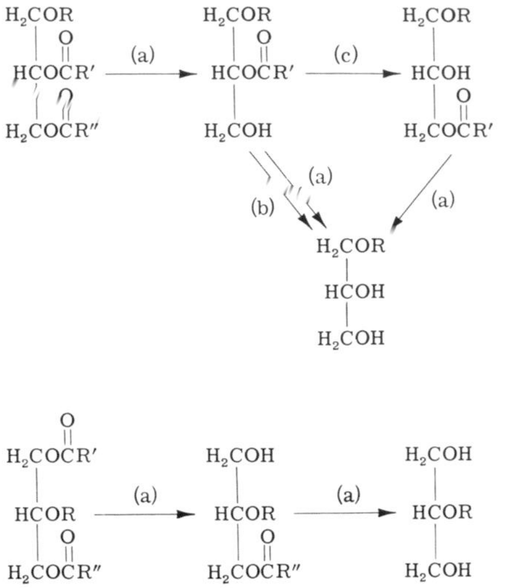

H_2COR H_2COR H_2COR

$HCOCR'$ (a)→ $HCOCR'$ (c)→ $HCOH$

H_2COCR'' H_2COH H_2COCR'

(b) (a)   (a)

H_2COR

$HCOH$

H_2COH

H_2COCR' H_2COH H_2COH

$HCOR$ (a)→ $HCOR$ (a)→ $HCOR$

H_2COCR'' H_2COCR'' H_2COH

Fig. 11. Deacylation of 1- and 2-isomeric forms of ether-linked glycerolipids by lipases. The small letters in parentheses above arrows designate: (a) pancreatic lipase, (b) lipases from adipose and heart tissues, and (c) acyl migration.

the glyceride lipases from plasma, adipose tissue, or heart do not show any specificity for the 2- or 3-acyl moieties of alkyl glycerolipids (Greten *et al.*, 1970). Similar studies with these lipases have not been reported for *O*-alk-1-enyl substrates.

2. Phospholipases and Phosphatases

In general, specificities of phospholipases (Fig. 12) for acyl, phosphate, or phosphorylbase moieties in ether-linked glycerolipids are identical to those established for phosphatidylcholine, phosphatidylethanolamine, phosphatidic acid, and the corresponding lyso-derivatives (van Deenen and de Haas, 1966). The reactions involving the ether-linked lipids as substrates are generally slower, but differences in results obtained with phospholipases by various laboratories are difficult to interpret since the assay techniques and other conditions used are not always identical. Investigations dealing with phospholipases and ether-linked substrates are summarized in Table I.

Acid and alkaline phosphatases are also capable of hydrolyzing free phosphate moieties in lipid substrates (Blank and Snyder, 1970). Alkaline phosphatase is highly specific in that it only hydrolyzes the phosphate moiety from glycerolipids that contain free hydroxyl or ketone groups at the 2-position of the glycerol moiety. In contrast, acid phos-

Table I

PHOSPHOLIPASES AND ETHER-LINKED SUBSTRATES

Enzyme	Substrate	Group hydrolyzed	Reference
Phospholipase A (3.1.1.4)	Alk-1-enylacylglycerylphosphorylethanolamine	2-Acyl	Marinetti *et al.* (1959) Gottfried and Rapport (1963) Hartree and Mann (1961)
	Alkylacylglycerylphosphorylethanolamine	2-Acyl	Snyder *et al.* (1970d)
	Alkylacylglycerylphosphorylcholine	2-Acyl	Snyder *et al.* (1970d)
Phospholipase C (3.1.4.3)	Alk-1-enylacylglycerylphosphorylethanolamine	Phosphorylethanolamine	Kiyasu and Kennedy (1960) Warner and Lands (1963) Ansell and Spanner (1965) Snyder *et al.* (1971a)
	Alk-1-enylacylglycerylphosphorylcholine	Phosphorylcholine	Warner and Lands (1963)
	Alkylacylglycerylphosphorylethanolamine	Phosphorylethanolamine	Snyder *et al.* (1970d)
	Alkylacylglycerylphosphorylcholine	Phosphorylcholine	Snyder *et al.* (1970d)
Phospholipase D (3.1.4.4)	Alk-1-enylacylglycerylphosphorylethanolamine or phosphorylcholine	Ethanolamine and/or choline	Hack and Ferrans (1959) Lands and Hart (1965) Slotboom *et al.* (1967)

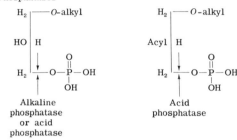

(I) Phospholipases

(II) Phosphatases

FIG. 12. Specificity of phospholipases (I) and phosphatases (II) for ether-linked phospholipids. The arrows indicate the position of enzymatic attack. The circled letters A₂, C, and D designate phospholipase type.

phatase cleaves free phosphate groups in glycerolipids irrespective of the chemical groupings at positions 1 and 2 of the glycerol portion (Fig. 12).

References

Ansell, G. B., and Metcalfe, R. F. (1971). *J. Neurochem.* **18**, 647.

Ansell, G. B., and Spanner, S. (1965). *Biochem. J.* **97**, 375.

Baumann, W. J. (1972). *In* "Ether Lipids: Chemistry and Biology" (F. Snyder, ed.), Chapter 3, pp. 51–79. Academic Press, New York.

Bergelson, L. D. (1969). *In* "Progress in the Chemistry of Fats and Other Lipids" (R. T. Holman, ed.), Vol. 10, pp. 239–286. Pergamon, Oxford.

Bergmann, H., Schneweis, K.-E., and Thiele, O. W. (1957). *Naturwissenschaften* **44**, 380.

Blank, M. L., and Snyder, F. (1970). *Biochemistry* **9**, 5034.

Blank, M. L., Wykle, R. L., Piantadosi, C., and Snyder, F. (1970). *Biochim. Biophys. Acta* **210**, 442.

Blank, M. L., Wykle, R. L., and Snyder, F. (1972). *Biochem. Biophys. Res. Commun.* **47**, 1203.

Bodman, J., and Maisin, J. H. (1958). *Clin. Chim. Acta* **3**, 253.

Cotman, C., Blank, M. L., Moehl, A., and Snyder, F. (1969). *Biochemistry* **8**, 4606.

Cymerman Craig, J., Hamon, D. P. G., Purushothaman, K. K., Roy, S. K., and Lands, W. E. M. (1966). *Tetrahedron* **22**, 175.

Davies, W. H., Heilbron, J. M., and Jones, W. E. (1933). *J. Chem. Soc., London* p. 165.

Day, J. I. E., Goldfine, H., and Hagen, P.-O. (1970). *Biochim. Biophys. Acta* **218**, 179.

Debuch, H. (1959a). *Hoppe-Seyler's Z. Physiol. Chem.* **314**, 49.

Debuch, H. (1959b). *Hoppe-Seyler's Z. Physiol. Chem.* **317**, 182.

Debuch, H. (1972). *In* "Ether Lipids: Chemistry and Biology" (F. Snyder, ed.), Chapter 1, pp. 1–24. Academic Press, New York.

Dorée, C. (1909). *Biochem. J.* **4**, 72.

Ellingson, J. S., and Lands, W. E. M. (1968). *Lipids* **3**, 111.

Ferrell, W. J., and Radloff, D. M. (1970). *Physiol. Chem. Phys.* **2**, 551.

Feulgen, R., and Voit, K. (1924). *Pfluegers Arch. Gesamte Physiol. Menschen Tiere* **206**, 389.

Garfinkel, D., and Hess, B. (1964). *J. Biol. Chem.* **239**, 971.

Gigg, J., and Gigg, R. (1967). *J. Chem. Soc. C* p. 431.

Gigg, R. (1972). *In* "Ether Lipids: Chemistry and Biology" (F. Snyder, ed.), Chapter 5, pp. 87–108. Academic Press, New York.

Goldfine, H. (1968). *Annu. Rev. Biochem.* **37**, 303.

Gottfried, E. L., and Rapport, M. M. (1963). *J. Lipid Res.* **4**, 57.

Greten, H., Levy, R. I., Fales, H., and Fredrickson, D. S. (1970). *Biochim. Biophys. Acta* **210**, 39.

Grigor, M. R., and Snyder, F. (1971). Unpublished data.

Hack, M. H., and Ferrans, V. J. (1959). *Hoppe-Seyler's Z. Physiol. Chem.* **315**, 157.

Hajra, A. K. (1969). *Biochem. Biophys. Res. Commun.* **37**, 486.

Hajra, A. K. (1970). *Biochem. Biophys. Res. Commun.* **39**, 1037.

Hajra, A. K., and Agranoff, B. W. (1968a). *J. Biol. Chem.* **243**, 1617.

Hajra, A. K., and Agranoff, B. W. (1968b). *J. Biol. Chem.* **243**, 3542.

Hanahan, D. J. (1972). *In* "Ether Lipids: Chemistry and Biology" (F. Snyder, ed.), Chapter 2, pp. 25–50. Academic Press, New York.

Hartman, F. C. (1968). *Biochem. Biophys. Res. Commun.* **33**, 888.

Hartman, F. C. (1970). *Biochemistry* **9**, 1776.

Hartree, E. F. (1964). *Metab. and Physiol. Significance Lipids, Proc. Advan. Study Course, Cambridge, Engl., 1963* p. 207.

Hartree, E. F., and Mann, T. (1961). *Biochem. J.* **80**, 464.

Horrocks, L. A. (1972). *In* "Ether Lipids: Chemistry and Biology" (F. Snyder, ed.), Chapter 9, pp. 177–272. Academic Press, New York.

IUPAC-IUB Commission on Biochemical Nomenclature (1967). The Nomenclature of Lipids. *J. Lipid Res.* **8**, 523.

Kapoulas, V. M., and Thompson, G. A., Jr. (1969). *Biochim. Biophys. Acta* **187**, 594.

Kapoulas, V. M., Thompson, G. A., Jr., and Hanahan, D. J. (1969). *Biochim. Biophys. Acta* **176**, 250.

Kates, M. (1972). *In* "Ether Lipids: Chemistry and Biology" (F. Snyder, ed.), Chapter 15, pp. 351–398. Academic Press, New York.

Kaufman, S. (1959). *J. Biol. Chem.* **234**, 2677.

Kennedy, E. P. (1957). *Fed. Proc., Fed. Amer. Soc. Exp. Biol.* **16**, 847.

Kennedy, E. P., and Weiss, S. B. (1956). *J. Biol. Chem.* **222**, 193.

Kiyasu, J. Y., and Kennedy, E. P. (1960). *J. Biol. Chem.* **235**, 2590.

Kleinig, H., Zentgraf, H., Comes, P., and Stadler, J. (1971). *J. Biol. Chem.* **246**, 2996.

Klenk, E., and Debuch, H. (1954). *Hoppe-Seyler's Z. Physiol. Chem.* **296**, 179.

Klenk, E., and Debuch, H. (1963). *In* "Progress in the Chemistry of Fats and Other Lipids" (R. T. Holman, W. O. Lundberg, and T. Malkin, eds.), Vol. 6, pp. 3–29. Pergamon, Oxford.

Kolattukudy, P. E. (1970). *Biochemistry* **9**, 1095.

Kossel, A., and Edlbacher, S. (1915). *Hoppe-Seyler's Z. Physiol. Chem.* **94**, 277.

Lands, W. E. M., and Hart, P. (1965). *Biochim. Biophys. Acta* **98**, 532.

McMurray, W. C. (1964). *J. Neurochem.* **11**, 315.

Malins, D. C., and Sargent, J. R. (1971). *Biochemistry* **10**, 1107.

Mangold, H. K., and Baumann, W. J. (1967). *In* "Lipid Chromatographic Analysis" (G. V. Marinetti, ed.), Vol. 1, pp. 339–359. Dekker, New York.

Marinetti, G. V., and Erbland, J. (1957). *Biochim. Biophys. Acta* **26**, 429.

Marinetti, G. V., Erbland, J., and Stotz, E. (1959). *J. Amer. Chem. Soc.* **81**, 861.

Murooka, Y., Seto, K., and Harada, T. (1970). *Biochem. Biophys. Res. Commun.* **41**, 407.

Norton, W. T., Gottfried, E. L., and Rapport, M. M. (1962). *J. Lipid Res.* **3**, 456.

Nozawa, Y., and Thompson, G. A., Jr. (1971). *J. Cell Biol.* **49**, 712.

Paltauf, F. (1972). *FEBS Lett.* **20**, 79.

Pfleger, R. C., Piantadosi, C., and Snyder, F. (1967). *Biochim. Biophys. Acta* **144**, 633.

Pfleger, R. C., Anderson, N. G., and Snyder, F. (1968). *Biochemistry* **7**, 2826.

Piantadosi, C. (1972a). *In* "Ether Lipids: Chemistry and Biology" (F. Snyder, ed.), Chapter IV, pp. 81–85. Academic Press, New York.

Piantadosi, C. (1972b). *In* "Ether Lipids: Chemistry and Biology" (F. Snyder, ed.), Chapter VI, pp. 109–120. Academic Press, New York.

Piantadosi, C., and Snyder, F. (1970). *J. Pharm. Sci.* **59**, 283.

Piantadosi, C., Ishaq, K. S., and Snyder, F. (1970). *J. Pharm. Sci.* **59**, 1201.

Piantadosi, C., Ishaq, K. S., Wykle, R. L., and Snyder, F. (1971). *Biochemistry* **10**, 1417.

Piantadosi, C., Ishaq, K. S., Blank, M. L., and Snyder, F. (1972). *J. Pharm. Sci.* **61**, 607.

Poulos, A., Hughes, B. P., and Cumings, J. N. (1968). *Biochim. Biophys. Acta* **152**, 629.

Rao, G. A., Sorrels, M. F., and Reiser, R. (1970). *Lipids* **5**, 762.

Rapport, M. M., and Franzl, R. E. (1957). *J. Neurochem.* **1**, 303.

Rapport, M. M., and Norton, W. T. (1962). *Annu. Rev. Biochem.* **31**, 103.

Rapport, M. M., Lerner, B., Alonzo, N., and Franzl, R. E. (1957). *J. Biol. Chem.* **225**, 859.

Rose, I. A., and O'Connell, E. L. (1969). *J. Biol. Chem.* **244**, 6548.

Schmid, H. H. O., Baumann, W. J., and Mangold, H. K. (1967a). *Biochim. Biophys. Acta* **144**, 344.

Schmid, H. H. O., Baumann, W. J., and Mangold, H. K. (1967b). *J. Amer. Chem. Soc.* **89**, 4797.

Slotboom, A. J., de Haas, G. H., and van Deenen, L. L. M. (1967). *Chem. Phys. Lipids* **1**, 192.

Snyder, F. (1969). *In* "Progress in the Chemistry of Fats and Other Lipids" (R. T. Holman, ed.), Vol. 10, Part 3, pp. 287–335. Pergamon, Oxford.

Snyder, F. (1971). *In* "Progress in Thin-Layer Chromatography and Related Methods" (A. Niederwieser and G. Pataki, eds.), Vol. 2, pp. 105–141. Ann Arbor Sci. Publ., Ann Arbor, Michigan.

Snyder, F., ed. (1972a). "Ether Lipids: Chemistry and Biology" Academic Press, New York.

Snyder, F. (1972b). *In* "Ether Lipids: Chemistry and Biology" (F. Snyder, ed.), Chapter 7, pp. 121–156. Academic Press, New York.

Snyder, F., and Malone, B. (1970). *Biochem. Biophys. Res. Commun.* **41**, 1382.

Snyder, F., and Piantadosi, C. (1968). *Biochim. Biophys. Acta* **152**, 794.

Snyder, F., Malone, B., and Wykle, R. L. (1969a). *Biochem. Biophys. Res. Commun.* **34**, 40.

Snyder, F., Malone, B., and Blank, M. L. (1969b). *Biochim. Biophys. Acta* **187**, 302.

Snyder, F., Piantadosi, C., and Wood, R. (1969c). *Proc. Soc. Exp. Biol. Med.* **130**, 1170.

Snyder, F., Wykle, R. L., and Malone, B. (1969d). *Biochem. Biophys. Res. Commun.* **34**, 315.

Snyder, F., Malone, B., and Blank, M. L. (1970a). *J. Biol. Chem.* **245**, 1790.

Snyder, F., Blank, M. L., Malone, B., and Wykle, R. L. (1970b). *J. Biol. Chem.* **245**, 1800.

Snyder, F., Rainey, W. T., Jr., Blank, M. L., and Christie, W. H. (1970c). *J. Biol. Chem.* **245**, 5853.

Snyder, F., Blank, M. L., and Malone, B. (1970d). *J. Biol. Chem.* **245**, 4016.

Snyder, F., Malone, B., and Cumming, R. B. (1970e). *Can. J. Biochem.* **48**, 212.

Snyder, F., Piantadosi, C., and Malone, B. (1970f). *Biochim. Biophys. Acta* **202**, 244.

Snyder, F., Blank, M. L., and Wykle, R. L. (1971a). *J. Biol. Chem.* **246**, 3639.

Snyder, F., Hibbs, M., and Malone, B. (1971b). *Biochim. Biophys. Acta* **231**, 409.

Snyder, F., Malone, B., and Goswitz, F. A. (1971c). Unpublished data.

Snyder, F., Wykle, R. L., Blank, M. L., Lumb, R. H., Malone, B., and Piantadosi, C. (1972). *Fed. Proc.* **31**, 454.

Soodsma, J. F., Piantadosi, C., and Snyder, F. (1970). *Cancer Res.* **30**, 309.

Soodsma, J. F., Piantadosi, C., and Snyder, F. (1972). *J. Biol. Chem.* **247**, 3923.

Stoffel, W., and LeKim, D. (1971). *Hoppe-Seyler's Z. Physiol. Chem.* **352**, 501.

Stoffel, W., LeKim, D., and Heyn, G. (1970). *Hoppe-Seyler's Z. Physiol. Chem.* **351**, 875.

Tabakoff, B., and Erwin, V. G. (1970). *J. Biol. Chem.* **245**, 3263.

Thiele, O. W. (1959). *Hoppe-Seyler's Z. Physiol. Chem.* **315**, 117.

Thompson, G. A., Jr. (1968). *Biochim. Biophys. Acta* **152**, 409.

Thompson, G. A., Jr., and Kapoulas, V. M. (1969). In "Lipids" (J. M. Lowenstein, ed.), *Methods in Enzymology*, Vol. 14, p. 668–678. Academic Press, New York.

Tietz, A., Lindberg, M., and Kennedy, E. P. (1964). *J. Biol. Chem.* **239**, 4081.

Tsujimoto, M., and Toyama, Y. (1922). *Chem. Umsch. Geb. Fette Oele Wachse Harze* **29**, 27.

van Deenen, L. L. M., and de Haas, G. H. (1966). *Annu. Rev. Biochem.* **35**, Part 1, 157.

Varanasi, U., and Malins, D. C. (1969). *Science* **166**, 1158.

Warner, H. R., and Lands, W. E. M. (1961). *J. Biol. Chem.* **236**, 2404.

Warner, H. R., and Lands, W. E. M. (1963). *J. Amer. Chem. Soc.* **85**, 60.

Wykle, R. L. (1970). Biosynthesis of alkyl glyceryl ethers by microsomal enzymes from tumors: Identification and characterization of intermediates containing ether bonds. Ph.D. Thesis, Univ. of Tennessee Medical Units, Memphis.

Wykle, R. L., and Snyder, F. (1969). *Biochem. Biophys. Res. Commun.* **37**, 658.

Wykle, R. L., and Snyder, F. (1970). *J. Biol. Chem.* **245**, 3047.

Wykle, R. L., Blank, M. L., and Snyder, F. (1970). *FEBS (Fed. Eur. Biochem. Soc.), Lett.* **12**, 57.

Wykle, R. L., Blank, M. L., and Snyder, F. (1971). *Fed. Proc., Fed. Amer. Soc. Exp. Biol.* **30**, 1243.

Wykle, R. L., Blank, M. L., Malone, B., and Snyder, F. (1972a). *J. Biol. Chem.* (in press).

Wykle, R. L., Piantadosi, C., and Snyder, F. (1972b). *J. Biol. Chem.* **247**, 2944.

Lipids in the Nervous System of Different Species as a Function of Age: Brain, Spinal Cord, Peripheral Nerve, Purified Whole Cell Preparations, and Subcellular Particulates: Regulatory Mechanisms and Membrane Structure

GEORGE ROUSER AND GENE KRITCHEVSKY

*Division of Neurosciences, City of Hope National Medical Center,
Duarte, California*

AND

AKIRA YAMAMOTO

*Second Department of Internal Medicine, Osaka University
Medical School, Osaka, Japan*

AND

CLAUDE F. BAXTER

*Neurochemistry Laboratories, Veterans Administration
Hospital, Sepulveda, California*

I. Introduction

General interest in lipids has increased a great deal in the last 10 years. The importance of lipid metabolism in health and disease has made a better knowledge of lipid metabolism and enzymology necessary. The lipid composition of whole organs and isolated subcellular particulates has become of great importance to those who study cell membranes. Membranology has become the common meeting ground for many chemists and biologists with different types of specialized training and experience. The lipid composition of the major organs of some species of higher animals has been defined with considerable accuracy. Among the vertebrates, most studies have been concerned with lipids of rat and mouse heart, kidney, lung, liver, and spleen with some attention paid to human, cattle, guinea pig, rabbit, frog, and a few other species. The lipids of invertebrates other than insects have received little attention.

Lipids of the nervous system have been investigated fairly extensively, but much of the early work is of limited value because inadequate analytical methods were used. The lipid classes occurring in the nervous system have now been rather well defined, and rather carefully evaluated methods of analysis have been described in detail (see Section II). Even so, adoption of the best available procedures for lipid analysis has been slow. Also, the analysis of samples of gray and white matter, in the belief that these would disclose all of the significant features of brain lipid composition, delayed understanding of the true nature of brain lipid composition changes with age in particular. Analysis of gray and white matter samples, particularly small samples taken at random, ignores the well-known differences in the time at which different areas of brain are myelinated. Myelination of some regions of brain appears to take place even in adult life.

The lipid composition of brain subcellular particulates has not been studied extensively, and a relatively small number of laboratories have contributed the available data. The study of subcellular particulates requires their isolation and characterization as well as their lipid (and now also protein) analysis. The expertise required in the several areas of laboratory investigation appears to have made subcellular particulate studies less attractive.

In this chapter, data relevant to the changes with age and species variations of the lipid composition of the nervous system are brought together and evaluated. Also, a scheme for membrane biosynthesis is presented, the factors that determine the lipid class composition of membranes are considered, and a model for membrane structure is given. The figures presented have not been published previously. The data used in graphic analysis done by the senior author were derived in part from unpublished data for human brain obtained by G. Rouser, G. Kritchevsky, and A. Yamamoto, and the data for different animal species were obtained by G. Rouser, G. Kritchevsky, C. F. Baxter, and G. Simon. This review which contains new data extends our previous reviews (Fleischer and Rouser, 1965; Rouser *et al.*, 1968b; Rouser and Yamamoto, 1969), the review of Eichberg *et al.* (1969) that was based on information published through 1967, and chapters in the recent volume on chemistry and brain development (Paoletti and Davison, 1971). The review of Eichberg *et al.* is recommended in particular for a good and still up-to-date consideration of metabolic pathways in brain that are not covered in this review and for references to some of the earlier literature not cited here. We have limited our considerations to lipid class composition. It is planned that the extensive literature on fatty acid composition will be considered in another review. Preliminary analysis of human brain fatty acid data obtained in this laboratory has been presented (Rouser and Yamamoto, 1968, 1969; Rouser *et al.*, 1970b). Also, lipid composition changes in pathological states are considered in detail elsewhere (Rouser and Kritchevsky, 1972). We have confined our citations largely to references with data pertaining to changes with age and species variations. Other references can be obtained by consulting the references cited.

II. Assessment of Methods for Accurate, Precise, Quantitative Lipid Analysis and the Reporting of Lipid Class Composition Data

The first studies of lipids of the nervous system were qualitative in nature. Lipid classes were isolated in purified form and characterized. Since the isolation procedures were not quantitative and the accuracy of earlier methods of analysis was uncertain, the presence of other lipid classes in significant amounts could not be excluded. Later, column chromatographic procedures were used to separate most lipid classes in quantitative yield and the major components of brain were shown to be cholesterol, cerebroside, sulfatide, phosphatidyl choline, phosphatidyl ethanolamine, phosphatidyl serine, and sphingomyelin with smaller amounts of phosphatidyl inositol, phosphatidyl inositol mono- and di-phosphates, phosphatidic acid, diphosphatidyl glycerol, various types of gangliosides, ceramide, triglyceride, sterol esters, and several uncharacterized acidic phospholipids (Rouser and Yamamoto, 1969; Rouser et al., 1961a,b,c,d, 1963, 1964, 1965a,b, 1967a, 1968b). Each lipid class was characterized by chromatographic migration in several different systems, by infrared spectrophotometric examination, and by hydrolysis to the proper amounts of characteristic components without contamination by components characteristic of other lipid classes. Subsequent studies demonstrated the presence of small amounts of ceramide dihexosides and glycosyldiglycerides, cerebroside esters, phosphatidyl glycerol, lysodiphosphatidyl glycerol, phosphatidyl glycerolphosphate, N-acyl phosphatidyl ethanolamine, and lysobisphosphatidic acid as well as traces of squalene. The known components account for over 99.9% of the total lipid weight extracted from brain, and the structural formulas for the most abundant lipid classes have been presented (Rouser and Yamamoto, 1968, 1969; Rouser et al., 1970b). Additional trace components may well be detected by isotope labeling. Although cholesterol sulfate was reported as present in brain, we have not been able to confirm this, even with the use of ^{35}S label that provides a very sensitive means of detection.

The same lipid classes occur in all vertebrate brains examined thus far and are found also in some invertebrates. Ceramide aminoethylphosphonate and ceramide phosphorylethanolamine occur in some invertebrate brains, and sphingomyelin may be absent. The quantitative differences among animal species are considered in Sections IV and V.

The first step in quantitative analysis of lipids of the nervous system is sample selection. The exact approach will depend upon the objectives of the investigation and must be conducted in the light of the morphological changes that take place in different regions of brain with increasing age. The detailed discussion by Prensky (1967) of the many morphological difference seen in different regions of brain at different ages and their significance for sample selection is highly recommended.

Brain development has been divided into four periods during which the main morphological changes are different and characteristic (McIlwain, 1959). Three completely different periods are apparent. In the first period, neurons and glial cells proliferate. In the second, there is outgrowth of dendrites and axons in particular. In the third period, myelination begins and is, at first, very rapid. Myelination of different regions of brain takes place at widely different ages and probably continues into the fourth decade in human brain (Yakovlev and Lecours, 1967). Before myelination begins, the regional differences in brain lipid composition are relatively small, but during and after the period of rapid myelination the differences are large. Thus, the most appropriate method of sample selection will depend upon the type of information sought.

The overall definition of changes with age in any one species can be accomplished only with representative samples of whole brain. This has been the method used for the study of brains of small animals. The changes with age are now recognized to occur throughout life and are rather well defined for several species (see Section IV). In contrast, changes with age in the brains of larger animals were studied mostly with samples of gray and white matter with the result that age changes were recognized only during the early period of development (the first postnatal year in humans) in most studies, whereas use of representative samples of whole brain later disclosed changes with age throughout life (see Section III). The full extent of changes with age can be determined for different regions of brain that can be dissected in their entirety in a reproducible manner. Cerebrum, cerebellum, brain stem, and certain nuclei dissected as described by Prensky (1967) fulfill these criteria, but they have not been examined. Changes with age can be made to appear very small indeed if, after myelination has progressed to the point that it is essentially complete in some areas, the grayest gray and whitest white matter samples are selected for analysis.

Species differences can be disclosed only by careful selection of samples and methods of data analysis (see Sections IV and V). Since large changes with age are apparent for all vertebrate species, it is necessary to compare species at the same stage of development. It is thus necessary to know when the period of rapid myelination begins and the period over which it extends, as well as the age of the animal, or to use representative samples of whole brain and the graphic analysis method described in Sections III and IV that depends upon plotting lipid class values against total lipid (that is a function of age). Species differences can be disclosed using representative samples of whole brain (Section IV) or subcellular particulates (Section V).

A very important method of sample selection that can disclose changes that may be obscured by other methods is well illustrated by the work of Bass (1971) on the effects of severe malnutrition on rat brain development. This investigator used electron microscopic examination of a subcortical area of white matter that is very homogeneous with regard to cell type and from which cells normally migrate into the cerebral cortex to show that malnutrition prevented the normal cell migration and subsequent development including myelination of that area of the brain. Bass used lipid analysis to define quantitatively the abnormalities seen by electron microscopy. Malnutrition was thus found to prevent a normal morphological change in a specific area of brain and to be associated with a large deviation from normal in the lipid composition of that area. The changes were not reversed upon return of the animals to a normal diet. This combination of morphological and chemical methods has an important place in neurochemistry. Without the knowledge of morphological abnormalities, a defect could go unrecognized because an abnormally low total lipid may not be associated with abnormal lipid class relationships (defined in Section III).

After the sample has been obtained, lipid is commonly extracted by addition of 19 volumes of chloroform–methanol (2:1) per gram of tissue followed by homogenization and filtration to remove the insoluble residue (Folch *et al.*, 1957). Nonlipid contaminants are then very commonly removed from the crude lipid extract by shaking the extract once with an aqueous solution of KCl (Folch *et al.*, 1957). The washed extracts are then used for lipid analysis. The upper phase is generally thought to contain all of the gangliosides and the lower phase all other lipids. One chloroform–methanol extraction does not remove all of the lipid from the tissue residue (Rouser *et al.*, 1963). Recoveries vary from 93 to 96% of the phospholipid, and acidic phospholipids are preferentially retained by the residue. As judged by the failure of acid hydrolysis to release fatty acids from the insoluble tissue residue, essentially complete extraction is obtained when two extractions with chloroform–methanol (2:1) are followed by one with chloroform–methanol (1:2) and then chloroform–methanol (7:1) containing 3% by volume 28% aqueous ammonia (Rouser *et al.*, 1963). The ammoniacal solution ensures extraction of acidic phospholipids. With whole brain, the chloroform/methanol mixtures extract essentially all of the lipid. With subcellular particulates, the ammoniacal solvent may be essential, particularly for mitochondria. With mitochondria, some diphosphatidyl glycerol is retained when chloroform–methanol 2:1 and 1:2 only are used (Rouser *et al.*, 1963). Similar results have been reported for purified cytochrome oxidase preparations from which all of the diphosphatidyl glycerol could be extracted only with chloroform–methanol–ammonia (Awasthi *et al.*, 1971). Most of the phospholipid of purified beef heart proteolipid is diphosphatidyl glycerol (Eichberg, 1969). Thus, diphosphatidyl glycerol is apparently bound very strongly by proteins of various organs.

Some investigators prefer to determine gangliosides after extraction with chloroform–methanol 1:1 and 1:2 (Vanier *et al.*, 1971). Suzuki (1965) found that gangliosides were not completely extracted with chloroform–methanol 2:1 only and recommended extraction with 2:1 followed by chloroform–methanol 1:2 containing 5% water. It appears that general agreement has been reached on the point that one extraction with chloroform–methanol 2:1 according to Folch does not remove all gangliosides from the tissue residue. Of special importance for extraction of gangliosides from subcellular particulates is the observation that, after removal of inorganic ions from the membrane preparations, gangliosides are not extracted completely with chloroform–methanol 2:1 unless salts are added to the solvent (Spence and Wolfe, 1967a). In our experience, complete extraction can also be obtained using the chloroform–methanol–ammonia mixture noted above.

A single KCl wash is most commonly used to remove nonlipid contaminants and gangliosides from the crude lipid extract, and the wash is assumed to be quantitative. Widely varying results are obtained, however, depending upon the nature of the material extracted. Also, if multiple washes are done, some acidic phospholipid and sulfatide may be removed from the lower phase. To obtain quantitative partition of gangliosides, one group very experienced in ganglioside analysis uses two partitions with 0.2% KCl followed by one partition with water (Vanier *et al.*, 1971). The partition with water after KCl was found by Suzuki (1965) to be essential for quantitative recovery from the lower phase of the least polar gangliosides. With ^{14}C-labeled choline, retention of 0.9% of the label in the lower phase was noted if the lipid extract was washed only once with 0.7% NaCl, but the amount was reduced to 0.09% by two additional washes (Hallinan *et al.*, 1966). It thus appears that the method of washing of the extract must be varied depending upon the objectives of the investigator, any one procedure not being entirely satisfactory for all purposes.

In the classical paper describing washing of lipid extracts with KCl and NaCl (Folch *et al.*, 1957), washing was also described with divalent ions (Ca^{2+} and Mg^{2+}). Divalent ions change the partition of a number of substances. Thus, gangliosides partition largely into the lower phase with Ca^{2+}, but with Na^+, K^+, and Mg^{2+} gangliosides partition into the upper phase (Kruger and Mendler, 1970; Quarles and Folch-Pi, 1965). Furthermore, erratic results suggested loss of gangliosides by adsorption onto the glassware used in partitioning with Ca^{2+} (Quarles and Folch-Pi, 1965). The sodium salt of triphosphoinositide partitions into the upper phase, whereas the calcium and magnesium salts partition into the lower phase (Dawson, 1965). In the presence of calcium, acidic phospholipids become linked through calcium to inorganic phosphate. Formation of this complex causes calcium and inorganic phosphate to enter the lower phase (Bader, 1964; Cotmore *et al.*, 1971) and has been shown to be responsible for the presence of dialyzable phosphate in polyphospho-inositide preparations (Kerr *et al.*, 1963). It thus appears that washing with aqueous solutions of calcium and magnesium salts cannot be recommended as a general procedure. Also, authors are urged to note the details of the procedure they used in addition to citing the classical reference to Folch because several different procedures were described in the paper.

Some investigators have taken the weight of the salt-washed lower phase as the weight of total lipid. The lower phase contains protein that is by definition proteolipid protein (Folch *et al.*, 1957). The protein can be removed by washing with an alkaline solution (Webster and Folch, 1961) or by evaporation to dryness to denature it, followed by extraction of the lipid and filtration to remove the insoluble residue. As an example, in one study, about 12% of the weight of the crude brain lipid extract was removed by washing three times with $0.1 M$ KCl and 7–9% of the weight of the washed extract was reported as denaturable protein (Mesdijian and Cornée, 1969). Many factors influence the amount of protein soluble in the lower phase (Lees, 1965). Thus, peptides may be present even after evaporation to dryness (De Konig, 1964). When inorganic ions are removed as in the preparation of some subcellular particulates, more protein enters the chloroform phase (Lees, 1968). Also relevant to subcellular particulate work is the observation that sucrose increases the amount of protein in the lower phase (Lees, 1966). The amount of protein is also influenced by the types of lipids in the lower phase. Some lipids increase and others decrease protein solubility (Lees, 1969). It is thus clear that taking the weight of the lower phase as lipid will provide an error of 7 to 20% or possibly even more depending upon the type of sample extracted.

Aside from protein, we have always found that about 5% of the weight of the lower phase is KCl when this salt is used to wash extracts of brain or subcellular particulates. This is to be expected since lipid in the original crude extract obviously causes many water-soluble compounds to enter the organic solvent phase and a high water content is not essential for solubility. The presence of protein and salt in the lower phase thus prevents use of the weight of the lower phase as an even moderately accurate measure of its lipid content.

The quantitative removal of nonlipid contaminants and complete separation of gangliosides from other lipids can be accomplished by partition chromatography on Sephadex G-25 (Rouser *et al.*, 1967b, 1969b, 1970b; Siakotos and Rouser, 1965). Lipids other than gangliosides are eluted with chloroform–methanol (19:1) saturated with water, gangliosides with chloroform–methanol (19:1 or 9:1) containing acetic acid and water, and nonlipid contaminants with methanol–water 1:1). The method is simple, easy to use, and avoids most of the problems encountered with the wash procedure. It has been applied with equal success to extracts from vertebrate and invertebrate animal organs and subcellular particulates. The reason for the improved quantitative separation of fractions is readily understood when it is realized that the partition chromatographic system is equivalent to washing the chloroform phase many times with water and the water phase many times with chloroform.

If the lipid extract is evaporated to dryness to denature protein, the lipid fractions from Sephadex are largely, if not entirely, free of protein. If the extract is not evaporated to dryness and solvent replacement is used to remove methanol and water (Rouser et al., 1967b, 1969a), about 1.5% of the weight of the first Sephadex column fraction is chloroform-soluble protein and somewhat more is present in the ganglioside fraction. Solvent replacement is recommended because it avoids decomposition reactions that occur when lipids are spread dry over a glass surface. These decomposition reactions are most extensive when nonlipid contaminants are completely removed. We have observed conversion of phosphatidyl serine to phosphatidic acid, phosphatidyl ethanolamine to an altered product (Siakotos and Rouser, 1965), and diphosphatidyl glycerol to many uncharacterized more polar substances when dry and spread over a glass surface. The Sephadex procedure is recommended for general use with samples from brain, spinal cord, and peripheral nerve as well as for subcellular particulates isolated from them.

A very rapid means for removal of nonlipid contaminants is still under study in the senior author's laboratory. The lipid extract is evaporated to dryness and, in order to avoid alteration of lipids, is immediately taken up in equilibrated lower phase obtained by mixing chloroform, methanol, and 2 N aqueous ammonia in the ratio 8:4:3. The solution is then washed once with equilibrated upper phase. The upper phase is removed and washed with 5 volumes of equilibrated lower phase to ensure complete recovery of sulfatide and acidic phospholipids. The two lower phases are combined for analysis. No more than minute traces of protein have been found in the lower phase, and quantitative recovery of most brain lipids has been established.

With the number and general concentration range of lipid classes established by satisfactory column procedures, other quantitative methods can be evaluated by comparison. Before the advent of chromatography, solvent precipitation and partition were used to obtain fractions that are known now to be mixtures of lipid classes. Thus, the data obtained in the early studies employing such procedures cannot be used to define lipid class composition. Even in this early period, however, lipid hexose, sulfate and phosphate, as well as cholesterol, could be determined with accuracy.

The combination of mild alkaline and acid hydrolysis to release water-soluble phosphate esters that are separated by chromatography and determined by phosphorus analysis has been used for lipid class analysis. The first hydrolytic procedure was shown to give erroneous lipid class values because plasmalogen was incompletely hydrolyzed and thus phosphatidyl ethanolamine values were low, sphingomyelin values were high, and an uncharacterized fraction was obtained (Pietruszko and Gray, 1960). The hydrolytic method evolved through a series of changes. The most recent method was reported by Wells and Dittmer (1966). As judged from the close correspondence by graphic analysis of rat brain values obtained by the method (Wells and Dittmer, 1967) with those obtained in our laboratories by chromatography of intact lipids (see Section VI), the modified hydrolytic method can provide accurate determinations of lipid classes of brain. The same conclusion was reached from comparison of the subcellular particulate lipid composition data of Eichberg *et al.* (1964) with our data (see Section V,E). Thus, only data obtained by the hydrolytic method after 1963 can be used to define lipid class composition accurately and precisely. Hydrolytic methods are less commonly used at present because thin layer chromatographic separation is more rapid and the fatty acid composition of each lipid class can be determined after TLC (thin layer chromatography) separation.

Column chromatography was the first method to provide accurate and precise values for brain lipid classes. The first column procedure to give accurate values for cerebroside was that of Radin *et al.* (1955). This was followed in 1961 by the introduction from the senior author's laboratory of complete and quantitative column chromatographic separation of brain lipids using combinations of diethylaminoethyl cellulose, silicic acid, silicic acid–ammonium silicate, and magnesium silicate columns (Rouser *et al.*, 1961a,b,c). The values reported in 1961 are very close to those obtained by the more recent TLC methods. Attempts to use aluminum oxide for quantitative column chromatography were made but were not successful. Lipids were altered by the adsorbent and incomplete separations were obtained.

A complete lipid analysis by column chromatography is possible only with a combination of different columns. Because the classical approach to column elution is slow, column chromatography has been replaced by TLC in most laboratories. The principles of modern high-speed, high-resolution liquid chromatography are now being applied in the senior author's laboratory. With the new approach, lipids are eluted rapidly with solvent mixtures more polar than those used previously, and peaks are detected and lipid classes determined chemically with Technicon autoanalyzers. Use of modern liquid chromatography principles shortens the time of analysis in some cases from hours to minutes and makes column chromatography competitive with TLC. In addition, the column methods can be automated. Thus, it appears that column chromatography will again be used in many laboratories for lipid analysis.

Habermann *et al.* (1961) described a method for phospholipid analysis with separation by one-dimensional TLC and direct determination of phosphorus in the presence of adsorbent. This method and modifications of it have been applied in many laboratories for brain lipid analysis. Two-dimensional TLC was applied to brain lipids somewhat later (Rouser *et al.*, 1964, 1965b, 1966) and spot aspiration rather than scraping was used to improve the speed and accuracy of determinations. One-dimensional TLC and silicic acid impregnated paper chromatography can provide satisfactory separation of some, but not all, lipid classes of brain and other parts of the nervous system. When the values obtained by column chromatography followed by TLC are compared to one-dimensional TLC, it is apparent that one-dimensional TLC with chloroform or a hexane-diethylether mixture is satisfactory for the separation of cholesterol which can then be scraped or aspirated from the plate and determined spectrophotometrically. Although correct values are sometimes obtained, recoveries tend to be low and variable. We thus prefer to separate cholesterol from other lipids by silicic acid column chromatography prior to spectrophotometric determination. Comparison of column-TLC with one-dimensional TLC only also shows that one-dimensional TLC with chloroform–methanol–water (65:25:4) as solvent is satisfactory for the separation of cerebroside and sulfatide from other lipids, and accurate and precise data (standard deviations in the 2–4% range) can be obtained by spectrophotometric determination of long-chain base after hydrolysis. Ceramides with normal and hydroxy fatty acids can be separated from each other and from other lipids by one-dimensional TLC with chloroform–methanol–28% aqueous ammonia (95:5:0.8) and accurate values obtained with the trinitrobenzenesulfonic acid method of Yamamoto and Rouser (1970).

One-dimensional TLC is less satisfactory for phospholipids. Since phosphatidyl choline and phosphatidyl ethanolamine are major lipid classes of the nervous system and one-dimensional TLC systems can resolve them from all but very minor components, one-dimensional TLC can be used for their determination with accuracy and precision. Difficulties are commonly encountered with the other phospholipids. Thus, the phosphatidyl serine and phosphatidyl inositol or sphingomyelin and phosphatidyl inositol spots may overlap, or the sphingomyelin and lysophosphatidyl ethanolamine spots may overlap. When brain samples are frozen and thawed, lysophosphatidyl ethanolamine formation may be accelerated and give rise to a falsely high value for sphingomyelin. One-dimensional TLC is of no value for the most minor phospholipid components of brain. These are acidic phospholipids that can be concentrated in the acidic lipid fraction from a diethylaminoethyl cellulose or triethylaminoethyl cellulose column and then determined accurately after separation by two-dimensional TLC (Rouser and Fleischer, 1967; Rouser *et al.*, 1963, 1967b, 1969b, 1970b).

Use of two-dimensional TLC greatly improves the accuracy of values for phosphatidyl serine, phosphatidyl inositol, sphingomyelin, lysophosphatidyl ethanolamine, lysophosphatidyl choline, diphosphatidyl glycerol, and phosphatidic acid since each is resolved from the other phospholipids. Also, sample size can be much larger for two-dimensional TLC as compared to one-dimensional TLC and, thus, the amounts of minor components can be determined with greater accuracy. The amounts of the phosphatidyl inositol mono- and diphosphates cannot be determined accurately in most cases since these lipids are hydrolyzed enzymatically very rapidly after death. The amounts of most of the other lipid classes of brain do not decrease so rapidly, although diphosphatidyl glycerol and phosphatidyl inositol levels may decrease 18 or more hours after death.

It is apparent that accurate and precise quantitative determination of all brain lipids began in 1961 and since that time column, paper, and thin layer chormatographic methods have evolved that can be used for accurate and precise analysis of some or all lipid classes of the nervous system.

The routine precision of spectrophotometric measurement is better with some methods than others. Phosphorus analysis is extremely precise and reproducible even in the presence of TLC adsorbent (Rouser *et al.*, 1966, 1970a) and standard deviations in the 1–2% range are obtained for components representing over 3% of the total, in the 2–5% range for components representing 1–3% of the total, and in the 10–20% range for some minor components representing less than 1% of the total phosphorus. Accuracy for minor components can be improved by the use of ion-exchange cellulose column chromatography to concentrate them in one fraction free of major components prior to two-dimensional TLC separation. In our experience, it is difficult to obtain similar high precision with most other methods, although very careful application may give results that are almost as precise. We have found that the carbohydrate reagents α-naphthol and anthrone (Yamamoto and Rouser, 1970) require more skill if precise results are to be obtained and accuracy can suffer from interfering substances that may increase or decrease the color yield. Also, accurate determination of the amounts of some glycolipids is possible only with a pure sample of the same glycolipid as a standard because different carbohydrates give different color yields. This difficulty is overcome by hydrolysis of glycosphingolipids to release long-chain base that is determined by the trinitrobenzenesulfonic (TNBS) procedure (Yamamoto and Rouser, 1970), since TNBS gives the same molar extinction coefficient with all long-chain bases.

We have obtained accurate, precise values for brain lipid classes after TLC separation by use of phosphorus assay for phospholipids, the hydrolytic TNBS assay for cerebroside, sulfatide, and gangliosides, the zinc chloride–acetyl chloride method for cholesterol, the hydroxamic acid method for sterol esters and free fatty acids after their conversion to fatty acid methyl esters, and the dinitrophenylhydrazone method for plasmalogens (Rouser *et al.*, 1966, 1970a,b; Yamamoto and Rouser, 1970). It is thus possible to do a complete lipid class quantitative analysis with only five different methods. The same methods are also used for characterization of lipid classes by determination of the phosphorus–amino group–ester–plasmalogen ratios or long-chain base–phosphorus–amide group ratios. Other methods may be chosen in other laboratories, and good analytical values obtained if the methods are carefully standardized and applied skillfully. Proof of the accuracy of methods of analysis is not generally reported, although presentation of evidence of precision (standard deviation, etc.) is more common.

We have found mistakes by the analyst to be a major source of error. Some individuals show a "drift," i.e., they will change a part of the procedure without determining whether or not the change(s) affect the accuracy and precision of results. The analyst may or may not be aware of the fact that he is drifting from the prescribed method. As an example, the isolation of pure phosphatidyl ethanolamine is easily accomplished by diethylaminoethyl cellulose column chromatography, and the method has been used successfully in many laboratories. The method depends, however, upon the use of the proper, relatively coarse grade of ion-exchange cellulose as demonstrated by many trials in the senior author's laboratory from which it was introduced. When the method was submitted, by request, to a biochemical preparations book, the investigators who checked the method noted on the one hand that the method could be "simplified" by substituting a finer grade of ion-exchange cellulose and on the other hand that the phosphatidyl ethanolamine fraction obtained by them was not pure. In the text, this result was described by the authors as a consequence of the substitution made. The checkers also noted that a sample of phosphatidyl ethanolamine obtained from another investigator who had used the proper grade of ion-exchange cellulose was pure. A further state of confusion was created by the fact that footnotes submitted by the author were not always distinguished from those contributed by the checkers (see Rouser, 1968).

One factor has emerged as of special importance in the use of the hydrolytic trinitrobenzenesulfonic acid (TNBS) procedure of Yamamoto and Rouser (1970) for glycosphingolipid and ceramide determination. The TNBS derivative is very sensitive to light at alkaline pH. Thus, TNBS should be added in the dark or in dim red light and the incubation with reagent at alkaline pH must be conducted in the dark with return of samples to light only after acidification. We have observed up to 50% loss in color yield by failure to avoid completely exposure to light. We have observed similar large fluctuations with carbohydrate reagents, and the wide range of values for glycolipids reported in the literature appears to be a reflection, at least in part, of similar difficulties in other laboratories.

The control of precision of glycolipid determinations on a routine basis is now conducted in the senior author's laboratory as follows. Each sample is run with eight spots and the standard deviation used as a measure of reproducibility within a run. The sample is then run again from 2 to 6 weeks later. If values for two separate runs differ by more than 5%, the sample is run a third time and the mean of the three determinations taken. This approach, although time-consuming, ensures that glycolipid values will be almost as accurate and precise as phospholipid values.

Total moles of ganglioside can be determined with the trinitrobenzenesulfonic acid reagent (Yamamoto and Rouser, 1970) that gives moles of long-chain base, or by determination of moles of fatty acid derived from gangliosides. Many investigators use the number of moles of sialic acid as a measure of total ganglioside, but this is not as informative because there are mono-, di-, and trisialogangliosides and their amounts vary in different regions of brain and with age. Individual gangliosides are generally separated by one-dimensional TLC and determined spectrophotometrically (MacMillan and Wherrett, 1969; Suzuki, 1965; Vanier *et al.*, 1971; Wherrett *et al.*, 1964), but complete resolution of all the different types of gangliosides is not obtained even when three solvent systems are used (Penick *et al.*, 1966). The common one-dimensional TLC method appears to be fairly accurate for the major types of gangliosides.

The polyphosphoinositides are degraded rapidly after death and thus they can be determined accurately only with samples frozen *in situ* (Dittmer and Douglas, 1969). Two methods have been used. The hydrolytic method (Dittmer and Douglas, 1969) is the most common, but separation of intact phospholipids on formaldehyde-treated paper has also been used (Palmer and Rossiter, 1965). Both methods appear to be satisfactory.

Lipid composition data for the nervous system has been presented in a number of ways. Reporting data as weight percentages of the total is not recommended. Weighing is subject to error from contamination by foreign substances and weight percentages add an unnecessary complication to data interpretation. The fatty acid composition of each lipid class is different and there are changes with age. Thus, weight percent values will reflect these differences and may prevent recognition of the precise relationships seen when values are expressed as molar percentages. The same is true for the relationship of cholesterol to polar lipids.

The expression of lipid composition data on the basis of protein or nucleic acid content has been suggested but is seldom used. The lipid to protein ratio (on a dry weight basis) is important to determine for isolated membranes such as myelin. The lipid to protein ratio for organelles such as nerve endings, nuclei, and mitochondria is not as meaningful because not all of the protein is present in the membranes of the organelles. Expression of lipid composition data for whole organs and regions of organs relative to total protein or nucleic acid presupposes useful and direct relationships that have not been established.

Lipid composition data is preferably reported in moles per unit fresh weight because precise relationships among the lipid classes have been defined by graphic analysis using this mode of expression (see Sections III and IV). Although samples can be stored without change in water content, fear of changes in water content have led some to express their data on a dry weight basis. Graphic analysis discloses lipid interrelationships to be more complex with values as percentage of the dry weight rather than fresh weight. The best solution to the problem appears to be reporting water content and all values necessary for calculation of data in either form regardless of the way the results are published.

Many authors have reported lipid class composition data as molar percentages of the total lipid. Full appreciation of the nature of changes with age and species differences is not possible with molar percentage values. The limitations are easily appreciated by consideration of a two-component system. When the sum of the two rises, the same percentage values can be obtained by an absolute increase in the amount of one or both components. With multicomponent systems, the situation is even more complex. Whether or not the amount of any particular lipid class increases as total lipid increases can be determined by examination of data expressed as moles per unit fresh or dry weight. The nature of the changes is very clear when the molar amount of a lipid class is plotted against total moles of lipid (see Sections III and IV).

Molar values for each different type of determination must be carefully standardized. Inorganic phosphate (K_2HPO_4) is satisfactory for phosphorus assay. We have made certain that glycolipid molar values match the phosphorus values by determining accurately the weight to mole conversion factor for a cerebroside standard. Moles of standard cerebroside are determined by measurement of its fatty acid content with pure fatty acids as standards. Chromatographically pure cholesterol and palmitaldehyde are available commercially.

III. Human Nervous System Lipid Composition Changes with Age

Human brain total lipid and galactolipid were reported (Bürger, 1956) to increase into the fourth decade and then to decline. This study was carried out with representative samples of whole brain. The paper appears to have gone almost entirely unrecognized, perhaps in part because of the older type of methodology used. Several investigations (see references quoted by Davison and Gregson, 1962) indicated that sulfatide determined as lipid sulfate increased throughout a major portion of the life of man and some animals. Later, studies employing gray and white matter samples disclosed changes mainly in the first year of life (Balakrishnan *et al.*, 1961; Cumings *et al.*, 1958; Fillerup and Mead, 1967; Lesch and Bernhard, 1967; Menkes *et al.*, 1966; O'Brien *et al.*, 1964; O'Brien and Sampson, 1965b; Pilz, 1968; Svennerholm, 1968; Svennerholm and Ställberg-Stenhagen, 1968). When representative samples of whole brain were analyzed by modern methods, lipid class and fatty acid composition changes were found to occur throughout life (Rouser *et al.*, 1967c, 1970b, 1971a,b; Rouser, 1971; Rouser and Yamamoto, 1968, 1969) in agreement with the earlier report of Bürger (1956).

The total lipid content of human brain appears to increase and then decrease (Fig. 1). The exact ages at which the rate of increase of lipid content changes cannot be determined with complete confidence with the data available. Large differences in total lipid content of different human brains at all ages are apparent from Fig. 1. The range is about ±14% of the mean value. Morphological examination of human brain has disclosed that myelination is completed at early ages in some regions, but, in other regions myelination is observed into the third, and possibly the

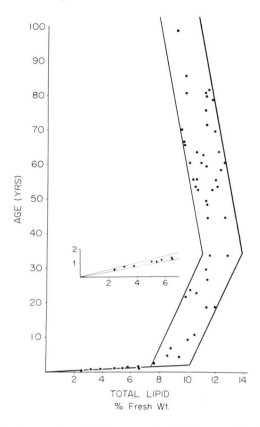

Fɪɢ. 1. Plot of human whole brain total lipid (minus gangliosides) against con-
ceptual age in years. Total lipid values were obtained from the weight of Sephadex
column fraction 1. Three periods are recognizable. The first period (up to about
1.5 years) is one of rapid development. The second is a period of less rapid increase,
and the third is a period of decline. The inset shows the first period on an expanded
plot. Large differences among individuals (± about 14% of the median value) are
apparent at each stage. See text for comments.

fourth, decade (Yakovlev and Lecours, 1967). It thus appears that the
rate for formation of new membranes is greater than the rate of loss by
cell death up into the fourth decade, after which the rate of loss exceeds
the rate of new membrane formation.

The amount of each lipid class and the fatty acid composition of each
lipid class of human brain changes continuously throughout life and
plots of the changes with age and equations relating the amount of each
lipid class to age have been published (Rouser *et al.*, 1970b; Rouser,
1971; Rouser and Yamamoto, 1968, 1969).

When a complete lipid analysis is available, it is possible to determine the relationship of the amount of any lipid class to that of another or to total lipid, total phospholipid, etc., by plotting the values against each other. If a scattergram is obtained there is no relationship, whereas a line or a curve demonstrates a direct or indirect relationship. The most convenient plots are those giving straight lines because equations for lines are easy to use and statistical evaluation is simplified. The definition of linear relationships can be done reliably only with values over the full range of variation. Data for a part of the range may suggest a linear relationship, although a curve is obtained when values over the entire range of variation are used.

Plotting of lipid class values as molar percentage of the total against millimoles per 100 gm fresh weight values for total lipid gives curves on arithmetic, semilogarithmic, and logarithmic paper. However, when lipid class values in millimoles per 100 gm fresh weight are plotted against total lipid in millimoles per 100 gm fresh weight, straight lines are obtained on arithmetic and logarithmic paper and curves are obtained on semilogarithmic paper. Thus, plots on arithmetic paper with values for lipid classes and total lipid expressed as millimoles per 100 gm fresh weight are preferable. Plotting of values expressed as moles per unit dry weight also give straight lines on arithmetic and logarithmic paper, but the relationships are more complex, and, thus, such plots are not as useful as those with values expressed as moles per unit fresh weight.

Different regions of one human brain differ in total lipid content and the relative amounts of the various lipid classes also differ as shown in Fig. 2. It is clear that the relationship of the amount of each polar lipid class relative to total polar lipid is linear on an arithmetic plot. The lines do not pass through the origin. Lines having intercepts on the total polar lipid axis are obtained for those lipid classes that increase in amount more rapidly than total polar lipid, i.e., values as molar percentage of the total increase. The reverse is true for lines with intercepts on the lipid class axis. Thus, it is clear that there is relatively more sphingomyelin, cerebroside, and sulfatide in particular in those regions of brain that contain more lipid, and that the same regions contain lower percentages of phosphatidyl choline and phosphatidyl ethanolamine. Plots of values for one lipid class against those for other lipid classes also give straight lines. It is thus clear that the level of each lipid class in human brain is related to the levels of the other lipid classes.

Since the relative amounts of some lipid classes increase whereas the relative amounts of others decrease as total lipid increases, some lipid classes clearly replace others (Rouser *et al.*, 1971a,b). Which lipid classes replace others was determined by summing values that increase with

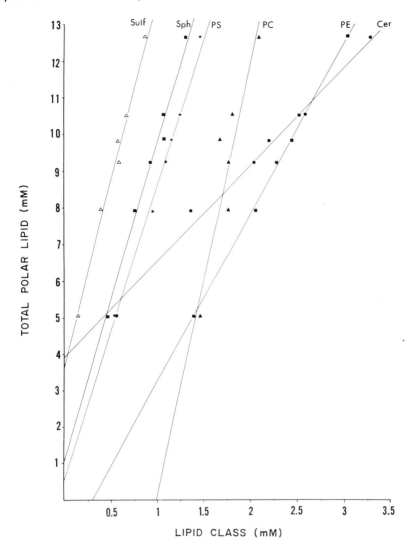

FIG. 2. Plot of normal human brain values (millimoles per 100 gm fresh weight) of lipid classes against total polar lipid (phospholipid plus cerebroside and sulfatide). The data were obtained from different regions of one brain. Note that values from different regions of the same brain form lines and that the lines for sulfatide, sphingomyelin, and phosphatidyl serine have similar slopes. The lines for cerebroside, sulfatide, sphingomyelin, and phosphatidyl serine represent increasing percentages as total lipid rises and the lines for phosphatidyl choline and phosphatidyl ethanolamine represent decreasing percentages. See text for further comments.

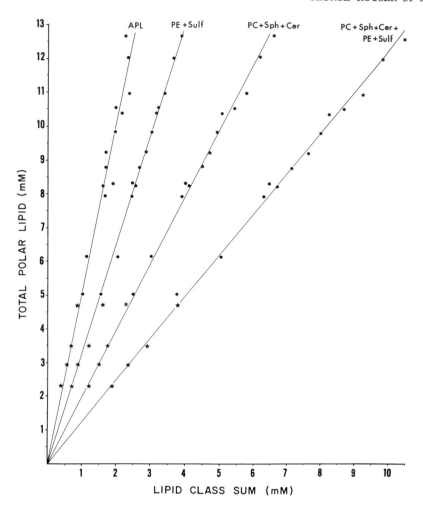

FIG. 3. Plot of sums of different lipid classes of human brain against total polar lipid (values as millimoles per 100 gm fresh weight) showing that four sums give straight lines passing through the origin. Solid circles are values from dfferent regions of two brains and stars are values obtained for representative samples of whole brains from four individuals in the early stages of development (25-week fetus and 1 day, 3 weeks, and 5 months postnatal age). Note that values for different regions of the same brain make the same lines made by values from representative samples of whole brains of different individuals. APL, acidic phospholipids; PE, phosphatidyl ethanolamine; Sulf, sulfatide; PC, phosphatidyl choline; Sph, sphingomyelin; Cer, cerebroside. See text for further comments.

those that decrease and noting which sums gave straight lines passing through the origin (Rouser *et al.*, 1971a,b). As shown in Fig. 3, four sums were found to give straight lines passing through the origin. These were: (1) cerebroside + sphingomyelin + phosphatidyl choline; (2)

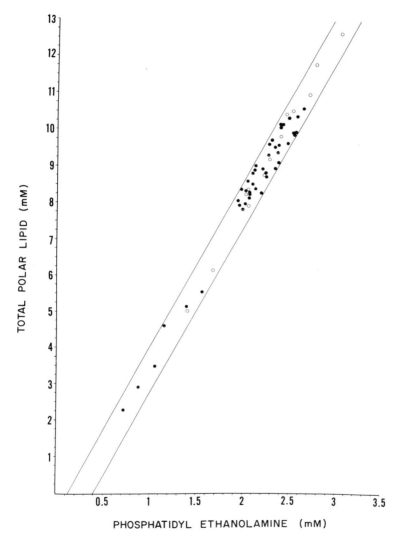

FIG. 4. Plot of human brain values (millimoles per 100 gm fresh weight) for phosphatidyl ethanolamine (plus lysophosphatidyl ethanolamine) against total polar lipid showing a relatively narrow range for all samples of whole brain (solid circles) as well as values for samples from different regions of the same brain (open circles). See text for comments.

phosphatidyl ethanolamine + sulfatide; and (3) what we have named substitution group II (the sum of all the acidic phospholipids, i.e., phosphatidyl serine, phosphatidyl inositol, diphosphatidyl glycerol, and miscellaneous minor components), as well as (4) what we have named substitution group I (the sum phosphatidyl choline + sphingomyelin + cerebroside + phosphatidyl ethanolamine + sulfatide) that is the sum of 1 + 2 above. Other sums did not give lines passing through the origin. It is thus apparent that, as the lipid content of human brain rises, cerebroside and sphingomyelin replace phosphatidyl choline; sulfatide replaces phosphatidyl ethanolamine; and acidic phospholipids replace each other. There are three different substitution groups in human brain, but only two in other organs in which phosphatidyl ethanolamine, phosphatidyl choline, and sphingomyelin substitute for each other. The values for substitution group I are (as percent of the total polar lipid): 63.3, 69.6, 72.7, 75.8, 78.6, 81.2, and 83.8%.

The relationships of the different lipid classes to total polar lipid of normal human whole brain defined by data from this laboratory are shown in Figs. 4–10. Most of the relationships were derived from data for representative samples of whole brain from 60 or more individuals and samples from different regions of three different brains. The figures present the progress in data analysis since our previous publications. The data are presented as ranges of variation that include the maximum random fluctuation with the methods used. The values for different regions of one brain fall into the same range as those from representative samples of whole brains from different individuals. When plotted against total polar lipid, the values for phosphatidyl ethanolamine, phosphatidyl serine, phosphatidyl inositol, cerebroside, and sulfatide give one line each within the range of experimental error. Thus, there is no indication of biological variability for the levels of these lipid classes. However, the ranges for phosphatidyl choline, sphingomyelin, and cholesterol are greater than the range of analytical error. These broader ranges appear to arise from biological variability. Two lines of evidence suggest that different human brains have reproducibly different levels of phosphatidyl choline, sphingomyelin, and cholesterol. First, on plots of molar amounts of cholesterol against the molar amounts of total phospholipid or total polar lipid, points tend to cluster around lines drawn at the two extremes and the mean of the range. This suggests that there are at least three subgroups. Second, plots of values for regions of one brain form one line in the center or on the right or left side of the normal range established by samples from whole brains of different individuals.

The relationships of the different lipid classes to total phospholipid are shown in Figs. 11–17. Plots of lipid class amounts against total phos-

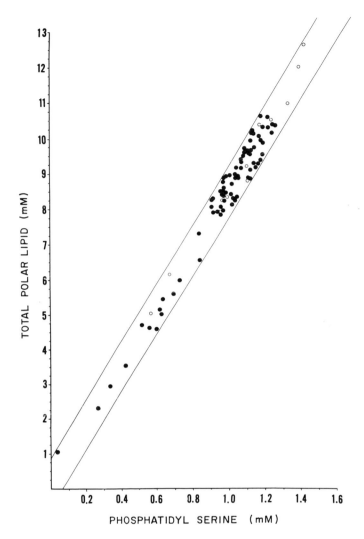

FIG. 5. Plot of values (millimoles per 100 gm fresh weight) for human brain phosphatidyl serine against total polar lipid. Note that the range of variation is relatively small (compare with Fig. 2). Symbols as for Fig. 4. See text for comments.

pholipid do not give the complete picture of the changes during development seen with total polar lipid plots, but they are useful for comparing different species (see Section IV) and for disclosing abnormal levels in pathological states. Within the range of measurement error, only one line (group) is seen on total phospholipid plots for phosphatidyl ethanolamine, phosphatidyl serine, phosphatidyl inositol, cerebroside, and sul-

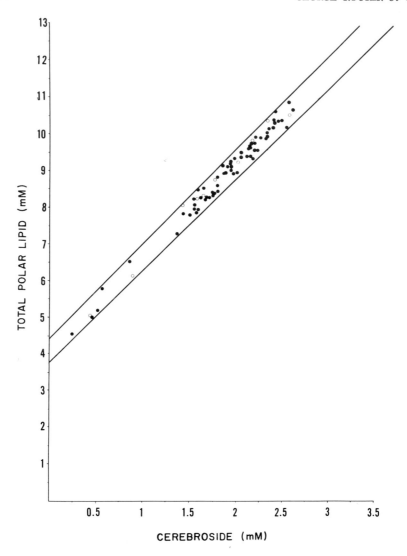

Fig. 6. Plot of values (millimoles per 100 gm fresh weight) of human brain cerebroside against total polar lipid. Symbols as for Fig. 4. See text for comments.

fatide (Figs. 11–14, 17). At least three subgroups (lines) appear probable for phosphatidyl choline and sphingomyelin (Figs. 15–16) as well as cholesterol. Graphic analysis thus indicates either genetic variability among humans for some brain lipid class levels or that environmental factors may influence brain development. Values obtained in this laboratory for samples of human spinal cord show the cord to differ from brain.

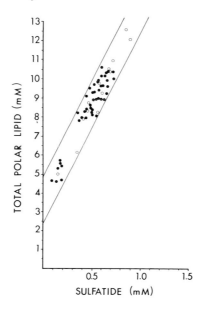

FIG. 7. Plot of values (millimoles per 100 gm fresh weight) of human brain sulfatide against total polar lipid. Symbols as for Fig. 4. See text for comments.

There is generally more sphingomyelin and less phosphatidyl choline in spinal cord, although the lipid class ranges for brain and cord overlap to a small extent. Both show the same relationships of phosphatidyl ethanolamine, phosphatidyl serine, phosphatidyl inositol, and sulfatide to total phospholipid.

All lipid classes give a broader range with three lines (subgroups) indicated when plotted against total lipid (that is, total polar lipid plus cholesterol). The probable explanation for this is that the three groups arise from the occurrence of different levels of substitution groups I and II. Individuals appear to differ with respect to the amounts of phosphatidyl choline and sphingomyelin that can be synthesized and thus the amounts of the choline lipids at any given total lipid level vary as the total amount of substitution group I varies. The amount of residual acidic phospholipid (substitution group II minus phosphatidyl serine and phosphatidyl inositol) goes up and down to exactly the same extent as the level of total choline lipid. Thus, it appears that, when the amounts of substitution groups I and II differ, the difference in substitution group I is accounted for by differences in the amounts of phosphatidyl choline and sphingomyelin, whereas the substitution group II requirement is met by varying amounts of residual acidic phospholipids (acidic phospholipid minus phosphatidyl serine and phosphatidyl inositol). Since the

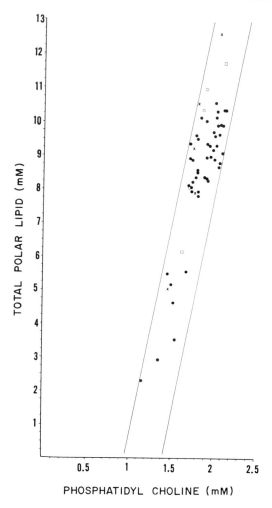

FIG. 8. Plot of values (millimoles per 100 gm fresh weight) of human brain phosphatidyl choline (+ lysophosphatidyl choline) against total polar lipid. Solid circles are values for representative samples of whole brains; open circles, open squares, and X's are values from different regions of three different brains. The range is somewhat larger than those shown in Figs. 4–6. See text for comments.

changes in substitution groups I and II exactly balance each other, one line only is obtained for phosphatidyl ethanolamine, phosphatidyl serine, phosphatidyl inositol, diphosphatidyl glycerol, cerebroside, and sulfatide on total phospholipid or total polar lipid plots. Three lines are obtained for these lipid classes when values are plotted against total lipid that includes cholesterol because there are three different levels of cholesterol.

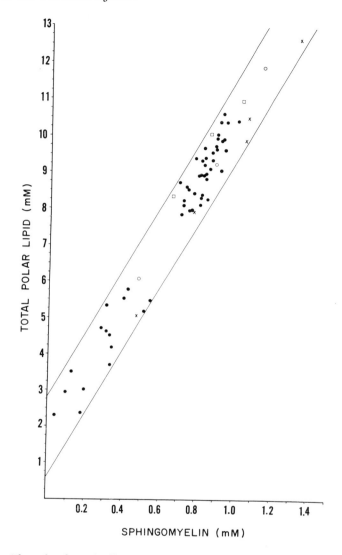

FIG. 9. Plot of values (millimoles per 100 gm fresh weight) for human brain sphingomyelin against total polar lipid. Symbols as for Fig. 8. See text for comments.

Cholesterol appears to bind to only certain polar lipids (phosphatidyl ethanolamine and acidic phospholipids, see Section V), and its level is thus determined by the amounts of these polar lipids.

Plots of lipid class values against age and against other lipid class values as well as lipid class versus total phospholipid and total polar lipid on both a fresh and dry weight basis were used to evaluate data

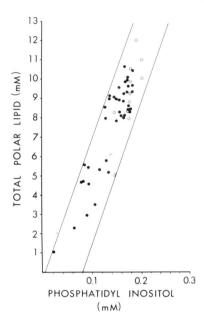

Fɪɢ. 10. Plot of values (millimoles per 100 gm fresh weight) for human brain phosphatidyl inositol against total polar lipid. Symbols as for Fig. 4. See text for comments.

from the literature. The only data for human brain phospholipids that failed to show wide variability and that were consistent with our data were reported by Svennerholm (1968), Pilz (1968), and Lesch and Bernhard (1967), all of whom who used one-dimensional TLC. The data of Svennerholm for two fetal whole brains and cerebral cortex and white matter of nine brains from individuals ranging in age from 1 day to 82 years were checked on lipid class versus lipid class and lipid class versus total phospholipid plots with values expressed as percentage of the dry weight since the water content of their samples was not reported. The data of Pilz and Lesch and Bernhard were less complete and could be checked only on lipid class versus lipid class plots. Data of Lesch (1969) could not be compared easily because values were presented as very small graphs of lipid content plotted against age. The only data for human brain cerebroside and sulfatide from the literature that was compatible with ours was that reported by Pilz (1968) and Lesch and Bernhard (1967). The data of Fishman *et al.* (1969) for human brain cerebroside plus sulfatide (estimated as lipid hexose) of six brains plotted against total phospholipid were in close correspondence to ours, a good straight line being obtained with a slope only slightly different

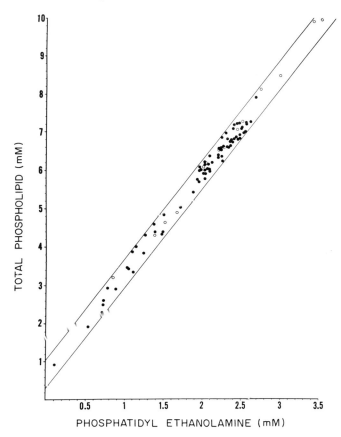

Fig. 11. Plot of values (millimoles per 100 gm fresh weight) for human brain phosphatidyl ethanolamine (+lysophosphatidyl ethanolamine) against total phospholipid. Symbols as for Fig. 4. See text for comments.

from that derived from our data. Some of the phospholipid data not compatible with ours were obtained by the first hydrolytic method to be reported. This method was later found to give incorrect values (see Section I). The major reason for the failure of column chromatographic data from some laboratories to agree with our data appears to be that the other investigators evaporated their samples to dryness, a procedure that altered lipids. Low sulfatide values in some studies can be traced to incomplete elution from magnesium silicate columns.

The total ganglioside content of human whole brain samples first increases and then decreases. As a function of age, total ganglioside as micromoles per 100 gm fresh tissue increases to about 6 months of age and then declines (Rouser and Yamamoto, 1968, 1969; Rouser *et al.*,

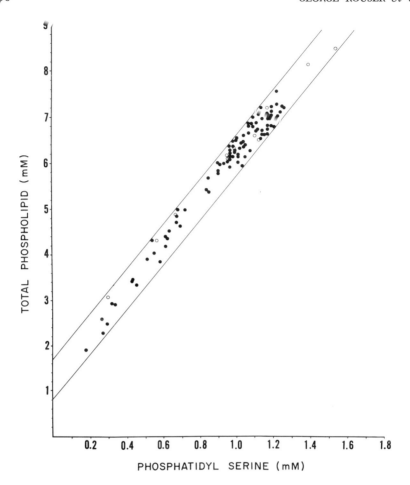

Fɪɢ. 12. Plot of values (millimoles per 100 gm fresh weight) for human brain phosphatidyl serine against total phospholipid. Symbols as for Fig. 4. See text for comments.

1970b, 1971b). The findings are in general agreement with those of Cumings *et al.* (1959) who reported human brain cerebral cortex and white matter neuraminic acid (grams per 100 gm dry tissue) first to increase and then decrease.

There are also changes in the pattern of ganglioside types with age. The nomenclature of Svennerholm and the abbreviations G for ganglioside, M for monosialo, D for disialo, and T for trisialo and the designation of different structures within a major group by numbers and letters is most commonly used. The changes noted first by Suzuki (1967) for the four major types of gangliosides in frontal cortex were a large post-

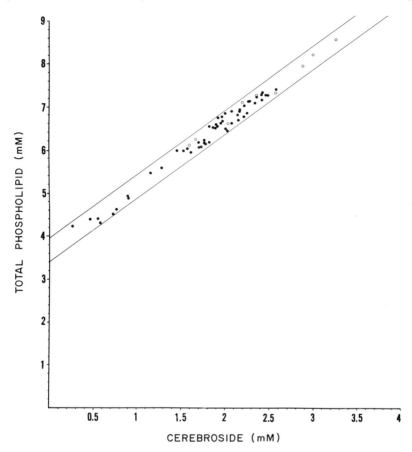

Fig. 13. Plot of values (millimoles per 100 gm fresh weight) for human brain cerebroside against total phospholipid. Symbols as for Fig. 4. See text for comments.

natal decline (as molar percentage of the total gangliosides) of G_{D1a} from birth to about 40 years of age with a fall in the relative amount of G_{M1} over the same period. These changes were balanced by relative increases in the amounts of G_{D1b} and G_{T1}. The findings were confirmed and extended by Vanier *et al.* (1971) who reported values for the fetal period of development. For the most part, the changes in the fetal period were the reverse of those seen in the postnatal period. Thus, in the frontal cortex, the molar percentage of G_{D1a} increased and the percentages of G_{T1} and G_{D1b} declined up to the time of birth. The percentage of G_{M1} fell to a low at 30 weeks and then rose to a peak at birth. The data of Suzuki (1967) showed a postnatal decline in G_{M1} that is less apparent in the data of Vanier *et al.* (1971) who suggested that Suzuki

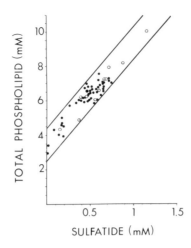

FIG. 14. Plot of values (millimoles per 100 gm fresh weight) for human brain sulfatide against total phospholipid. Symbols as for Fig. 4. See text for comments.

may have lost some G_{M1} prior to analysis. Vanier *et al.* (1971) noted that, in frontal white matter, the molar percentage of G_{M1} increased up to about 1 year of age and then remained rather constant (to 30 years), whereas there was a rather steady rise in G_{D1b} and G_{T1} from the first to the thirtieth year of life and a continuous decline in the molar percentage of G_{D1a} from birth to 30 years.

IV. Animal Nervous System Lipid Composition Changes with Age and Comparison to Humans

It is desirable to know whether or not species differ with respect to lipid class relationships during development. Clear quantitative differences are the presence of ceramide aminoethylphosphonate or ceramide phosphorylethanolamine and the absence of sphingomyelin in some (but not all) invertebrate species (Rouser *et al.*, 1968b). Ceramide aminoethylphosphonate and ceramide phosphorylethanolamine have not been found in vertebrate organs. For other lipid classes it is necessary to distinguish true quantitative species differences from individual variations within a species and differences arising from comparison of different stages of development.

Lipids of brain and other parts of the nervous systems of vertebrates and invertebrates have been studied in a number of laboratories (Avrova, 1971; Benton *et al.*, 1966; Bernhard *et al.*, 1969; Berry *et al.*, 1969; Dalal and Einstein, 1969; Davison and Wajda, 1959; Dekaban *et al.*, 1971;

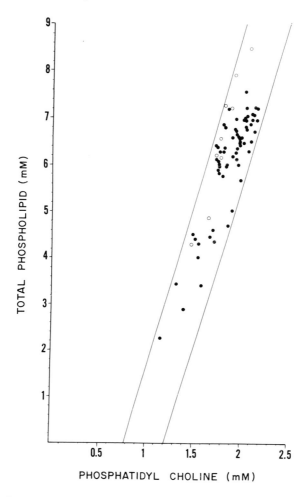

FIG. 15. Plot of values (millimoles per 100 gm fresh weight) for human brain phosphatidyl choline (+ lysophosphatidyl choline) against total phospholipid. Symbols as for Fig. 4. The broad range appears to arise from the presence of distinct groups of individuals having different phosphatidyl choline levels. See text for comments.

De Rooij and Hooghwinkel, 1967; Dvorkin and Gasteva, 1969; Erickson and Lands, 1969; Folch-Pi, 1955; Freysz *et al.*, 1963, 1966; Galli and Cecconi, 1967; Galli and Fumagalli, 1968; Hauser, 1968; Honnegger and Freyvogel, 1963; Hrachovec and Rockstein, 1959; Idler and Wiseman, 1968; Ishizuka *et al.*, 1970; Kishimoto *et al.*, 1965; Kishimoto and Radin, 1959; Kreps *et al.*, 1963, 1968; Lafranchi, 1938; Lenaz *et al.*, 1969; Lesch, 1969; McColl and Rossiter, 1950; McMurray *et al.*, 1964; Medda and

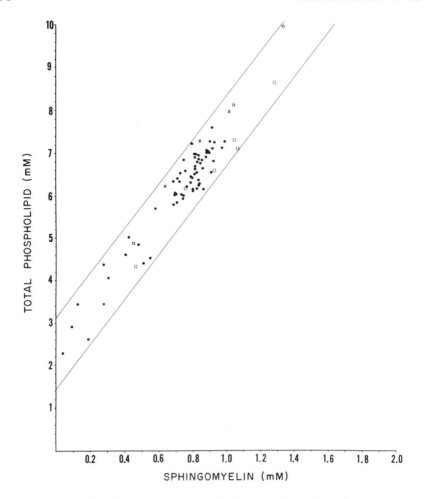

FIG. 16. Plot of values (millimoles per 100 gm fresh weight) for human brain sphingomyelin against total phospholipid. Symbols as for Fig. 8. The broad range appears to arise from distinct groups of individuals having different sphingomyelin levels. See text for comments.

Bose, 1967; Paoletti *et al.*, 1965; Patterson *et al.*, 1945; Porcellati, 1963; Prensky *et al.*, 1971; Pritchard and Cantin, 1962; Radin, 1970; Reinišová and Michalec, 1966; Reva and Rudenko, 1969; Roukema *et al.*, 1970; Rouser *et al.*, 1968b; Roots, 1968; Schengrund and Rosenberg, 1971; Sheltawy and Dawson, 1969; Spence and Wolfe, 1967a; Tsuyuki and Naruse, 1964; Vernadakis *et al.*, 1968; Wells and Dittmer, 1967; Williamson and Coniglio, 1971; Witting *et al.*, 1968; Yamakawa and Nishimura, 1966).

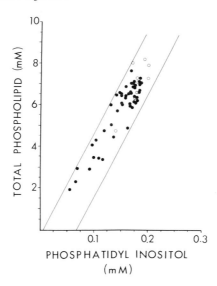

FIG. 17. Plot of values (millimoles per 100 gm fresh weight) for human brain phosphatidyl inositol against total phospholipid. Symbols as for Fig. 4. See text for comments.

Many species comparisons have been made with samples from animals of unknown age and without regard to the continuous nature of the increase of lipid with age. Rabbit brain total lipid was reported to increase steadily from birth to 620 days of age (the period of study) by Hrachovec and Rockstein (1959). Similar results were reported by Davison and Wajda (1959) whose data indicate a fall in lipid content at the end of the second year of life. Kishimoto et al. (1965) recognized that total lipid, cholesterol, and cerebroside plus sulfatide increased throughout the life span of the rat. Since the reports on the continuous nature of human brain lipid composition changes with age appeared (see Section III), it has become generally recognized upon reappraisal of the data for whole animal brain lipid at different ages that brain lipids change throughout life in other species (see, e.g., Ansell, 1971; Prensky et al., 1971). The continuous nature of the changes is perhaps best appreciated when data are plotted on semilogarithmic paper (Rouser and Yamamoto, 1968). Also, the amount of myelin isolated from rat brain was shown to increase through 425 days, which was the period of study in one case (Davison, 1969), and from 25 to 540 days in another (Rawlins and Smith, 1971). A threefold increase in the amount of myelin isolated from mouse brain at 26 months as compared to 3 months of age was reported by Sun and Samorajski (1972).

The general features of the lipid class composition changes with age in all vertebrate species are an increase in the relative amount of cerebroside, sulfatide, and sphingomyelin and a decrease in the relative amount of phosphatidyl choline and phosphatidyl ethanolamine. Also, the amounts of the di- and triphosphoinositides increase in rat brain from birth to 30–40 days of age (Sheltawy and Dawson, 1969).

The changes with age of gangliosides and the enzymes of ganglioside metabolism have been reviewed recently (Tettamanti, 1971). The ganglioside content of animal brains has not been studied extensively. There is some uncertainty in evaluation of the data because Lowden and Wolfe (1964) reported that hypercapnia caused a decrease in cat brain sialic acid content. Such changes were not found with rat brain (Holm, 1968). From the rather limited data for different species (Witting *et al.*, 1968; Ishizuka *et al.*, 1970; Avrova, 1971) it appears that vertebrates may differ in the types of brain gangliosides with some of the lower vertebrates having rather large amounts of tetra- and pentasialogangliosides.

The total ganglioside content of human brain appears to increase up to about 6 months postnatally and then declines (see Section III). A similar rise up to about 20 days and then a fall through at least 50 days of age is apparent for rat brain (Spence and Wolfe, 1967b; Suzuki, 1967). The data of Pritchard and Cantin (1962) show very clearly the early rise in rat brain cerebral cortex total gangliosides as do the rat brain data of Roukema *et al.* (1970), Vanier *et al.* (1971), Wells and Dittmer (1966), and Kishimoto *et al.* (1965).

The distribution of ganglioside types as a function of age has been determined for rat brain (Suzuki, 1967; Vanier *et al.*, 1971). For whole brain, Suzuki found an increase of G_{D1a} as molar percentage of the total ganglioside from birth up to about 20 days followed by a continuous decline through the 50-day period of study. During the same period, G_{T1} decreased sharply and then increased slightly with G_{D1b} following a similar pattern. The molar percentage of G_{M1} decreased to 9–10 days and then rose. The data of Vanier *et al.* are somewhat different. They observed the molar percentage of G_{D1a} of rat cerebellum to rise only up to about the sixth day and then to remain relatively constant. Very little change was noted in G_{T1} or G_{D1b} and the rise of G_{D1a} was balanced by a fall in G_{M1}. Vanier *et al.* (1971) suggested that the differences might be attributable to a loss of G_{M1} during sample preparation in Suzuki's studies. Schengrund and Rosenberg (1971) determined chicken brain ganglioside distribution in the prehatching period and found a large decline in the molar percentage of monosialoganglioside balanced largely by a fall of disialoganglioside with trisialoganglioside remaining constant up to about 12 days after which a decline was noted.

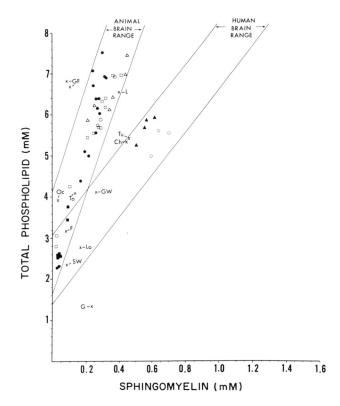

Fig. 18. Plot of values (millimoles per 100 gm fresh weight) for sphingomyelin against total phospholipid of different animal species with the normal human brain range (see Fig. 16) shown. Symbol designation: solid circles, whole mouse brain; open circles, whole bovine brain; open triangles, different regions of mouse and rat brains; solid triangles, whole rat brain data of Galli *et al.* (1970) to show that these values fall within the range for humans whereas other rat brain values do not; open squares, whole rat brain data from the authors' laboratory and that reported by Wells and Dittmer (1967); solid squares, inbred Beagle dogs; X's whole brain data for other species (from the authors' laboratory) designated as: Ch, chicken; F, frog; G, *Glycera;* GF, goldfish; GW, gray whale; L, lizard; Lo, lobster; Oc, octopus; SW, sperm whale; To, toad; and Tu, turtle. Note that the range labeled "animal brain" is characteristic for rat and mouse brains as well as some other species, but that *Glycera* has relatively more sphingomyelin and goldfish less than the other species. Some species fall in the human brain range. See text for further comments. The values of Kreps *et al.* (1968) for molluscs, when plotted, clearly placed the octopus in the animal brain region in agreement with our data. Absence of sphingomyelin at low total phospholipid levels is predicted by the range lines and shown by the data of Kreps *et al.* Their data place squid in the human brain range. The data of Prensky *et al.* (1971) place the pig in the human brain range. The data of Galli and Fumagalli (1968) place the stingray, lemon shark, nurse shark, and skipjack in the animal brain range. Other data from the literature (see text for references) were checked with values expressed on a dry weight basis (no figure shown). The data place sturgeon, carp, and frog in the range with less sphingomyelin than human brain, whereas values for rabbit, pigeon, tortoise, and some rats fall in the human brain range in keeping with data checked on fresh weight plots.

The changes in ganglioside patterns in three species (man, rat, and chicken) demonstrate that the pattern of each species changes with age, and, while the changes are similar, they are quantitatively different (i.e., species differ).

Desmosterol represents a large proportion of the total brain sterol at birth in several species (see reviews by Paoletti *et al.*, 1965; Paoletti, 1971). The percentage in chicken brain falls from about 10 to zero by 30 days of age. In rat and mouse brains the percentage at birth is even higher (24 to 30) and the percentage falls to or near zero by 30 days of age. A decline is also noted in human and guinea pig brains. Various sterols will no doubt be found in many invertebrate brains (for which data are not available) because a number of different sterols have been found in other tissues and whole organisms. Thus, Idler and Wiseman (1968) found seven sterols in the Alaskan king crab. Cholesterol (62.3%) and desmosterol (31.1%) were the major sterols and small to trace amounts of 22-dehydrocholesterol, brassicasterol, 24-methylenecholesterol, β-sitosterol, and fucosterol were also detected. Cholesterol (93.8%) and desmosterol (6.1%) were found in the North Atlantic queen crab by the same investigators. Cholesterol (54.5%) and brassicasterol (36.7%) were reported as the major sterols in a crab (Kritchevsky *et al.*, 1967). The changes with age in the amount of cholesterol relative to total phospholipid and total glycolipid are considered in Section V,C in which changes in whole brain and myelin are compared.

Differences among individuals of the same species and species variations in the lipid class distribution of brain were investigated by plotting values for lipid classes against each other and against total polar lipid and total phospholipid. The latter plots are shown in Figs. 18–24. The data obtained in the authors' laboratory and data for phospholipids, cerebroside, and sulfatide from the literature published after 1963 were used (see Section I for discussion of methods and the reasons for not using data published prior to 1963). Data from the literature were compared with our data on lipid class versus lipid class and lipid class versus total phospholipid or total lipid on a fresh or dry weight basis depending upon the data reported. Despite the use of different methods of analysis, good general agreement was noted.

The first general conclusion to be emphasized is that the lipid class distribution among animals of the same species is highly variable. Thus, brains of rats and mice frequently have less cerebroside, sulfatide, and sphingomyelin and correspondingly more phosphatidyl choline and phosphatidyl ethanolamine than human brain, but some rodent brains have the same high sphingolipid levels found in human brain. This is clearly shown by the rodent brain data obtained in the authors' laboratory as

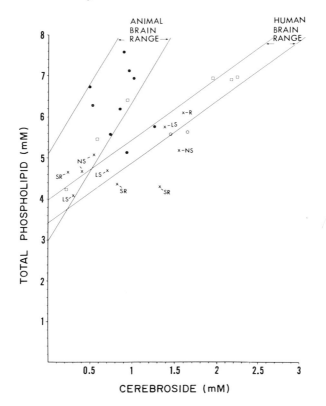

FIG. 19.   Plot of values (millimoles per 100 gm fresh weight) for cerebroside against total phospholipid of several animal species with the normal human range (see Fig. 13) shown. Symbols: solid circles, mouse brain; open squares, rat brain (Wells and Dittmer, 1967); X's data of Galli and Fumagalli (1968) for SR, stingray; LS, lemon shark; NS, nurse shark; and R, rat. Below 3 mmoles of total phospholipid, rat and mouse brain values are zero (points not shown). Also, all invertebrate brains not containing cerebroside have total phospholipid values below 3 mmoles. This suggests that cerebroside is not detectable because the total lipid level is low. Some rat and mouse values are in the human brain range whereas others are lower. Values for lemon shark and nurse shark and the stingray also appear to be in or near the human brain range. The skipjack (not shown) falls in the lower animal brain range. Several laboratories reported the sum of cerebroside and sulfatide. When tested against the human and mouse brain ranges, the data of Folch-Pi (1955) for mouse brain fell in the same range as data from our laboratory. The data of Prensky *et al.* (1971) for the pig place the range for this species just above and parallel to the human range whereas the sheep brain range (data from Patterson *et al.*, 1971) overlaps the human brain range but extends somewhat beyond it (higher values for glycolipid in some cases). There appear to be two phases for sheep brain. The first is a slow rise of glycolipid (up to about 120 days of age) followed by the second phase of more rapid increase of glycolipid. The values for this second period overlap the human brain range.

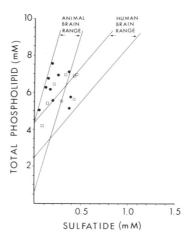

FIG. 20. Plot of values (millimoles per 100 gm fresh weight) for sulfatide against total phospholipid of rat and mouse brains with the human brain range shown. Symbols and comments as for Fig. 19.

well as in those of Wells and Dittmer (1967) and Galli and Fumagalli (1968). All of the values reported by the latter investigators fell in the human brain range. Another important feature of the variability is that rats and mice having the lower sphingolipid levels show a sizable range of variation in their amounts in contrast to the lack of biological variation in humans (see Section III). We have observed that some animals of the same inbred strain of mice have different lipid class levels and similar results were obtained with brains from inbred beagle dogs. Variations within an inbred strain suggest that some environmental factor such as diet may play a role in determining the lipid class distribution of brain.

Aside from the large variations among animals of the same species, the absence of any phylogenetic trend for lipid class distribution is quite striking. The concept of a phylogenetic trend consisting of a decreasing amount of sphingomyelin, cerebroside, and sulfatide with increasing amounts of phosphatidyl choline and phosphatidyl ethanolamine as animals progressively lower on the phylogenetic scale are examined has been accepted by many investigators. These conclusions are clearly incorrect. This is shown by graphic analysis that makes species comparisons possible without ambiguity. The conclusions drawn by other investigators were based on examination of tables of percentage values. This form of comparison did not separate differences among individuals of the same species and differences in the stage of development from true species variations. Also, more data are available now than previously.

The relative amount of sphingomyelin clearly does not show a phylo-

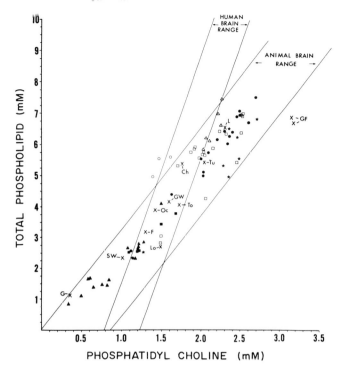

Fig. 21. Plot of values (millimoles per 100 gm fresh weight) for phosphatidyl choline (+ lysophosphatidyl choline) of animal species with the human brain range shown. Symbols for species: solid circles, mouse; open circles, bovine; open squares, rat; solid squares, Beagle dog; open triangles, values for different regions of rat and mouse brains; solid triangles, data for squid, octopus, *Helix,* and *Unio crassa* (Kreps *et al.,* 1968); stars, pig (Prensky *et al.,* 1971); X's, other species designated as indicated in the legend for Fig. 18. The range for rat and mouse brain is also the range for the other species shown except goldfish that has higher and bovine lower phosphatidyl choline. The data for different brain regions place the squid and octopus in the animal brain range whereas lemon and nurse sharks, stingray, and bovine brains appear to be in the human brain range. The data for goldfish brain reported by Roots (1968) falls to the left of the animal brain range shown, in keeping with our data. Other data from the literature were evaluated using ranges determined for values on a dry weight basis. These placed frog, sturgeon, and carp in the animal brain range (higher phosphatidyl choline than human brain) and pigeon, tortoise, rabbit, and some rats in the human brain range.

genetic progression (Fig. 18). Thus, the level of sphingomyelin in rabbit brain is clearly the same as or higher than that of human brain. The data of Dalal and Einstein (1969) recalculated as percentage of the total phospholipid place sphingomyelin of whole rabbit brain at about 21% in older animals, whereas it is never more than 15.6% in human brain.

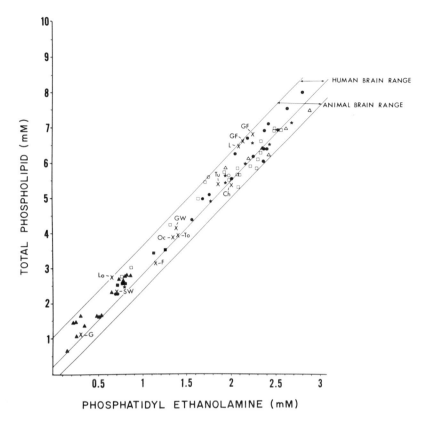

FIG. 22. Plot of values (millimoles per 100 gm fresh weight) for phosphatidyl ethanolamine (+ lysophosphatidyl ethanolamine) against total phospholipid of animal species with human brain range shown. Symbols as for Fig. 21. Note that the human and animal brain ranges overlap and that the range of variation for rat and mouse brain is the same as the range for all other animal species. Other data checked on a plot from values on a dry weight basis showed the same overlap of ranges. Thus, all vertebrate and invertebrate species were found to fall in the range shown for animal brain.

The data of Davison and Wajda (1959), although obtained by a less reliable method (column chromatography on aluminum oxide), suggest that rabbit brain sphingomyelin can be as high as 35% of the total phospholipid. Also, the data of Galli *et al.* (1970) indicate that rat brain may have sphingomyelin levels as high as in human brain. In addition, our data for *Glycera*, a bloodworm and the lowest form of animal in our series, demonstrates sphingomyelin to be very high (about 20% of the total phospholipid).

The complete absence or occurrence at a low level of sphingomyelin, cerebroside, and sulfatide in brain can be explained in several ways. The

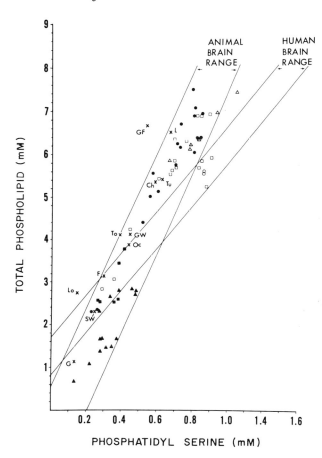

Fig. 23. Plot of values (millimoles per 100 gm fresh weight) for phosphatidyl serine against total phospholipid of animal species with the human brain range shown. Symbols as for Fig. 21. Some rat and mouse brain values fall in the human brain range whereas others do not. The animal brain range is the extent of variation for rats, mice, and most other species, but lobster, goldfish, sturgeon, carp, skipjack, and frog have less phosphatidyl serine and fall outside of the range. Data for some species were compared with ranges established from values on a dry weight basis.

relationships shown in Figs. 18–20 predict that these lipids may be absent at low total phospholipid levels. The data of Kreps *et al.* (1968) demonstrate that this situation exists in the octopus, since in the cerebral ganglion about 3.2% sphingomyelin was found at a total phospholipid level of about 2.80 mmoles per 100 gm fresh weight, whereas the level is zero in the optic ganglion that has only about 1.5 mmoles phospholipid per 100 gm fresh weight. This is in keeping with the low levels of

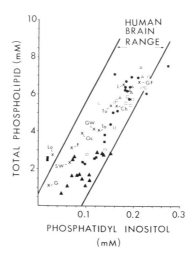

Fig. 24. Plot of values (millimoles per 100 gm fresh weight) for phosphatidyl inositol against total phospholipid of animal species with the human brain range shown. Symbols as for Fig. 21. The range for all animal species established from values on a fresh weight as well as a dry weight basis showed complete overlap with the human brain range.

sphingomyelin found in the brains of humans, rats, mice, and other species at early ages and a rise in the percentage of sphingomyelin as the total content increases. As shown in Fig. 18, the sphingomyelin levels of chicken, turtle, lobster, sperm whale, and gray whale are all in the human brain range.

A similar situation is found with cerebroside and sulfatide. The ratio of the sum of these glycolipids to total phospholipid in rabbit brain can be as high as 0.67 (Dalal and Einstein, 1969) but is not more than 0.40 in human brain. Rats and mice may have cerebroside and sulfatide levels as high as those of human brain, and we have found chicken brain to have levels of these glycolipids equal to that of human brain.

It seems probable that cerebroside and sulfatide are low in the brains of fish and most invertebrate species for one of two reasons. One is that the total lipid level is lower, perhaps because the animals studied are generally younger or because no appreciable amount of myelin is made at any age. The values of cerebroside and sulfatide reported by Reinišová and Michalec (1966) show that these glycolipids can represent about the same percentage of the total lipid in mammals, birds, reptiles, amphibians, and fish, but that the levels per gram fresh weight are highest in mammals, somewhat lower in birds, and still lower in amphibian and fish brains. The extent to which age differences influenced the comparisons was not determined. These authors reported detection of cerebroside and sulfatide in cockroach and crayfish brains, but quantitative data were not presented. The other reason that cerebroside and sulfatide are lower in some animal brains is that some species use exceptionally large amounts of phosphatidyl choline, sphingomyelin, or phosphatidyl ethanolamine. Both the goldfish and skipjack have higher phosphatidyl choline levels than were found in the other species for which there are data. Thus, less cerebroside, sulfatide, and sphingomyelin are required. Some species of flies have an exceptionally large relative amount of phosphatidyl ethanolamine, and sphingomyelin, cerebroside, and sulfatide are absent. We have found this to be the case with the blowfly (63.3% phosphatidyl ethanolamine + lysophosphatidyl ethanolamine). As noted above, *Glycera* (a bloodworm) has an exceptionally high sphingomyelin percentage that can account for the absence of cerebroside and sulfatide. It thus is not certain whether or not species lacking these glycolipids have lost the ability to synthesize them. A study of other organs of the same species may disclose the presence of glycolipid and thus prove that they can indeed synthesize glycolipids.

The presence of ceramide phosphorylethanolamine in some invertebrate species indicates that a mutation occurred making possible the transfer of the ethanolamine phosphate moiety of cytidine diphosphate ethanolamine to ceramide as well as diglyceride. Although this lipid has not been reported to occur in any vertebrate species, its presence in some unstudied species seems possible. Ceramide aminoethylphosphonate occurs in some invertebrates, but the presence of this lipid is not restricted to invertebrates because it is also present in some fungi (Hendrix and Rouser, unpublished data).

Species show the least variability for phosphatidyl ethanolamine and phosphatidyl inositol as indicated in Figs. 22 and 24. The range of phosphatidyl ethanolamine values for many species is the same as that for rat and mouse brains, and the range of human brain covers about one-half of the animal brain range. In contrast, many animal species have lower levels of phosphatidyl serine at high total phospholipid values and higher levels at low total phospholipid values as compared to human and bovine brains. Fish are exceptional in having very low phosphatidyl serine levels. There are no differences apparent for any vertebrate species for the amounts of substitution groups I and II.

It is apparent that some animal species have brain lipid compositions like that of the human, and thus, selection of the proper strain of a particular species can provide an animal model for collection of data most directly relevant to humans. Our data for bovine brain shows this species to be like humans in every respect.

Data are not available for extensive species comparisons of spinal
cord composition. The data for 30-day-old pig (Berry *et al.,* 1969),
cat (Reva and Rudenko, 1969), and adult human (Rouser and Wade,
unpublished data) spinal cords indicate that the three species differ in
the amounts of most lipid classes, but the comparisons cannot be made
graphically and thus neither age differences nor individual variations
within each species can be evaluated. Adult human and cat (values in
parentheses) spinal cords contained as percentage of the total phospholipid respectively: phosphatidyl ethanolamine, 34 to 36% (18%); phosphatidyl choline, 20 to 21% (28%); sphingomyelin, 18 to 20% (22%); phosphatidyl serine, 16 to 17% (17%); phosphatidyl inositol, 1.8% (5.4%). Pig
brain values for sphingomyelin were lower (13%) and the phosphatidyl
choline values higher (42%). These differences are probably largely a
reflection of the younger age (30 days) of the pigs. A comparison of
fetal and adult human cords showed the typical differences found in
brain, that is, an increase in cerebroside, sulfatide, sphingomyelin, and
phosphatidyl serine, and a decrease in phosphatidyl ethanolamine with
age. Of special interest was the complete absence of sulfatide from both
25- and 40-week-old fetuses with cerebroside being readily detectable
and making up 8% of the weight of the total lipid of the 40-week-old
fetus. Sheep spinal cord (Patterson *et al.,* 1971) has more cerebroside
plus sulfatide than human brain and appears to be similar to human
spinal cord in its glycolipid content.

The basis for the quantitative differences among animal species for
brain lipid class composition is of interest. Since brain lipid class differences are found among species (man, bovine, mouse, rat, frog) for
which no species differences are apparent for the composition of liver,
lung, heart, and kidney (Baxter *et al.,* 1969; Rouser *et al.,* 1969a; Simon
and Rouser, 1969), it is possible that differences in membrane lipid-
binding proteins account for part of the species differences. The basic
protein of myelin does not occur in other membranes of brain (Agrawal
et al., 1970) and, at least in some species, is not found in early brain
myelin (Einstein *et al.,* 1970). This suggests that the change in lipid
composition of myelin with age seen in some species may be the result
of different lipid-binding affinities of different proteins that change in
amount with age. The relative amounts of the lipid classes of myelin
from brain, spinal cord, and peripheral nerve is different (see Section V)
and this is associated with the presence of different amounts of myelin
proteins (Wolfgram and Katorii, 1968a,b).

In addition to differences in the amounts of lipid-binding proteins
with different affinities for lipid classes, it also seems probable that some
individual and species differences arise from differences in the balance
between biosynthetic and degradative enzyme levels, but there is no

information available on relative enzyme levels. A rise in the percentage of sphingomyelin with age had been noted for human aorta (Rouser and Solomon, 1969; Eisenberg *et al.*, 1969) and some animal species. This is associated with a decline with age of the sphingomyelinase level and a rise in the amount of degradative enzymes for glycerolphospholipids (Eisenberg *et al.*, 1969). Species differ from each other in the extent to which sphingomyelin substitutes for phosphatidyl choline and phosphatidyl ethanolamine. The relative amount of sphingomyelin also increases with age in the lens of the eye and there are species differences (see Section V,C). The lens is particularly interesting to compare with brain because both have a relatively large proportion of plasma membrane. It is not surprising therefore that the lens has a high sphingomyelin content (see Section V,C) since, according to our concept of lipid class replacement, sphingomyelin should substitute more extensively for phosphatidyl choline when the relative amount of plasma membrane is large. The age changes in brain appear to differ somewhat from those of aorta and the lens in that, in brain, the changes in man appear to arise entirely from changes in the proportions of membranes rather than their lipid class distribution, although changes in lipid class distribution of membranes do occur in some species (see Section V,D). Species differences appear to arise particularly in highly differentiated organs that show large changes with age (brain, aorta, lens of the eye, etc.).

In conclusion, it is to be emphasized that species can be compared for similarities in brain lipid class distribution by graphic analysis without knowledge of the age of each animal or the developmental time scale of each species. The range of variability for each species should be established by examination of an adequate number of analyses of whole brains from individual animals. Also, data for different regions of the same brain should be obtained so that the slope of the line made when the values are plotted can be used to determine whether or not it follows that of human or other species.

V. Conclusions Derived from Studies of Lipid Composition of Isolated Whole Cell and Subcellular Particulate Preparations of the Nervous System

A. Evaluation of the Possibility of Lipid Loss or Gain by Subcellular Particulates During Isolation

Lipid loss or gain by subcellular particulates during isolation is generally recognized as possible, but does not appear to have been evaluated. Accurate and precise definition of composition changes of membranes and organelles is essential if the relationships of lipid to protein are to be defined and explained and the factors regulating the lipid class composition of membranes determined. The data for brain particulates are so limited that it is necessary to derive conclusions largely from the data for other membranes. Wolman *et al.* (1966) observed loss of about 50% of the lipid of myelin into water after treatment with salt solutions. All lipid classes appeared to be lost to about the same extent. Loss of 50% of the lipid from myelin was brought about when myelin was incubated in a detergent solution (Dobiašová and Radin, 1968) and, although all lipid classes were lost, phosphatidyl ethanolamine appeared to be lost to the greatest extent. Cholesterol, galactolipid, and protein were lost to a greater extent than phospholipid from myelin incubated in various salt solutions (Leitch *et al.*, 1969). Lipid exchange *in vitro* between labeled lipid micelles (of phosphatidyl choline and cerebroside) and brain particulates (myelin and mitochondria) was studied and found to take place to a small extent (Dobiašová and Radin, 1968). Similar results were reported for exchange of lipids with rat heart mitochondria (Dobiašová and Linhart, 1970). Net uptake of lipid by the cellular particulates was not determined. Roeske and Clayton (1968) observed that labeled sterol introduced *in vitro* into a homogenate of insect muscle was distributed in the subcellular fractions in a manner similar to that found when labeled sterol was administered *in vivo*. Exchange of sterol incorporated *in vivo* into mitochondria was small when the labeled mitochondria were added to an unlabeled homogenate. The studies show that lipid can exchange between subcellular particulates during isolation, but net gain or loss was not determined.

Lipid loss and gain *in vitro* have been observed with particulates incubated in solutions of plasma lipoproteins. Rat liver plasma membranes were observed to lose 47–54% of their cholesterol without loss of phospholipid or protein when incubated in a cholesterol-depleted plasma lipoprotein solution (Graham and Green, 1969). Conversely, the cholesterol content of rat liver mitochondria incubated in a plasma lipoprotein solution was almost doubled (Bruckdorfer *et al.*, 1968; Graham and Green, 1970). The mechanism of these gains and losses was determined with red blood cells. The exchange of intact phospholipid molecules is best studied with red blood cells and their ghosts because they do not have the biosynthetic and degradative enzymes found in other membranes. The rate of exchange of phospholipids determined by isotope labeling is influenced in most membranes by phospholipases that produce lysophospholipids that have different protein binding affinities from the parent molecules.

Plasma contains the enzyme phosphatidyl choline-cholesterol acyltransferase that transfers a fatty acid from phosphatidyl choline to cholesterol to give cholesterol ester and lysophosphatidyl choline, although this enzyme was not detected in rat brain (Eto and Suzuki, 1971). Thus, when plasma or serum is allowed to stand, the free cholesterol content is reduced. About 30% of the cholesterol of red blood cells from normal persons is lost when the cells are exposed to incubated serum (Murphy, 1962). If fresh plasma is heated to destroy the enzyme, red blood cells do not lose cholesterol on incubation. The loss of cholesterol is not accompanied by loss of phospholipid. Phospholipid (25–35% of the total) and cholesterol (25–35%) is lost from red blood cells incubated in plasma depleted of glucose (Cooper and Jandl, 1969; Reed and Swisher, 1966). The phospholipid loss is not reversible, but cells that have lost only cholesterol regain it when incubated in heated serum. Cells depleted of cholesterol were found to be osmotically more fragile and spherical, but these properties returned to normal when cholesterol was restored. When phospholipid loss was observed, all phospholipid classes appeared to be lost to the same extent. Cholesterol and phospholipid loss from red blood cells also takes place upon incubation in buffered albumin solution containing paramercuribenzoate (Jacob, 1967). In one study, the weight of lipid lost appeared to be balanced by a gain of protein (Langley and Axell, 1968).

The changes observed in human red blood cell lipid content in various pathological states can be explained by the simultaneous occurrence of altered plasma lipid levels and abnormal activity of the phosphatidyl choline-cholesterol acyltransferase. Plasma phospholipids and free and esterified cholesterol are greatly elevated in some hyperlipidemic states, but red cell cholesterol and phospholipid content are usually normal when the level of the acyl transferase is normal. The hyperlipemia of liver disease is associated with an increase in erythrocyte cholesterol (up to about twice the normal level) with total phospholipid being normal or increased, the relative amount of phosphatidyl choline being above normal and the levels of phosphatidyl ethanolamine and sphingomyelin being lower than normal (Nye and Marinetti, 1967; Neerhout, 1968a,b; Boon *et al.*, 1969; Cooper, 1969). The erythrocyte cholesterol increase appears to arise from the abnormally high ratio, in plasma, of free to esterified cholesterol brought about by bile acid inhibition of the phosphatidyl choline-cholesterol acyltransferase. There is thus an excess of both free cholesterol and phosphatidyl choline in plasma, and both lipids are transferred to the red blood cells. The plasma and erythrocyte lipid alterations in liver disease are similar to those of patients with a hereditary deficiency of the acyltransferase. The above-normal levels of phosphatidyl choline and cholesterol in the erythrocytes of these patients are lost upon incubation *in vitro* in plasma from normal individuals and, conversely, cells from normal individuals incubated in patients' plasma gain cholesterol (Norum and Gjone, 1968). Similar changes of cholesterol content during *in vitro* incubation were reported for erythrocytes of patients with "spur" cell liver disease (Cooper, 1969). Changes in erythrocyte lipid content occur in Zieve's syndrome. Very large increases of erythrocyte cholesterol and phospholipid (mainly phosphatidyl choline) may be observed. In one patient, the increase of cholesterol and phospholipid was more than twofold (Westerman *et al.*, 1968). Patients with abetalipoproteinemia (acanthocytosis) have low total plasma lipid, but the patients' erythrocytes have normal total phospholipid and acyl transferase.

It is clear that the abnormalities of erythrocyte lipids are largely confined to cholesterol, phosphatidyl choline, and sphingomyelin. These are the red cell lipids that exchange with plasma or lipoprotein solutions *in vitro* and *in vivo* (Cooper, 1969; Norum and Gjone, 1968; Westerman *et al.*, 1968; Murphy, 1965; Basford *et al.*, 1964; Ashworth and Green, 1964; Bruckdorfer and Green, 1967; Sakagami *et al.*, 1965a,b; Reed, 1968). Total exchange of cholesterol was reported, but the exchangeable phospholipids may not always exchange completely.

As much as 25% loss of cholesterol and phospholipid from normal human red blood cells was encountered as the result of treatment of the cells with hypotonic solutions to prepare ghosts, and up to 50% loss of phospholipids and cholesterol was obtained by washing with aqueous solutions containing ethylenediaminetetraacetate (Turner and Rouser, unpublished data). All phospholipid classes were lost to very nearly the same extent. Another feature of the loss of lipid from red cell ghosts is its variability, i.e., the membranes of red cells from some subjects lost more lipid than those of other subjects when ghosts were prepared by the same procedure.

The data suggest that, in general, membranes may lose lipid to or gain lipid from some aqueous solutions; that the loss may be variable even when the same method is employed; that the ratio of cholesterol to phospholipid may be changed by selective loss or gain of cholesterol; and that the relative proportions of the phospholipids (and perhaps cerebroside and sulfatide as well) may not change appreciably even when there is a large loss of lipid.

Subcellular particulates isolated from most organs contain small amounts of lysophospholipids (principally lysophosphatidyl ethanolamine and lysophosphatidyl choline) and free fatty acids. Some enzymatic degradation of lipids during isolation is to be expected and thus the finding (Lunt and Rowe, 1968) that the combined yield of unesteriﬁ₊₊l fatty acid from subcellular fractions of rat brain was greater than that from unfractionated tissue is not surprising. The presence of large amounts of lyso compounds arising from exposure to high levels of lipases and phospholipases was reported for pancreas organelles (Meldolesi *et al.*, 1971). A relatively low level of the products of enzyme degradation of phospholipids does not ensure, however, that the lipids have not been altered by degradative enzymes since both lysophospholipids and free fatty acids can be selectively transferred from organelles to other proteins including albumin (Fleischer and Fleischer, 1967; Meissner and Fleischer, 1972). Thus, enzymatic degradation followed by avid sequestering of lyso compounds and free fatty acids by proteins added to the isolation medium is a means of lipid loss that will require attention in future studies.

The values reported from different laboratories for lipid to protein ratio of the same membrane isolated from the same species are quite variable. Values ranging from 25 to 50% lipid have been reported for retinal rod outer segments (Adams, 1967, 1969; Anderson and Maude, 1970; Borggreven *et al.*, 1970; Eichberg and Hess, 1967; Nielsen *et al.*, 1970; Poincelot and Zull, 1969). If the higher value is correct, loss of up to one-half the total lipid is indicated. This is in agreement with the results obtained with erythrocyte ghosts as is the fact that closely similar values were obtained in two laboratories for lipid class percentages when total lipid was 25% and 50% respectively of the dry weight (Anderson and Maude, 1970; Nielsen *et al.*, 1970). The variability may be explained, however, by loss of protein to different extents, or, at least in part, to true biological variability.

The range of values reported in the literature for myelin total lipid is 60–80% of the dry weight. There are typically light and heavy myelin fractions and in a sucrose gradient myelin spreads to give a rather wide band (Adams and Fox, 1969). The differing densities suggest differences in lipid content. The lipid content of myelin of six human brains (stored in the frozen state) was determined by Dr. Elie Shneour in the senior author's laboratory by the method described by Norton (1971). Lipid content as percentage of the dry weight was determined by weighing lipid separated from protein by Sephadex column chromatography. Values of 59, 63, 70, 81, 89, and 90% of the dry weight were obtained. If the commonly quoted 75% value is correct, then loss of one-half of the lipid without loss of protein would result in preparations having about 66% lipid. Since loss of the basic protein from myelin has been observed to arise from standing for 2 hours *in vivo* prior to isolation as well as during *in vitro* incubation (Dickinson *et al.*, 1970), and since this protein commonly makes up about 30% of the total protein (Eng *et al.*,

1968), its selective loss without lipid loss would give about 85% lipid. Thus, the results obtained in our laboratory as well as those reported in the literature correspond fairly well to the expectations based upon the findings with red cell ghosts and the observed loss of the basic protein of myelin *in vivo* and *in vitro.*

Subcellular particulates isolated from brain by the commonly used procedures have low total ganglioside contents (Wiegandt, 1967; Lapetina *et al.,* 1967). Failure to recover gangliosides completely (loss during isolation) appears to have been documented by Spence and Wolfe (1967b), although Hamberger and Svennerholm (1971) did not find gangliosides in their supernatant fractions. Spence and Wolfe (1967b) described isolation from neonatal rat brain of a membrane with a high content (7–9% of the dry weight) of ganglioside. Membranes perhaps corresponding to those of dendrites have been isolated by dissection (Derry and Wolfe, 1967) and found to have a high ganglioside content. Thus, either loss of gangliosides during isolation or the failure to isolate the proper fractions or both factors seem to be responsible for the findings. Gangliosides appear to be located primarily in the dendritic processes rather than in the nerve cell body or the axonal membranes. In keeping with these conclusions, we have found only traces of ganglioside in bovine peripheral nerve, and the olfactory nerve of the garfish that is a good source of nonmyelinated axons and hence neuronal plasma membranes (Easton, 1971) does not appear to contain gangliosides (Holton and Easton, 1971). Gangliosides are, like lysophosphatidyl choline and lysophosphatidyl ethanolamine, water soluble and, like free fatty acids, are acidic. Since lysophospholipids and free fatty acids are all bound strongly to albumin to which they will transfer from membranes, it seems possible that a similar transfer can take place with gangliosides. The large number of polar groups and the high water solubility of gangliosides suggest that they might also simply leave membranes and exist free in solution.

In summary, the available data suggest that lipid loss from membranes during isolation by some methods does occur and that it should be carefully evaluated in future studies. Except for cholesterol and gangliosides, however, lipid loss or gain may not have distorted the lipid class distribution of brain particulates to any major extent.

B. Lipids of Neurons, Glial Cells, and Capillaries (Endothelial Cells) of Brain

The lipid composition of purified preparations of neurons (cell bodies mainly devoid of plasma membrane extensions), astrocytes, oligodendroglia, and capillaries (endothelial cells) of brain have been reported (Cremer *et al.*, 1968; Derry and Wolfe, 1967; Fewster and Mead, 1968; Freysz *et al.*, 1968; Hamberger and Svennerholm, 1971; Hemminki, 1970; Johnston and Roots, 1970; Norton and Poduslo, 1971; Poduslo and Norton, 1972; Raine *et al.*, 1971; Siakotos *et al.*, 1969a; Tamai *et al.*, 1971a,b). The data are summarized in Table I. Neurons and astrocytes were found to have closely similar lipid compositions and the composition did not change significantly with age during the period when whole brain changes are large (Norton and Poduslo, 1971). Both types of cells have low levels of cerebroside and sulfatide. In contrast, the oligodendroglia that form myelin have high cerebroside and sulfatide levels. Also, cholesterol (weight percentage of the total lipid) of oligodendroglia is about twice as high as that of neurons and astrocytes. This is in keeping with the findings of Jones *et al.* (1971) that neuron-enriched fractions showed less *in vitro* isotope incorporation into cholesterol than did glial-enriched fractions. Cerebroside and sulfatide were not detected in brain capillaries, and capillaries have a greater percentage of the total phospholipid as sphingomyelin than neurons or astrocytes.

The lipid composition of the different cell types suggests that only myelin-forming cells contain an appreciable amount of cerebroside and sulfatide and that changes in lipid composition with age are largely, if not entirely, restricted to myelin and other membranes of the cells that form myelin. From the data, it appears that subcellular particulates from neurons and astrocytes must have very low levels of cerebroside and sulfatide, whereas the levels from oligodendroglia should be high. Thus, subcellular particulate preparations differing in the relative contributions made by oligodendroglia and other cells should have different glycolipid and phospholipid distributions.

C. Lipids of Membranes of the Eye

Membranes of the eye are of interest in comparison with those from the central nervous system. Data for various parts of the eye from several species are available (Anderson *et al.*, 1969, 1970; Anderson, 1970; Broekhuyse, 1968, 1969, 1971; Broekhuyse and Veerkamp, 1968; Feldman *et al.*, 1965, 1966a,b; Handa and Burton, 1969; Klein, 1968; Klein and Mandel, 1968; Plazonnet *et al.*, 1969; Windeler and Feldman, 1970). Rod outer segments are thought to be extensions of a nerve cell plasma membrane (Porter and Bonneville, 1968) and most of the lipid of the lens is present in a plasma membrane extension of epithelial cells (a thin layer of cells at the periphery of the lens).

Data are available for frog (Eichberg and Hess, 1967) and bovine rod

Table I

LIPID COMPOSITION OF BRAIN WHOLE-CELL PREPARATIONS

Lipid class	Neurons			Astrocytes[a,b]	Mixed glial[c,d]	Oligodendro-glia[a,f]	Endothelial cells[a,h]
	(1)[a,b]	(2)[c,d]	(3)[a,e]				
Total lipid	34.4–46.2 pg/cell[i]			177–309 pg/cell		15.6–25.9% dry wt.	NR
Cholesterol	10.0–11.5	35.5	9.0 ±2.5	12.4–17.0	35.8	29.6–31.5	NR
Cerebroside	⎰ 1.4–2.6	2.8	ND[j]	⎰ 1.2–2.2	3.2	9.5–11.4	ND
Sulfatide	⎱	0.6	ND	⎱	0.8	4.2–4.4	ND
Sphingomyelin	2.6–3.5	4.8		3.0–4.6	5.3	5.0–6.2	17.0–21.2
Phosphatidyl choline	36.1–44.2	28.4	46.7 ±3.2	33.3–39.2	25.4	13.2–14.8	32.6–34.3
Phosphatidyl ethanolamine	17.4–19.3	19.9	28.3 ±3.3	16.9–22.0	22.6	16.9–17.1	23.5–25.2

Phosphatidyl serine	3.4–4.1	4.5	8.7 ±1.2	4.6–5.7	4.8	7.8–12.7	10.0–11.0

Phosphatidyl serine	3.4–4.1	4.5	8.7 ±1.2	4.6–5.7	4.8	7.8–12.7	10.0–11.0
Phosphatidyl inositol	4.4–5.6	3.4	NR[k]	3.6–4.2	1.9	0.7–1.9	4.3–4.8
Diphosphatidyl glycerol	3.8–4.8[l]	NR	NR	3.5–4.2[l]	NR	NR	1.0–1.5
Uncharacterized	NR	NR	NR	NR	NR	2.1–11.0	ND
Phosphatidic acid	NR	NR	NR	NR	NR	NR	0.2–0.9

[a] Lipid class values as weight percentages of the total lipid.
[b] Range for rat brain data from Norton and Poduslo (1971). See also Davison et al. (1966) and Freysz et al. (1968).
[c] Lipid class values as molar percentages of the total lipid.
[d] Range for rabbit brain data from Hamberger and Svennerholm (1971).
[e] Range for pig brain data from Tamai et al. (1971a).
[f] Range for bovine brain data from Fewster and Mead (1968). The data of Poduslo and Norton (1972) for calf brain oligodendroglia show very different weight ratios for cholesterol to galactolipid to phospholipid (i.e., 14:10:62) as compared to 30:14.5:42 reported by Fewster and Mead.

[g] Lipid class values as molar percentages of the total phospholipid.
[h] Range for human and bovine brain data from Siakotos et al. (1969a).
[i] pg/cell, picograms per cell.
[j] ND, not detected.
[k] NR, not reported.
[l] Range for rat brain data from Freysz et al. (1968).

outer segments (Adams, 1967, 1969; Anderson and Maude, 1970; Borg-greven *et al.*, 1970; Nielsen *et al.*, 1970; Poincelot and Zull, 1969). Cerebroside and sulfatide were not detected. As can be seen in Table II, a striking feature of the composition of this membrane is its low sphingomyelin content with a correspondingly higher phosphatidyl choline content than plasma membranes from cells in other organs. The composition is in good agreement with that expected from the lipids of whole brain prior to onset of myelination. We found sphingomyelin values (as molar percentage of the total polar lipid) to be 1.2 for newborn whole human brain and 1.1–1.2 for newborn whole mouse brain. As noted in Section V,B, neurons have very low levels of sphingomyelin in all of their membranes. Thus, one of the most characteristic features of plasma (cell surface) membranes from most cells, i.e., a relatively high level of sphingomyelin, is not seen in neuronal plasma membranes. Also, it appears that rod outer segments may contain less cholesterol (4.3 weight % of the total lipid; Eichberg and Hess, 1967) than other neuronal plasma membranes; however, the low level may be a reflection, at least in part, of the age of the animal.

The similarity of the phospholipid compositions of frog and bovine rod outer segments indicates that little species variability is to be expected. About 23% by weight glycolipid was reported for the frog membranes (Eichberg and Hess, 1967), but glycolipid values were not reported for bovine membranes. Since some neuronal processes of vertebrates in general are rich in gangliosides, their presence in rod outer segments of other species may be expected. Although more data are needed for evaluation of species differences, as shown in Table II, the close correspondence of whole retinal lipid class composition of man, dog, pig, sheep, cattle, and rabbit (Anderson *et al.*, 1970) suggests that species variations in rod outer segment composition will prove to be small for vertebrates. The variable total lipid content of rod outer segments discussed in Section V,A should be evaluated carefully.

Lipids in the lens, retina, iris, choroid, cornea, sclera, and vitreous body of cattle have been compared by Broekhuyse and Veerkamp (1968). Lens, iris, choroid, cornea, and sclera were all found to have similar compositions with a rather high sphingomyelin level (14–18%) that is rather characteristic of plasma membranes of epithelial cells and that is similar to that of oligodendroglia, but is in contrast to the low level of sphingomyelin in whole retina, rod outer segments, and neurons in general. The first report of human lens phospholipids (Feldman *et al.*, 1966a) indicated a very high level of sphingomyelin (up to about 70% of the total phospholipid) and a low level of phosphatidyl choline (under 5%). Subsequently, more detailed work (Broekhuyse, 1969) has

Table II

Lipid Composition of Membranes of the Eye[a]

Lipid class	Rod outer segment		Retina[b]						Humans lens cortex[c]		
	Frog[d]	Bovine[e]	Dog	Pig	Human	Sheep	Bovine	Rabbit	20 yr	32 yr	66 yr
Sphingomyelin	1.8	1.3–4.2	4.4	3.7	4.3	3.4	2.1	4.4	40.7	46.5	58.0
Phosphatidyl choline	49.4	36.6–41.2	48.1	47.4	48.1	47.5	43.4	46.5	9.4	7.0	5.5
Phosphatidyl ethanolamine	30.2	38.1–43.0	30.0	32.3	31.7	30.8	34.1	34.7	21.8	20.0	11.7
Phosphatidyl serine	9.5	11.2–14.5	8.9	8.1	8.6	9.7	10.0	7.4	5.7	8.5	6.2
Phosphatidyl inositol	1.4	1.5–2.5	4.6	5.5	4.4	5.2	5.6	4.3	0.8	0.4	0.1
Phosphatidic acid	3.0	0.4	NR[f]	NR	NR	NR	NR	NR	NR	NR	NR
Diphosphatidyl glycerol	1.3	0.2	NR	NR	NR	NR	NR	NR	1.4	0.7	0.3
Lysophosphatidyl ethanolamine[g]	—	—	—	—	—	—	—	—	8.6	8.4	7.6
Uncharacterized	—	—	—	—	—	—	—	—	5.2	6.1	5.8

[a] Values as molar percentage of the total phospholipid.
[b] Data from Anderson (1970).
[c] Data from Broekhuyse (1969).
[d] Data from Eichberg and Hess (1967).
[e] Range of values reported by Nielsen *et al.* (1970), Anderson and Maude (1970), and Borggreven *et al.* (1970).
[f] NR = Not reported.
[g] Lysophosphatidyl ethanolamine values when reported were added to phosphatidyl ethanolamine values (as were lysophosphatidyl choline and phosphatidyl choline values) except for human lens in which the level of lysophosphatidyl ethanolamine was reported to be exceptionally high.

shown that lipids of the lens change throughout life with the percent of sphingomyelin rising and the percentages of phosphatidyl choline and phosphatidyl ethanolamine in particular decreasing (Table II). Although the percentage of sphingomyelin rises in all species (Broekhuyse, 1971), it appears that the extremely high level of the human lens is not found in other species. Also, the high lysophosphatidyl ethanolamine level reported for human lens was not found in other species. The human lens contains a much larger amount of ganglioside than does bovine lens (Windeler and Feldman, 1970). Species differences are thus apparent for lens lipid composition. The nature of the changes is similar to that in aorta in which the percentage of sphingomyelin increases with age in all species thus far studied, with species differences in the amounts of the lipid classes being apparent.

D. CHANGES WITH AGE OF BRAIN SUBCELLULAR PARTICULATE LIPID COMPOSITION

The lipid composition of the different membranes in brain and other parts of the nervous system must be evaluated with regard to changes with age that are disclosed by analysis of whole brain and different regions of one brain (Section IV). Evaluation of the subcellular particulate data reported in the literature is complicated by several factors. The electron microscopic appearance of subcellular particulates is an essential morphological criterion, but photographs documenting preparations are seldom presented. Thus, it is not always possible to judge the values reported in the literature in the most critical manner. The determination of the levels of characteristic enzymes is also an important part of characterization, but the complexities of brain fractionation have made such determinations infrequent. It is now apparent that electrophoretic separation of proteins can be very useful in characterization of myelin in particular, but the method has not been used by many investigators. Also, seemingly small differences in isolation methods may cause loss of lipid which is difficult to evaluate because detailed procedures are not described in some cases. The limitations of a particular analytical method may be known, but the care with which it is applied and the influence of undescribed modifications cannot be evaluated. The wide range of values reported in the literature for the composition of the same particulate from the same species is an indication that methodology may not have been controlled with sufficient care. The lipid class composition of neurons and astrocytes is similar, but very different from that of oligodendroglia (Section V,B), and thus differences in the contribution of the different cell types to the preparation isolated can give rise to variability in composition.

Different laboratories employing different methods of lipid analysis have reported lipid composition data in different ways. We have evaluated the data by compilation in the form reported in the literature and conversion of the values (when possible) to molar percentages of the total lipid (phospholipid + glycolipid + cholesterol), molar percentages of the total polar lipid (phospholipid + glycolipid), and molar percentages of the total phospholipid. Each method of expression was found to have certain advantages and to disclose differences not as readily seen with the others. Unfortunately, the data available are not adequate to give clear answers to some of the most basic questions.

The lipid class composition of myelin isolated from mouse brain was found to change with age (Horrocks, 1968). Galactolipid (cerebroside + sulfatide) increased throughout the period of study (from 14 to 82 days of age). During the same period, the percentage of phosphatidyl choline decreased progressively. The myelin changes are those typical of whole brain. Data in the same publication indicate that the lipid composition of the microsome fraction did not change appreciably with age. Data for rat brain (Cuzner and Davison, 1968) recalculated as molar ratios from the data originally presented as micromoles per brain indicate that the galactolipid to total phospholipid ratio increases with age in microsomes, nuclei, and mitochondria which are derived from all cell types, but not in nerve endings that are derived from neurons. This is to be expected from the data for whole cells (Section V,B). The cholesterol to total phospholipid ratios were somewhat variable, but the data indicate a general rise that was greatest for myelin. The changes reported for the phospholipid composition of chicken brain particulates from the prehatching and posthatching periods (Kreps *et al.*, 1966) indicate that the relative proportions of phospholipids of microsomes, nuclei, and mitochondria change with age. The major changes were a rise in sphingomyelin and a decrease in phosphatidyl choline, as expected from whole brain composition data. Data for the desmosterol content of rat brain also indicate that the relative amount declines with age in all subcellular particulates (Smith *et al.*, 1967). It is clear that cholesterol and desmosterol can replace each other in membranes and that cholestanol can replace cholesterol (Stahl *et al.*, 1971). These replacements are similar to the replacement of tetrahymanol by ergosterol in *Tetrahymena pyriformis* (Conner *et al.*, 1971). It thus appears that lipid class proportions change in most, if not all, particulates with increasing age in some species. More work on subcellular particulates other than myelin is essential for more complete definition of the nature of the changes with age.

Data for rabbit brain and spinal cord myelin (Dalal and Einstein, 1969) demonstrate large changes with age throughout the period of study (1 to 170 days). Thus, as molar percentages of the total lipid of brain myelin, galactolipid rose from 0.4 to 22.5%; total phospholipid decreased (from 57 to 40%); sphingomyelin increased (from 5 to 10%); phosphatidyl choline decreased (from 26.9 to 12.2%) as did phosphatidyl ethanolamine (from 21.1 to 15.2%). A striking feature was a gradual increase of cholesterol from 4.6 to 37.8%. Brain and spinal cord myelins gave slightly different quantitative lipid analyses. Cord myelin appeared to contain more sphingomyelin, but the difference is difficult to evaluate because sphingomyelin and phosphatidyl inositol were determined together. Dekaban *et al.* (1971) noted a less striking increase in the cholesterol to total phospholipid ratio of rabbit cerebral pallium.

In one study (Eng and Noble, 1968), no appreciable change in the cholesterol content of purified rat brain myelin was apparent in the 15- to 90-day period of development, and only a relatively small increase of galactolipid (from 20 to 24%) and a decrease of phosphatidyl choline (from 15 to 9%) were reported with little or no change in the percentages of the other phospholipids. In another study (Cuzner and Davison, 1968) different results were obtained. The molar percentage of cholesterol of rat brain myelin was observed to increase from 24 to 40.5% for the day of birth to adulthood (over 100 days) and large changes in galactolipid and phosphatidyl choline content were found. A parallel rise of cholesterol and cerebroside + sulfatide is also apparent from the data of Radin (1970) for whole rat brain. Such large differences in rat brain myelin and whole brain composition data suggest methodological problems and/ or strain differences. Some of the variability has been traced to a membrane, the myelinlike fraction, that has a low cerebroside content (Agrawal *et al.*, 1970). This fraction is particularly high in some conventional myelin preparations from young animals.

It seems probable that the amount of cholesterol in brain myelin, at least in some rats, increases with age in a manner similar to that of rabbit brain and spinal cord myelin, since such changes are apparent from the data for whole rat brains. There may be large strain differences, however, because it appears from data for human brain myelin (O'Brien and Sampson, 1965a; Eng *et al.*, 1968; Gerstl *et al.*, 1967) that the cholesterol content does not change appreciably with age. The finding is in keeping with our data for whole human brain in which the molar percentage of cholesterol is constant throughout postnatal life (range 39–44 moles % of the total lipid). The galactolipid content of human brain myelin does not appear to change with age (Eng *et al.*, 1968; Gerstl *et al.*, 1967). It appears that myelin can increase in amount with or without appreciable change in lipid class composition depending upon the species, and strain differences are indicated.

In summary, although more data are required for a clear understanding, changes with age of the lipid class composition of all subcellular particulates can be expected for some species. Wide species and strain differences appear to exist with regard to the time that some lipid classes such as cholesterol reach their maximum levels.

E. Species Differences and the Characteristic Compositions of Each Type of Membrane

Whole brain data demonstrate species differences (see Section IV) that are also apparent from subcellular particulate data. Before the nature of species variations could be assessed, we found it necessary to convert all the data to a uniform basis as noted in Section V,D. The data used were from Agrawal *et al.* (1970), Banik *et al.* (1968), Banik and Davison (1967), Clausen (1969), Clausen and Berg Hansen (1970), Cuzner *et al.* (1965a,b), Cuzner and Davison (1968), Dalal and Einstein (1969), Davison *et al.* (1966), Eng *et al.* (1968), Eng and Noble (1968), Eto *et al.* (1970, 1971), Gerstl *et al.* (1967), Hamberger and Svennerholm (1971), MacBrinn and O'Brien (1969), Norton (1971), Norton and Autilio (1965), Nussbaum *et al.* (1963), O'Brien *et al.* (1967), O'Brien and Sampson (1965a), Singh *et al.* (1971), Smith (1969), Smith *et al.* (1970), and Soto *et al.* (1966).

Myelin preparations from brain, spinal cord, and nerve may differ in composition. Bovine optic nerve myelin is closely similar in composition to bovine brain myelin (MacBrinn and O'Brien, 1969) whereas bovine spinal root myelin contains more sphingomyelin and less cerebroside and sulfatide than spinal cord myelin (O'Brien *et al.*, 1967). As noted in Section III, the range of levels for whole human brain and spinal cord phosphatidyl choline and sphingomyelin overlap, with some spinal cords containing relatively more sphingomyelin and less phosphatidyl choline than whole brain. In keeping with the overlapping range for human brain and spinal cord is the report of Dalal and Einstein (1969) who found rabbit brain and spinal cord myelins to be very similar in composition. That myelin of the peripheral nervous system is in general higher in sphingomyelin content than brain and spinal cord myelin is indicated by the data for squirrel monkey spinal cord and brachial plexus myelins presented by Horrocks (1967). Not enough data are available to consider spinal cord and peripheral nerve myelin from the standpoint of species variations. The following comparisons are thus restricted to brain particulates.

The data for the lipid class composition of the subcellular particulates from adult brains of different species are shown in Tables III–VI. Only adult brain values are comparable since composition changes with age in some species (Section V,D). The phosphatidyl choline and phosphatidyl ethanolamine values include the small amounts of the lyso compounds when these were reported. The sum of cerebroside and sulfatide was considered most often because the two lipid classes are most commonly determined together as total galactolipid. Species were divided into groups when the range of values reported for one species gave a mean that was clearly different from the mean of values for other species. In some cases, the ranges for different groups overlap to some extent. Uncertainties are indicated by question marks. Most of the data for rat brain myelin place cerebroside + sulfatide and sphingomyelin percentages below those of human and bovine preparations, but the values in one report (Eng and Noble, 1968) place the percentages of these lipids in the higher range. The mouse brain myelin galactolipid and sphingomyelin values reported by Horrocks (1968) and Singh *et al.* (1971) are also in the human range. Whole brain data (Section IV) demonstrate large individual differences in galactolipid levels of rats and mice and indicate that some rats and mice have glycolipid levels in the human brain range.

Species do not appear to differ in the amount of cholesterol in adult brain myelin (Table III). Three groups are apparent for galactolipid (cerebroside + sulfatide) content. Two of these groups (II and III, Table III) are firmly established. The values for frog myelin appear to establish a group with less glycolipid, but there is uncertainty because the age of the animals used and the developmental time scale of the frog are not known. The total phospholipid level is higher in those species with lower galactolipid levels. In rat, mouse, and frog myelins, the sphingomyelin percentage is in the lower group when the galactolipid percentage is lower, and the percentages of phosphatidyl choline and phosphatidyl ethanolamine are in the higher group. The pigeon is different in that the percentage of sphingomyelin is in the lower group whereas glycolipid is in the higher group. No particular characteristic combinations of acidic phospholipid values are apparent for the different species. The data for myelin as well as for whole brain (Section IV) do not support the conclusion drawn from some early studies of whole brain that there is a gradual fall in the percentages of the galactolipids and sphingomyelin as animals progressively lower on the vertebrate scale are examined.

Table III: Species Differences in Lipid Class Composition of Adult Brain Myelin[a,b,c,d]

Lipid class	Molar percentage of the total lipid			Molar percentage of the total phospholipid		
	Group I	Group II	Group III	Group I	Group II	Group III
Chol	41.3 (37.2–49.4) all	—	—	100.6 H,B,M,RA	96.0 R	83.2 DF,F
Cer + Sulf	8.6 (?) F	16.1 (14.2–17.1) DF,M,R,RA	19.8 (15.0–23.0) B,GP,H,M,P,R,RA	17.4 F	37.2 (32.5–41.6) DF,F,M,R,RA	51.2 B,GP,H,M,P,R,RA
TPL	38.7 (30.7–40.8) B,GP,H,M,P,R,RA	43.0 (36.2–50.2) R,M	49.6 (49.2–50.1) DF,F	—	—	—
Sph	3.0 (1.5–4.6) M,F,P,R	5.9 (4.6–7.9) B,DF,GP,H,R(?),RA	—	7.4 (4.6–9.4) M,F,P,R	16.1 (11.6–18.6) B,GP,H,R(?),RA	—
PC	9.4 (7.8–11.4) B,GP,H,P,RA	12.9 (10.3–18.0) DF,M,R,RA	19.3 (?) F	24.0 (18.4–33.4) B,GP,H,P,RA	30.1 (24.9–35.9) DF,F,M,R,RA	—
PE	13.6 (9.0–15.9) B,GP,H,P,RA	18.8 (15.7–22.3) DF,F,M,R,RA	—	36.9 (31.3–31.4) B,GP,H	44.0 (39.3–48.5) DF,F,M,P,R,RA	—
PS	3.4 (0.6–5.4) B,DF,GP,H,M,P,R,RA	6.8 (5.9–8.8) B,GP,H,R(?),RA	—	9.7 (4.6–15.6) DF,F,GP,M,R,RA	19.0 (18.0–23.9) DF,F,M,P,R,RA	—
PI	1.0 (0.6–1.2) B,DF,GP,H,P,RA	2.5 (1.8–3.1) R	—	2.4 (1.7–3.1) DF,F,GP,H,P,RA	5.4 (4.5–6.7) R	—
DPG	0.5 (0.0–1.0) F,GP,H	2.2 (1.1–3.2) DF,F,P,R,RA	—	0.5 (0.0–1.8) F,GP,H	3.2 (2.6–4.4) R	7.6 (6.4–8.8) DF,P,RA
PA	—	—	—	1.4 (0.5–3.0) B,F,GP,H	—	—

[a] Data from Agrawal *et al.* (1970); Cuzner *et al.* (1965a,b); Cuzner and Davison (1968); Dalal and Einstein (1969); Davison *et al.* (1966); Eichberg *et al.* (1964); Eng and Noble (1968); Eto *et al.* (1971); Hamberger and Svennerholm (1971); Herschkowitz *et al.* (1968b); Horrocks (1968); Norton and Autilio (1965); Siakotos *et al.* (1969b); Singh *et al.* (1971).

[b] The range for each lipid class is shown in parentheses and the species falling into each group are shown below the range.

[c] Abbreviations: B, bovine; DF, dogfish; F, frog; GP, guinea pig; H, human; M, mouse; P, pigeon; R, rat; RA, rabbit; Chol, cholesterol; Cer, cerebroside; Sulf, sulfatide; TPL, total phospholipid; Sph, sphingomyelin; PC, phosphatidyl choline; PE, phosphatidyl serine; PI, phosphatidyl inositol; DPG, diphosphatidyl glycerol; PA, phosphatidic acid.

[d] Polyphosphoinositides are concentrated in myelin (Eichberg and Dawson, 1965).

Table IV

SPECIES DIFFERENCES IN THE LIPID CLASS COMPOSITION OF ADULT BRAIN MICROSOMES[a,b]

Lipid class	Molar percentage of total lipid			Molar percentage of total phospholipid		
	Group I	Group II	Group III	Group I	Group II	Group III
Chol	40.7	55.8	—	77.6	90.2	123
	(38.3–42.6)	(53.8–57.8)		H,P,R,RA	M	DF,F
	GP,H,M,P,R,RA	DF,F		2.4	13.0	30.0
Cer + Sulf	1.1	6.8	13.5	DF,F	GP,H,P,R,RA	(M?)
	(tr–1.1)	(5.6–7.8)	(?)			
	DF,F	GP,H,P,R,RA	(M?)			
TPL)	44.9	52.4	—	—	—	—
	(41.1–46.5)	(50.1–54.5)				
	DF,F,M	GP,H,P,R,RA				
Sph	2.9	5.9	—	6.6	12.0	—
	(2.0–3.9)	(5.0–7.9)		(4.4–7.5)	(10.5–15.2)	
	GP,M,R	DF,F,H,P,RA		GP,M,R	B,Ch,DF,F,H,P,RA	

PC	17.2 (12.4–22.3) DF,F,H,M,P,R,RA	?	—	36.9 (27.9–39.7) DF,F,M,P,R,RA	43.6 (40.8–47.1) B,Ch,GP,H	—
PE	10.0 (9.3–10.8) DF,H	16.5 (12.4–19.5) F,M,P,R,RA	—	24.9 (20.2–28.8) B,Ch,DF,GP,H	34.2 (31.6–42.0) F,M,P,RA,R	—
PS	5.8 (5.1–6.9) DF,F,H,R	10.0 (?) P	—	12.4 (10.9–15.2) B,Ch,DF,F,GP,H,R,RA	19.9 (?) P	—
PI	3.3 (1.8–4.1) F,DF,H,R	? ?	—	6.3 (3.3–8.9) All (?)	? P ?	—
DPG	0.5 (0.0–1.2) B,DF,GP,H	1.4 (1.1–1.8) R	2.9 (2.6–3.2) F,RA	0.4 (0.0–0.5) B,GP,H	3.0– (2.0–3.6) DF,R	6.1 (5.8–6.4) F,RA
PA	—	—	—	0.7 (0.0–1.4) GP,HB	?	—

[a] Data from Cuzner *et al.* (1965a,b, 1966); Cuzner and Davison (1968); Cumings *et al.* (1968); Davison *et al.* (1966); Eichberg *et al.* (1964); Horrocks (1968); Kreps *et al.* (1966); Mandel and Nussbaum (1966); Rouser *et al.* (1970b); Rouser and Siakotos (unpublished data).
[b] See footnote c of Table III for abbreviations; tr, trace.

The percentage of cholesterol in microsomes of most species (Table IV) is in the same range and about equal to the percentage found in myelin. The data for dogfish and frog microsomes (Cuzner *et al.*, 1965a) indicate a group with a very high (55.8 molar %) cholesterol content. The possibility should be considered that the high values may have been the result of cholesterol uptake from other membranes during isolation, particularly since the values for cholesterol in myelin of the two species were like those from other species. The galactolipid percentages for microsomes are less than one-half those of myelin. Since the galactolipid content of neurons and astrocytes in very low and that of oligodendrocytes is high (Section V,B), it appears that the microsome preparations are generally derived mostly from oligodendrocytes. Rat and rabbit brain microsomes have as much galactolipid as microsomes from human brain, whereas in myelin the galactolipid percentage is usually lower than that found in human brain myelin. Some of the species differences noted for myelin composition are not seen in microsome preparations.

Mitochondrial preparations give two very different lipid composition analyses (Table V). Type I preparations have a lower percentage of sphingomyelin and a higher percentage of diphosphatidyl glycerol than Type II preparations. In Type I preparations, cholesterol is about 7 moles % of the total lipid whereas in Type II preparations the value is about 20%. The galactolipid level is less than 1% of the total lipid in Type I preparations and as high as 20% in Type II preparations. The differences can be explained by contamination of Type II preparations with microsomes and/or myelin. This is clearly the case for the Type II preparations of Kreps *et al.* (1966) who analyzed a crude mitochondrial fraction and Gerstl *et al.* (1969) who noted that their mitochondrial preparations contained myelin. The data reported by Mandel and Nussbaum (1966) and Hamberger and Svennerholm (1971) are included with Type II preparations because of their high sphingomyelin levels. The high level of diphosphatidyl glycerol and the low level of phosphatidyl ethanolamine in the report of Mandel and Nussbaum (1966) suggest that the preparation may have been highly purified, but that some phosphatidyl ethanolamine was converted to lysophosphatidyl ethanolamine that was included in the sphingomyelin value. The values reported by Hamberger and Svennerholm (1971) fall into the Type II category with high sphingomyelin and cholesterol values, but rabbit brain may indeed have a higher sphingomyelin level since whole rabbit brain does have a high level of sphingomyelin (see Section IV). The data for Type I mitochondrial preparations do not disclose any striking species differences and it may well be that more data will demonstrate species differences among vertebrates to be small in general.

Table V

SPECIES DIFFERENCES IN LIPID CLASS COMPOSITION OF ADULT BRAIN MITOCHONDRIA[a]

Lipid class	Type I preparations				Type II preparations							
	Guinea pig[b]	Rat[c]	Human[d]	Bovine[d]	Bovine[e]	Bovine[f,g]	Bovine[f,h]	Human[f,g]	Human[f,h]	Chicken[i]	Rat[j,m]	Rabbit[k]
Sphingomyelin	3.7	1.9	3.3	ND[l]	17.3	11.4	16.9	9.5	14.3	8.7	7.1	7.0
Phosphatidyl choline	40.0	38.1	37.5	36.1	28.7	41.0	35.6	40.1	32.3	37.2	42.9	45.8
Phosphatidyl ethanolamine	32.7	40.8	29.0	35.8	27.2	41.0	36.4	37.7	44.7	31.3	20.9	36.2
Phosphatidyl serine	5.9	6.3	5.3	6.3	11.3	{6.5	{10.9	{11.9	{17.5	13.5	6.2	6.0
Phosphatidyl inositol	5.5	NR[m]	4.3	5.4	3.0					5.2	4.4	5.2
Diphosphatidyl glycerol	11.1	7.8	9.7	9.2	4.6	ND	NR	ND	NR	2.8	8.5	NR
Phosphatidic acid	0.6	NR	0.9	0.8	0.7	NR	NR	NR	NR	NR	ND	NR

[a] Phospholipids as molar percentages of the total phospholipid.
[b] From Eichberg *et al.* (1964).
[c] From Cuzner *et al.* (1966).
[d] From Rouser and Siakotos (unpublished data).
[e] From Parsons and Basford (1967).
[f] From Gerstl *et al.* (1969).
[g] From gray matter.
[h] From white matter.
[i] From Kreps *et al.* (1966).
[j] From Mandel and Nussbaum (1966).
[k] From Hamberger and Svennerholm (1971).
[l] ND, not detected.
[m] NR, not reported.
[n] See also Seminario *et al.* (1964).

Table VI
LIPID CLASS COMPOSITION OF BRAIN NUCLEI, MITOCHONDRIA, NERVE ENDINGS, SYNAPTIC VESICLES, AND PLASMA MEMBRANES[a,b]

Lipid class	Nuclei[c]	Mitochondria[c]	Nerve endings[c]			Synaptic vesicles[c]			Plasma membranes[c]			Ribosomes[c]
									NE	N	SC	
	(1)	(2)	(3)	(5)	(4)	(3)	(3)	(4)	(6)	(7)	(7)	(8)
Sph	4.0	2.2	5.3	8.1	6.2	12.3	10.1	10.6	3.8	10.0	9.0	9.7
PC	52.6	37.9	39.3	40.9	38.2	40.7	42.0	45.6	44.9	45.9	44.2	43.0
PE	22.9	34.6	33.6	38.8	33.8	25.1	35.1	24.9	36.2	34.4	32.6	21.8
PS	5.4	6.0	12.9	9.6	13.8	10.2	13.3	13.2	}15.2	10.4	14.5	10.6
PI	7.9	5.0	4.0	2.7	4.8	5.9	4.1	5.1		NR	NR	4.0
DPG	0.3	9.5	1.6	NR	1.7	0.0	0.6	ND	NR	NR	NR	6.5
PA	0.8	0.8	0.7	NR	1.6	2.3	1.4	0.5	NR	NR	NR	ND

	(9)	(9)	(5)	(9)	(5)	(9)	(5)	(6)
Chol	30.0	7.0	25.8	37.6	32.0	34.5	36.9	48.0
Cer + Sulf	7.0	<1	NR	2.3	2.8	5.9[d]	0.8	—
TPL	63.0	92.0	74.2	60.1	65.2	59.6	62.3	—

[a] Phospholipid values are expressed as molar percentage of the total phospholipid except for neuronal plasma membrane and Schwann cell plasma membrane expressed as percentage of the phospholipids shown. Cholesterol, galactolipid, and total phospholipid values are expressed as molar percentage of the total lipid.

[b] Abbreviations: Sph, sphingomyelin; PC, phosphatidyl choline; PE, phosphatidyl ethanolamine; PS, phosphatidyl serine; PI, phosphatidyl inositol; DPG, diphosphatidyl glycerol; PA, phosphatidic acid; Chol, cholesterol; Cer + Sulf, cerebroside + sulfatide; TPL, total phospholipid; N, neuron; NE, nerve ending; SC, Schwann cell; NR, not reported; ND, not detected.

[c] Key to numbers in parentheses above each column of data:

(1) Mean of bovine values from Siakotos et al. (1969a).
(2) Mean of values from Type I preparations in Table V.
(3) Guinea pig brain values from Eichberg et al. (1964).
(4) Bovine brain values from Rouser and Siakotos (unpublished data).
(5) Rabbit brain values from Hamberger and Svennerholm (1971).
(6) Rat brain values from Cotman et al. (1969).
(7) Squid giant axon values from Camejo et al. (1969).
(8) Rat brain values from Mandel and Nussbaum (1966).
(9) Rat brain values from Lapetina et al. (1968).

[d] The true glycolipid level is probably less than 1 mole % of the total lipid.

The data available for highly purified preparations of nuclei, nerve-ending particles, synaptic vesicles, nerve-ending plasma membranes and other types of plasma membranes are shown in Table VI. The data are not adequate to define the range of variation in any one species or species variations. The close correspondence of phospholipid values for guinea pig and bovine brain nerve endings and synaptic vesicles indicates that species differences may well prove to be small in general for these particulates. The data of Cuzner and Davison (1968) shown in Table VI indicate that nuclei probably contain less cholesterol (30%) than microsomes (about 41%). Nerve endings and plasma membranes, like myelin, appear to contain 32–48% cholesterol. Nuclei appear to contain 7% galactolipid (Cer + Sulf) which is also the percentage found for microsomes of some species. The galactolipid content of highly purified nerve endings and their subfractions is much lower (probably less than 2% of the total lipid).

When the data for purified whole cell preparations of neurons, astrocytes, and oligodendroglia (Section V,B) as well as for membranes of the eye (Section V,C) and brain subcellular particulates are evaluated for a general picture of species differences, a definite pattern emerges and a tentative proposal can be made. The data suggest that vertebrate species are closely similar when neurons and neuronal membranes are compared and that the lipid composition of whole neurons and their membranes does not change appreciably with age. These conclusions are supported by the failure to find changes with age in the lipid composition of neuron and astrocyte preparations, the close similarity of the lipid composition of whole retina and rod outer segments of different species, and the close correspondence of the lipid composition of whole brains of different species prior to the onset of myelination. The latter is illustrated in Figs. 18–24 by the convergence of the lipid class ranges of different species at lower total phospholipid levels and the close correspondence of the values for human, mouse, dog, and frog brains prior to onset of myelination (Table VII).

In contrast to the constancy of neuron lipid composition, the composition of the myelin-forming cells may change with age, and species differences are apparent as judged from the differences in myelin composition (Table III). Changes with age and species differences are readily apparent for the lens of the eye that is derived from an epithelial cell layer. It thus appears that species differences among vertebrates are found when lipid composition changes with age are found. The data for lipids of the nervous system are in keeping with the findings for other organs. Thus, the lipid composition of aorta changes with age, and species differences are apparent (Rouser and Solomon, 1969; Eisenberg

Table VII

Lipid Composition of Whole Human, Mouse, Dog, and Frog Brains
Prior to Onset of Myelination[a]

	Human[b]	Mouse[c]	Dog[c]	Dog[c]	Human[c]	Frog[d]
Total phospholipid	2.30	2.30	2.32	2.54	2.92	2.99
Sphingomyelin	0.04	0.03	0.03	0.03	0.09	0.08
Phosphatidyl choline	1.15	1.13	1.08	1.21	1.38	1.26
Phosphatidyl ethanolamine	0.72	0.71	0.71	0.77	0.89	1.14
Phosphatidyl serine	0.27	0.29	0.36	0.38	0.34	0.30
Phosphatidyl inositol	0.06	0.04	0.02	0.02	0.09	0.07

[a] All values mmoles/100 gm fresh weight from Rouser *et al.* (unpublished data).
[b] Midterm fetus.
[c] First postnatal day.
[d] Age unknown but cerebroside and sulfatide were trace components only.

et al., 1969), whereas the lipid class composition of heart, kidney, and liver does not change appreciably after birth and the vertebrate species thus far examined are closely similar (Rouser *et al.,* 1969a; Simon and Rouser, 1969).

The data available for brain subcellular particulate lipid composition is grossly inadequate to define with certainty the characteristic features of most membranes and the range of values for different species.

The data for different membranes of brain indicate gradients of lipid composition in the order: myelin; microsomes and nuclei; mitochondria. Myelin contains the highest levels of cholesterol, cerebroside, sulfatide, and sphingomyelin and lower levels of phosphatidyl choline and phosphatidyl ethanolamine. Mitochondria contain a higher level of diphosphatidyl glycerol that is a trace or very minor component in other membranes.

The gradient concept of membrane lipid class composition has gradually evolved from studies of organs other than brain. The uncertainty regarding the extent of purification led at first to the working hypothesis that the presence of diphosphatidyl glycerol in preparations other than those of mitochondria indicated contamination with mitochondria. It was apparent, however, that microsomes from heart contain a high level of diphosphatidyl glycerol that cannot be accounted for by mitochondrial contamination (Rouser *et al.,* 1968b). Thus, while diphosphatidyl glycerol is a characteristic component of mitochondria and found in only small amounts in microsomes of most organs, it is present in large amount in microsomes of organs in which mitochondria contribute most of the lipid (see Section VI for a more complete explanation of the type of equilibrium that appears to exist). The concept of a gradient dependent upon the relative proportions of different membranes in an organ was thus indicated. Mitochondria from different organs also have different contents of sphingomyelin, phosphatidyl serine, and phosphatidyl inositol (Rouser *et al.*, 1968b; Fleischer *et al.*, 1967b). Thus, bovine kidney, heart, and liver mitochondria have about 4, 2, and 1% sphingomyelin respectively. The values obtained for sphingomyelin of bovine kidney, heart, and liver microsomes were 20, 13, and 1–5% respectively. Thus, there are large gradients for the lipid composition of different membranes from the same organ as well as the same membrane from different organs. The gradients appear to be determined by the relative proportions of the different membranes in each organ. The phospholipids showing the largest gradients in all organs thus far examined are phosphatidyl choline, sphingomyelin, and diphosphatidyl glycerol. The phosphatidyl ethanolamine levels of membranes other than those of mitochondria are not very different. The sphingomyelin gradient is commonly plasma membrane > microsomes > nuclei > mitochondria. A similar but reverse trend is apparent for phosphatidyl choline, but the gradient is somewhat different in different organs (see Section VI). Diphosphatidyl glycerol is highest in mitochondria, and the gradient is so steep in organs that are not rich in mitochondria that all other membranes usually contain a very low percentage of this lipid.

The gradient concept with transfer of lipids from one membrane to another, particularly when in close contact, is in keeping with the findings of Suzuki *et al.* (1967) and Suzuki (1970) who noted the presence of a small amount of ganglioside in myelin and of Norton and Turnbull (1970) and De Vries *et al.* (1972) who found the percentages of cerebroside and sulfatide in their axon preparations to be as high as or higher than the percentages in myelin.

VI. Membrane Biosynthesis and the Regulatory Mechanisms of Lipid Metabolism That Determine Membrane Lipid Class Composition

A. NORMAL INDIVIDUALS

In this section, information on membrane lipid composition, metabolism, and structure is brought together to give an overall picture of the way membrane lipid composition is determined and cellular membranes are formed. The fatty acid composition of lipid classes is not considered.

Metabolism of polar (membrane) lipid classes, their transport, and their entrance into membranes can be viewed as follows:

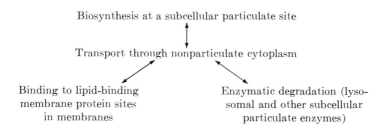

Biosynthesis at a subcellular particulate site

Transport through nonparticulate cytoplasm

Binding to lipid-binding
membrane protein sites
in membranes

Enzymatic degradation (lysosomal and other subcellular
particulate enzymes)

In general, hormones appear to have little direct effect upon the balance since administration of hormones or removal of endocrine organs does not appear to change the polar lipid composition of membranes appreciably (Johnson and Cornatzer, 1969), and sex-related differences are not apparent.

There is general agreement that lipid is synthesized de novo mainly in the endoplasmic reticulum. Some de novo lipid biosynthesis as well as exchange of polar groups has now been rather well established for mitochondria of various organs (Butschak, 1970; Stanacev *et al.*, 1969; Sribney, 1968; Jungalwala and Dawson, 1970; Davidson and Stanacev, 1971; Sarzala *et al.*, 1970; Kaiser and Bygrave, 1968; Bosmann and Case, 1969; Fujino and Nokano, 1969; Tombropoulos, 1971; Kaiser, 1969; Hajra *et al.*, 1968; Hildebrand *et al.*, 1970; Fang and Marinetti, 1970; Stoffel and Schiefer, 1968; Bygrave, 1969; Bygrave and Bücher, 1968; Davidson and Stanacev, 1970; Stuhne-Sekalec and Stanacev, 1970; Vorbeck and Martin, 1970; Zborowski and Wojtezak, 1969; Shephard and Hübscher, 1969; Beattie, 1969). In addition, phospholipase A_1 and A_2 degradation of glycerolphospholipids to lysophospholipids and reacylation of lysophospholipids appears to take place in most membranes. Exchange reactions in which one polar group replaces another make possible alteration of the relative proportions of lipid classes by a membrane that has little or no de novo biosynthetic activity.

Lipid is transported as a lipoprotein complex between membranes within cells, from one cell to another and thus throughout an organ, and from one organ to another via blood. Transport of lipid as soluble lipoprotein (present in the supernatant fraction) from one membrane to another has been demonstrated with rat liver microsomes and mitochondria (Beattie, 1969; Wirtz and Zilversmit, 1968, 1969; 1970; Wirtz *et al.*, 1970; McMurray and Dawson, 1969; Akiyama and Sakagami, 1969; Blok *et al.*, 1971). Similar transport in lipid exchange studies has been reported for potato and cauliflower membranes (Ben Abdelkader and Mazliak, 1970).

In brain, studies with ^{35}S-labeled sulfatide have indicated that sulfatide is synthesized in the endoplasmic reticulum and transported as soluble lipoprotein (isolated from the supernatant fraction) to myelin (Herschkowitz *et al.*, 1968a, 1969). Several soluble lipoproteins that occur in the nonparticulate phase of the cytoplasm and soluble fractions of nuclei and mitochondria have been reported (Koppikar *et al.*, 1971; Napier and Olson, 1965). The sulfatide-containing lipoproteins of rat brain account for about 2% of the total lipid and have lipid class compositions distinctly different from those of microsomes or myelin with a much higher percentage of phosphatidyl choline and a lower percentage of phosphatidyl ethanolamine than myelin, although the galactolipid content (17.7 moles % of the total lipid) is like myelin (Herschkowitz *et al.*, 1968b). Phosphatidyl serine was found in soluble lipoprotein and thus the soluble lipoproteins are distinctly different from plasma lipoproteins that do not contain this phospholipid. Three different soluble lipoproteins were separated by agar gel electrophoresis (Herschkowitz *et al.*, 1968b).

All types of lipids are bound to protein for transport. Steroid binding follows the polarity rule, i.e., it depends upon the type and number of polar groups (Westphal, 1961; Ganguly *et al.*, 1967). The observation that addition of plasma to a rat liver supernatant caused labeled mevalonate conversion mainly to squalene rather than cholesterol was traced to the occurrence in plasma of a protein with a high binding affinity for squalene (Onajobi and Boyd, 1970). Ritter and Dempsey (1970) observed that reduction of $\Delta^{5,7}$-cholestadienol to cholesterol by a microsome reductase was facilitated by a soluble liproprotein that binds the sterol. In general, it appears that target tissues concentrate steroid hormones because they contain proteins with high binding affinity for the steroids. Also, steroids are transported intracellularly to their sites of action as steroid-protein complexes.

Lipid transport from one region of brain to another has been demonstrated. Thus, cholesterol synthesized from mevalonate injected into one area of brain was observed to spread throughout the brain after several weeks and, at equilibrium, to be highest in concentration in the most heavily myelinated areas that contain more cholesterol (Gautheron *et al.*, 1969). Only about 24% of rat brain cholesterol was reported to be exchangeable with plasma cholesterol and only 2.5% was found to turn over by *in situ* biosynthesis (Chevallier and Giraud, 1966; Chevallier *et al.*, 1968; Chevallier and Petit, 1966).

Sterol and phospholipid exchange involving all membranes of brain is strongly indicated by recent data. A large accumulation of desmosterol is induced in myelin by the drug *trans*-1,4-bis-(2-chlorobenzylaminomethyl) cyclohexane dihydrochloride, and desmosterol is reduced to cholesterol after administration of the drug is discontinued (Fumagalli *et al.*, 1965). Banik and Davison (1971) demonstrated that myelin has a low level of 7-dehydrocholesterol reductase and thus it appears likely that desmosterol is transferred from myelin to other membranes prior to reduction to cholesterol. Exchange of phospholipids of myelin with other membranes was demonstrated by the finding that the altered fatty acid composition of rat brain myelin brought about by feeding a diet deficient in essential fatty acids was reversed when animals were returned to a normal diet (Galli *et al.*, 1971a,b; White *et al.*, 1971). These data are in agreement with the earlier reports that isotopic label is lost from some myelin lipids with phosphatidyl choline turnover being the most rapid and the turnover of cerebroside, cholesterol, sphingomyelin, and phosphatidyl ethanolamine being very slow (Smith, 1968; Smith and Eng, 1965; Ansell and Spanner, 1971). A somewhat surprisingly rapid rate of turnover was also noted for proteolipid protein of myelin.

Lipid exchange among organs takes place via lipid transported in blood. Relatively little is known about phospholipid exchange, but the data of Ansell and Spanner (1971) suggest that brain choline comes from blood as lipid (phosphatidyl choline or lysophosphatidyl choline). Many studies have been conducted on cholesterol exchange among organs (reviewed by Dietschy and Wilson, 1970). The disappearance of labeled cholesterol from blood is at first rapid and then very slow and this has given rise to the two-pool concept, i.e., one pool that exchanges rapidly and another that exchanges slowly. Brain and spinal cord are in the slowly exchangeable group. Although labeled cholesterol enters the brain of a rat well past the rapid stage of myelination and the label is heaviest in the most heavily myelinated areas (Chevallier and Petit, 1966), the amount is rather low. Svanberg (1970) injected labeled cholesterol into the yolk sacs of newly hatched chickens and followed the distribution of the label for 9 days by whole body autoradiography. No radioactivity was observed in the brain or spinal cord, but peripheral nerve was heavily labeled. Thus, cholesterol in brain and cord was apparently derived from *in situ* biosynthesis, whereas cholesterol of peripheral nerve was taken up to a great extent from blood. The turnover of cholesterol in brain, spinal cord, and peripheral nerves of adult animals is very low. When a nerve is sectioned, cholesterol esters appear, and it has been found that the cholesterol of the cholesterol esters is derived from the free cholesterol of the intact nerve (Simon, 1966). When mouse peripheral nerve is sectioned and allowed to go through the cycle of degeneration and regeneration, labeled cholesterol introduced prior to sectioning is still present (Rawlins *et al.*, 1970). Thus, peripheral nerve behaves as a closed system once cholesterol has entered it, and little or no biosynthesis or degradation of cholesterol is apparent. In hypercholesterolemic monkeys, the cholesterol level is increased in the eye, heart, aorta, peripheral arteries, lungs, liver, spleen, pancreas, kidney, testis, skin, tendon, muscle, and adipose tissue but the level in brain and jejunum does not increase (Armstrong *et al.*, 1969). Khan and Folch-Pi (1967) observed that labeled cholesterol persisted in rat brain subcellular particulates and in particular in the mitochondrial fraction. Cholesterol in the nervous system is thus a very stable unit. This was originally interpreted to indicate that myelin is metabolically stable. It now appears that myelin itself is not metabolically stable (as noted above), although some of its components are degraded very slowly (Davison, 1971).

Lipid is synthesized for the most part in the endoplasmic reticulum and is then transported to other membranes. Thus, differences in the relative amounts of membranes can play a part in determining the lipid class composition of the cell because endoplasmic reticulum and mitochondria do not synthesize or alter by exchange reactions all lipid classes to the same extent, and the total number of binding sites for lipids is determined in part by other membranes that do not synthesize appreciable amounts of lipid de novo. It is thus not surprising that organs can be divided roughly into four groups with different relative proportions of membranes (Rouser *et al.*, 1971b; Rouser, 1971). Three of the groups are characterized by having as the most abundant membrane either plasma membrane, mitochondria, or endoplasmic reticulum. In the fourth group there is no clear predominance of any one membrane. As an example, the same lipid class composition is found for heart and brown fat of the rat and both organs have mitochondria as the predominant membrane. Brain and other parts of the nervous system fall into the high plasma membrane group, a characteristic feature of both neurons and glial cells being the proliferation of many extensions of their surface membranes.

Two types of intracellular lipoproteins distinct from plasma lipoprotein have been recognized. One type is water soluble and is clearly a transport protein. The other type is found in cell membranes, is not water soluble, and shows strong self-aggregation tendencies. The lipid class composition of these lipoproteins is very different from that of plasma lipoproteins. The phospholipids of plasma lipoproteins and the lipovitellins of eggs are mainly phosphatidyl choline and sphingomyelin located on the surface of the particulate, and the less polar lipids are triglyceride and cholesterol (free and esterified) located inside the lipoprotein particle. The intracellular lipoproteins that transport lipid to membranes contain, in addition to phosphatidyl choline and sphingomyelin, large amounts of phosphatidyl ethanolamine and acidic phospholipids, free cholesterol, and little or no esterified cholesterol. The cholesterol of these lipoproteins is intimately associated with the phospholipid in contrast to its presence in an internal core in plasma lipoproteins and lipovitellins. Three different proteins have been found in myelin. One is acidic, another basic, and the third (and generally most abundant) is essentially neutral. The basic protein has been isolated in water-soluble form and its amino acid sequence determined (Eylar, 1970; Carnegie, 1971). The neutral Folch-Lees (proteolipid) protein has been isolated in pure form with retention of both water and chloroform solubility (Tenenbaum and Folch-Pi, 1966). This is of considerable significance because it suggests that this myelin protein could move in the water-soluble form through the nonparticulate phase of the cytoplasm from the site of biosynthesis (endoplasmic reticulum) to myelin. If so, water-soluble forms of the three myelin proteins should appear in the supernatant fraction of a brain homogenate. It is therefore of interest that Herschkowitz *et al.* (1968b) separated three distinct lipoprotein bands by acrylamide gel electrophoresis of the supernatant fraction of rat brain.

The water-soluble forms of the basic protein and proteolipid protein do not bind as much lipid *in vitro* as is found in myelin (Palmer and Dawson, 1969; Braun and Radin, 1969). This suggests the possibility of a conformational change leading to greater lipid binding upon insertion of protein into myelin. Large differences in the helical content in different solvents have been noted for proteolipid protein (Sherman and Folch-Pi, 1970) and methods have been devised to prepare this protein in the α-helical or β-type structure (Anthony and Moscarello, 1971). The helix content is low in polar solvents (water and methanol) and high in less polar solvents such as chloroform. Thus, it is reasonable to suppose that this protein can fold to become a tighter, more globular molecule when it inserts into the myelin structure which is a less polar phase than water, and that the conformational change leads to more extensive lipid binding.

From the above, the details of membrane formation can be visualized as follows:

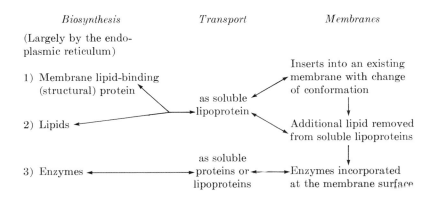

If membranes are formed by insertion of new units into existing membranes, mitochondria should grow and then divide. Growth in size followed by growing across of one of the central cristae and division appears to have been demonstrated rather conclusively in the insect fat body (Larsen, 1970). Also, anaerobically grown yeasts lacking typical mitochondria appear to form their mitochondria by enlargement of a small, promitochondrial particulate (Luck, 1963; Roodyn and Wilkie, 1968). Thus, one general method of membrane formation appears to be by insertion of newly synthesized lipoprotein and enzyme molecules into an existing membrane rather than by extension of the membrane where the lipoprotein unit is synthesized.

It is important to note that the scheme for membrane biosynthesis outlined above appears to have been proven for replication of lipid-containing animal viruses (Acheson and Tamm, 1967; Compans *et al.*, 1964; Morgan *et al.*, 1961). The virus particle is assembled first as a core composed of nucleic acid coated with a protein that is synthesized by enzymes of the endoplasmic reticulum. The core remains attached to the endoplasmic reticulum until the virus coat protein has moved from the endoplasmic reticulum to the host cell plasma membrane into which it inserts without causing any change in structure that can be seen with the electron microscope. The core particles then move to the modified plasma membrane surface to which they attach. The virus particle is formed by budding from the host cell surface during which process the core becomes covered with its lipoprotein coat. The virus utilizes host-cell lipids, and its lipid composition is usually (but not invariably) closely similar to that of the plasma membrane of the host cell.

The differences in lipid class composition of different membranes can be visualized as the result in part of the biosynthesis of lipid classes to different extents by different membranes. Thus, the characteristically high diphosphatidyl glycerol level of mitochondria presumably arises because more of this lipid is synthesized by this organelle which also appears to synthesize little or no phosphatidyl ethanolamine and less phosphatidyl choline than endoplasmic reticulum. Some of the lipid class distribution changes caused by mitochondria appear to arise from exchange reactions rather than de novo biosynthesis. Since there is little or no de novo biosynthesis of lipids at some membrane surfaces, lipid must be transported to them.

B. CHANGES IN HEREDITARY NEUROPATHOLOGICAL STATES

Detailed documentation and evaluation of changes in brain lipids in hereditary neuropathological states in which there are degradative enzyme deficiencies for lipid classes is not presented here to avoid inclusion of much information and discussion that is not directly related to the problems selected for detailed consideration. The general nature of the changes in lipid composition of brain and other organs caused by degradative enzyme deficiencies is, however, very informative with regard to regulatory mechanisms of lipid metabolism. Also, the ways in which the new knowledge of normal lipid class relationships can be used to detect pathology are important. Thus these areas are considered in a general way. Pertinent literature is reviewed in recent publications (Rouser and Yamamoto, 1969; Brady, 1970; O'Brien *et al.*, 1971).

Thus far, deficiencies for enzymes degrading sphingolipids have been recognized. One or more enzyme deficiencies are known for each type of sphingolipid. There are no reports of cases with deficiencies for degradative enzymes acting on glycerolphospholipids or any known examples of biosynthetic enzyme deficiencies for any of the polar lipids.

Niemann-Pick disease is known to be caused by a genetically determined reduction in the level of sphingomyelinase, the enzyme that hydrolyzes sphingomyelin to ceramide and phosphorylcholine. In the most severe infantile form, the enzyme is almost completely absent and sphingomyelin accumulates in large amount in all organs. In brain, myelination does not proceed normally, the total lipid level is below normal, and sphingomyelin accounts for an abnormally large amount of the total lipid. Graphic analysis (see Sections III and IV) was used to demonstrate that the amounts of cerebroside and sulfatide are abnormally high, that the amount of phosphatidyl choline is abnormally low, and that there are normal proportions of the other phospholipids (Rouser and Kritchevsky, 1972). Thus, failure to degrade one sphingolipid appears to result in a metabolic backup leading to replacement of phosphatidyl choline by sphingolipids. In Tay-Sachs disease that is caused by a deficiency of hexoseaminidase that degrades gangliosides and metachromatic leukodystrophy caused by a deficiency of the sulfatase that removes sulfate from sulfatide, there are large accumulations of ganglioside and sulfatide, respectively. In both diseases, as in Niemann-Pick disease, cerebroside and sulfatide are present in abnormally high proportions and the relative amount of phosphatidyl choline is abnormally low. A similar abnormal lipid class distribution is seen in phenylketonuria (phenylalanine hydroxylase deficiency) and is thus not limited to hereditary abnormalities of the enzymes of lipid metabolism.

Lipid deposits in the sphingolipid disorders appear first in lysosomes. The highest levels are found in the reticuloendothelial system and in cells with a long life span (such as neurons). The lysosomal localization probably accounts for the relatively normal composition of erythrocytes and some isolated membrane preparations from the nervous system in the sphingolipid disorders.

In the clinically milder forms of the sphingolipid disorders, the enzyme deficiency is not as great, and abnormalities of lipid class distribution in brain may be small or undetectable whereas they may be easily seen in other organs. In brain, it appears that cell degeneration and death caused by the milder enzyme deficiencies may decrease lipid biosynthesis and thus bring biosynthesis and degradation into a normal or nearly normal balance. Brain function may be normal in some of the adult forms of the sphingolipid disorders despite abnormally high lipid levels in liver and spleen. In these cases, decreased biosynthesis appears to compensate for decreased degradation in brain, whereas in spleen in particular, the inability of the phagocytic cells to degrade ingested blood cell lipids results in accumulation of excess lipid.

In liver and spleen in Niemann-Pick disease, there is a large accumulation of lysobisphosphatidic acid that is normally a very minor component (Rouser *et al.*, 1968a). This accumulation may be a metabolic backup phenomenon and if so may arise through the degradation pathway for sphingosine (conversion via sphingosine phosphate to fatty aldehyde and ethanolamine phosphate).

Gaucher's disease is caused by the deficiency of glucocerebrosidase, the enzyme that removes glucose from glucocerebroside. In the milder chronic form there are no neurological symptoms and brain lipids are normal, although cerebroside accumulates in the spleen. In the acute infantile form with neurological involvement and death within the first few months of life, brain lipids are also entirely normal. Normal brain lipid levels may be explained by the release of a relatively small amount of glucocerebroside by degradation of ganglioside with the probability that depression of biosynthesis and recycling of glucocerebroside maintain a normal lipid class balance. It appears that the enzymes that remove carbohydrate residues from glycolipids also hydrolyze the same linkages in glycoproteins and polysaccharides. This appears to be the major reason for the simultaneous accumulation of all three groups of substances in several disorders that may be referred to most properly as glycosidase deficiencies. Which of these accumulates to the greatest extent in any particular organ can thus be related to the extent to which substances with the particular carbohydrate linkage occur. Abnormal function in infantile Gaucher's disease may thus depend upon abnormal levels of glycoproteins and/or polysaccharides.

The realization that abnormalities of lipid class distribution in brain may be small or absent when degradative enzyme deficiencies are mild, or when the deficiency is for a glycolipid bond that is present in small amount only in brain, promises to be of value in the demonstration of other enzyme deficiencies. Thus, in Farber's disease, abnormal lipid and polysaccharide levels have been found in organs and the disorder is fatal within the first few years of life. The total lipid level of brain is below normal and the increase in the relative proportions of cerebroside, sulfatide, and sphingomyelin and the decrease of phosphatidyl choline seen in the sphingolipid disorders is apparent (Rouser and Kritchevsky, 1972). In addition, a very minor glycolipid spot not present in normal brain was detected by thin layer chromatography. When the lipids of other organs were examined, abnormal lipid class distributions were found. An abnormally low level of phosphatidyl ethanolamine was found in kidney, lung, and liver. This was accompanied in kidney by an increase of sphingomyelin and ceramide tri- and tetrahexosides and an increase of the ceramide polyhexosides only in lung and liver. The increase in ceramide polyhexoside with the TLC mobility of kidney and red blood cell globoside (ceramide tetrahexoside) was greatest in kidney. The findings point to a deficiency of a degradative enzyme for a carbohydrate linkage, perhaps for a glucose-galactose bond.

Other hereditary neuropathological states appear to have a hereditary enzyme deficiency as only one of two or more components necessary to bring about the clinical abnormality. This appears to be the case for Alzheimer's disease (see chapters in the book edited by Wolstenholme and O'Connor, 1970). Symptoms usually appear after 40 years of age and are associated with progressive brain degeneration leading to death within 2 to 5 years. We have found the total lipid content and lipid class distribution of brain to be normal or almost so. Because abnormal accumulation of glycoprotein and polysaccharide have been reported, we examined the kidney, an organ normally high in glycolipid, for a glycolipid abnormality.

A very small glycolipid spot was detected by TLC. The glycolipid spot was not seen in normal kidney or in kidneys from patients with the known disorders of lipid metabolism. This raised the possibility that a mild deficiency for a carbohydrate linkage common to glycolipid, glycoprotein, and polysaccharide could be one of the factors involved in development of the disorder. In addition to a metabolic abnormality, virus infection and physical trauma have been associated with onset of Alzheimer's disease. From the data, we have formulated a working hypothesis, i.e., that a relatively mild deficiency of a degradative enzyme for a carbohydrate linkage coupled with trauma to the nervous system combine to cause Alzheimer's disease. Trauma could arise from a blow on the head, virus infection, or vascular disease.

The lipid class relationships defined in Section III may be of value in detecting biosynthetic and degradative enzyme deficiencies. Biosynthetic defects can be expected to result in the lowering of the amount of the lipid class affected. This should result in a compensatory increase in the amounts of the lipid classes in the same substitution group. Alternatively, in some organs, a compensatory increase in the levels of enzymes for an alternate pathway may give rise to normal levels of all lipid classes. The approach to the detection of biosynthetic defects is clear. As in all cases, the first step is demonstration of an abnormal lipid class pattern. It is then necessary to show that degradative enzyme deficiencies do not exist and that there is a biosynthetic deficiency. The enzyme changes can be determined by *in vitro* enzyme assay or by *in vitro* or *in vivo* isotope incorporation rates.

Deficiencies of biosynthetic enzymes should be easily detectable in blood cells and isotope incorporation rates can be determined from leukocyte cultures. Leukocytes and erythrocytes may be very useful for distinguishing abnormal lipid patterns caused by degradative enzyme deficiencies from similar patterns caused by deficiencies of biosynthetic enzymes since only the latter should be readily apparent in blood cells. It seems probable that some biosynthetic defects have already been encountered but not recognized as such because methods of lipid analysis and interpretation of data were inadequate. Cases diagnosed as Niemann-Pick disease on the basis of an abnormally high sphingomyelin level but without a sphingomyelinase deficiency may prove to be examples of biosynthetic defects for glycerol phospholipids.

Detection of deficiencies for degradative enzymes acting on glycerol phospholipids has not been possible previously but seems to be feasible now. Such deficiencies should lead to accumulation of lipid in lysosomes. Also, more than one lipid class may be affected since some of the enzymes are not specific for one lipid class. Moreover, the lipid may not remain in its native form. The high polyunsaturated fatty acid content of glycerol phospholipids suggests that carbon chains may undergo autoxidation and polymerization. Several types of pathology have been reported in which relatively insoluble, lipid-containing deposits referred to as lipofuscin or ceroid are found. These may be representatives of the undetected glycerol phospholipid degradative enzyme deficiencies. Detection of such deficiencies should be possible with leukocytes by enzyme assay or determination of isotope incorporation rates. The relative binding affinities for different lipids to membrane lipid-binding proteins appears to be quite different. Both *in vitro* and *in vivo*, cholesterol, phosphatidyl choline, and sphingomyelin are quite generally found to move most rapidly from one membrane to another and thus appear to be less firmly bound (see Section V,A). Phospholipids with a net negative charge at physiological pH (acidic phospholipids) appear to bind most tightly to membranes, and phosphatidyl ethanolamine appears to occupy an intermediate position. The replacement of phosphatidyl choline by cerebroside and phosphatidyl ethanolamine by sulfatide that takes place during myelination (see Section III) can be explained as arising from such rapid formation of binding sites for lipids in myelin that biosynthesis of phosphatidyl choline and phosphatidyl ethanolamine is not adequate and thus the less firmly bound cerebroside and sulfatide can enter and replace them (see Section III for the way lipid class substitution has been defined).

VII. Membrane Structure

Although polar lipids are thought to bind directly to proteins, cholesterol has been visualized as being bound to polar lipids rather than to protein. Thus, the relationship of cholesterol to polar lipids is of considerable interest. Finean (1953) proposed that one molecule of cholesterol is bound to one of phospholipid or glycolipid. The molar ratio of total phospholipid to cholesterol to galactolipid has been noted to be approximately 2:2:1, but this is far from exact. It appears that the maximum number of cholesterol molecules normally bound to polar lipid can be determined only with data for membranes maximally loaded with cholesterol rather than with data for whole brain or other organs or subcellular particulates not maximally loaded with cholesterol (Rouser, 1971; Rouser *et al.*, 1971a,b). Maximum loading appears probable for myelin, the mammalian red blood cell, and plasma (cell surface) membranes of some other cell types.

Eng and Smith (1966) proposed that the molar amount of cholesterol is equal to the molar sum of phosphatidyl ethanolamine + sphingomyelin + cerebroside + sulfatide. This suggestion was made because they supposed that cholesterol would bind to the lipids they had found by isotope turnover studies to be the most stable metabolically. When we checked the correlation with data reported in the literature for myelin, it was found to hold fairly well as did the ratio of cholesterol to phosphatidyl choline + sphingomyelin + cerebroside + acidic phospholipids (Rouser *et al.*, 1971b) as shown in Table VIII. Since it seems most probable that cholesterol will bind to the same lipid classes in all membranes, the two relationships, if correct, should hold for all membranes that are fully loaded with cholesterol. When the relationships were tested with the data of Turner and Rouser (1970) for the lipids of human erythrocytes, they clearly did not hold (Table VIII). Thus, both relationships appear to be more or less fortuitous approximate correlations.

Rouser (1971) and Rouser *et al.* (1971b) proposed that a maximum of

Table VIII

RELATIONSHIP OF MOLES OF CHOLESTEROL TO MOLES OF POLAR LIPID SUMS OF ADULT BRAIN MYELIN AND ERYTHROCYTES[a,b]

Species	Cholesterol	PC + Sph + Cer + APL	PE + Sph + Cer + Sulf	2(PE + APL)	Cholesterol ÷ 2(PE + APL)	References[c]
A. Myelin						
Human	41.1	40.1	39.5	44.5	0.95	1, 2
Bovine	42.3	40.6	41.1	41.9	1.01	3, 4
Rabbit	38.9	42.1	42.4	34.6	1.07	4, 5
Pigeon	44.7	38.8	37.8	40.8	1.03	4
Dogfish	36.9	36.0	42.5	60.8	0.61	4
Rat	41.1	36.8	39.2	51.6	0.80	4,6–10
Mean (all species)	40.9	39.2	40.3	40.4[d]	1.02[c]	—
B. Erythrocytes						
Human	46.8	38.3	26.9	48.7	0.96	11
Animal	37.4	—[e]	—[e]	36.6	1.02	12

[a] Values as molar percentages of the total lipid. Myelin data for adult animal brains only.

[b] Abbreviations: PE, phosphatidyl ethanolamine; Sph, sphingomyelin; Cer, cerebroside; Sulf, sulfatide; PC, phosphatidyl choline; APL, acidic phospholipids.

[c] Data from: (1) Gerstl *et al.* (1967); (2) Eng *et al.* (1968); (3) Norton and Autilio (1965); (4) Cuzner *et al.* (1965a); (5) Dalal and Einstein (1969); (6) Cuzner and Davison (1968); (7) Eng and Noble (1968); (8) Davison *et al.* (1966); (9) Cuzner *et al.* (1965b); (10) Agrawal *et al.* (1970); (11) Turner and Rouser (1970); (12) Nelson (1967).

[d] Excluding dogfish and rat.

[e] Unable to calculate because glycolipid values not available.

two molecules of cholesterol can bind to one of phosphatidyl ethanolamine and the acidic phospholipids, i.e., that one-half the maximum molar amount of cholesterol is equal to the sum of phosphatidyl ethanolamine + acidic phospholipids (phosphatidyl serine, phosphatidyl inositol, diphosphatidyl glycerol, and all minor acidic phospholipids). The sum is readily calculated by subtraction of the phosphatidyl choline and sphingomyelin values from the value for total phospholipid. As shown in Table VIII, this relationship correctly estimates the percentage of cholesterol in myelin of several species. With an error of ±4% in the estimation of cholesterol and ±4% for the sum of the phospholipids, the expected range of the ratio is 0.92 to 1.08 and this was the range found for four species. Dogfish and rat brains appear to be underloaded with cholesterol. An increase in the percentage of cholesterol with age has been noted for rat brain (Section IV) and the lower than predicted cholesterol values for rat brain myelin can thus be explained as arising from the use of animals that have not attained the maximum cholesterol content. The relationship holds equally well for erythrocytes of man and all mammalian species for which accurate data are available (Table VIII). The ratios shown in Table IX indicate that the relationship also holds for plasma membranes of other cell types and for virus particles that obtain their lipid from the plasma membrane of the host cell. The range for plasma membranes is commonly between 0.5 and 1.0, but frog rod outer segments that are believed to be extensions of plasma membranes of neurons have a low percentage of cholesterol. The data suggest that the proposal that the maximum molar amount of cholesterol is equal to twice the sum of phosphatidyl ethanol amine and acidic phospholipids is correct.

Most models of cell membrane structure visualize lipid as occurring entirely between two layers of protein or inserted into a protein layer. A recently proposed model (Rouser, 1971; Rouser *et al.*, 1971b) places one-half of the lipid between protein layers and the other half external to the structural protein layers with the lipid molecules lying over the protein rather than perpendicular to it as in the classic Davson-Danielli model. With this arrangement, lipid-lipid and lipid-protein interactions are through both polar and apolar bonds. The lipid can be viewed as rows of bilayers lying over the protein rather than perpendicular to it. Because phospholipases can attack membrane lipids and the polar groups of some antigenic lipids must be available at the cell surface for reaction, models were proposed such as those of Vanderkooi and Green (1970, 1971) and Vanderkooi and Sundaralingam (1970) depicting lipid molecules inserted between protein molecules with some polar groups exposed.

Table IX

RATIO OF CHOLESTEROL TO TWICE THE LEVEL OF PHOSPHATIDYL ETHANOLAMINE
PLUS ACIDIC PHOSPHOLIPIDS OF PLASMA MEMBRANES AND VIRUS COAT
LIPIDS[a]

Species	Cell or organ	Cholesterol ÷ 2(PE + APL)	References[c]
Mouse	L-cells (fibroblasts)	0.96[b]	
		0.73	1
Bovine	Kidney	0.99	2
Hamster	Kidney	0.89	2
		0.91	3
Monkey	Kidney	0.72	3
SV5 virus	Grown in BK cells	0.86	2
	Grown in BHK cells	0.98	2
		1.01	3
	Grown in MK cells	0.71	3
Vesicular stomatitis virus	Grown in L-cells	0.52	4
	Grown in CE cells	0.52	4
Influenza virus	Grown in presence of vitamin A	0.97	5
	Incomplete virus	0.46	6
Sendai virus	—	0.51	7
Newcastle disease virus	—	0.63	7
Guinea pig	Pancreas	0.52	8
Rat	Intestinal brush border	0.54	9
		0.50	
	Liver	0.49	10
		0.56	11
		0.59	12
		0.67	13
		0.82	14
Frog	Retinal rod outer segments	0.13	15

[a] Abbreviations: PE, phosphatidyl ethanolamine; APL, acidic phospholipids. BK, bovine kidney; BHK, baby hamster kidney; MK, monkey kidney; CE cells, chick embryo cells.

[b] Two different methods gave different ratios.

[c] References: (1) Weinstein and Marsh (1969); (2) Klenk and Choppin (1970); (3) Klenk and Choppin (1969); (4) McSharry and Wagner (1971); (5) Blough and Weinstein (1967); (6) Blough and Merlie (1970); (7) Blough and Lawson (1968); (8) Meldolesi *et al.* (1971); (9) Millington and Critchley (1968); (10) Stahl and Trams (1968); (11) Dod and Gray (1968); (12) Keenan and Morré (1969); (13) Pfleger *et al.* (1968); (14) Skipski *et al.* (1965); (15) Eichberg and Hess (1967).

There are three main lines of evidence that indicate that some lipid is located external to the lipid-binding (structural) membrane protein and that lipid-requiring enzymes are then attached to the lipid (that may move to coat the enzyme on all sides). The most direct evidence comes from the observation of erythrocyte lipid loss to aqueous solutions (see Section V,A for references). About one-quarter of the total lipid of human red blood cells can be lost to the medium when cells are incubated *in vitro* and about one-half of the lipid can be washed from red cell ghosts and myelin with aqueous solutions without apparent loss of protein.

The second line of evidence comes from the nature of the lipid interaction with enzymes requiring lipid for activity. Lipid-requiring enzymes are specific for lipids with the proper polar groups. Thus, it seems that lipid probably interacts with the enzyme through both ionic groups and apolar bonds of carbon chains. This means that the lipid lies over the protein. To achieve such an orientation with most membrane models requires that the enzyme be inserted into the membrane. This destroys the model. In contrast, if the framework of the membrane is visualized as structural, lipid-binding protein coated on both sides with lipid and the lipid molecules lying over the protein (rather than projecting away from it), the lipid external to the structural protein is in the proper position to form active complexes with enzymes that become attached to the membrane surface, and the complex is freely available to interact with the substrate for the enzyme.

The third line of evidence indicating some lipid to be external to the structural protein comes from attempts to visualize the mechanism at the membrane of biosynthesis of molecules formed by a long sequence of enzyme reactions that require lipid. This of course involves considerations similar to the second line of evidence. The sequence of reactions involved in the biosynthesis of the complex bacterial cell envelope lipopolysaccharide provides a good example. The steps in the biosynthesis have been reviewed and a model of the structure of the biosynthetic apparatus presented recently (Rothfield and Romeo, 1971). There are two types of lipid requirements for this sequence. One is for interaction with phosphatidyl ethanolamine, presumably to attain the proper alignment of enzymes and substrates, and the other is for a glycolipid that supplies carbohydrate units to the growing polysaccharide chain. The entire sequence can be visualized easily if some lipid is external to the structural protein and the enzymes and substrates are attached to this surface lipid so that the growing chain of the lipopolysaccharide can pass from one enzyme to the next and be attached to lipid in the process, as depicted in the model of Rothfield and Romeo (1971).

The appearance of membranes when examined by high resolution electron microscopy is of fundamental importance in studies of membrane structure. The staining of membranes was at first thought to be due to interaction of the fixative (and counterstain) with lipid. It has been shown, however, that similar results can be obtained with membranes from which all of the lipid has been removed. Fleischer *et al.* (1967a) showed that typical unit membranes can be seen in lipid-depleted mito-chondria, and Napolitano *et al.* (1967) showed that all of the lipid of rat sciatic nerve could be removed with retention of the typical main and interperiod lines of myelin when the nerve was treated with glu-taraldehyde prior to extraction of lipid and was then exposed to osmium tetroxide in carbon tetrachloride. These data are in keeping with data on lipid loss during preparation of tissue for electron microscopic exami-nation. Bahr (1956) noted that both lipids and proteins of organs react with osmium tetroxide.

It has become apparent that fixation with osmium tetroxide is required for retention of lipid when tissue is prepared for electron microscopic examination. At best, with most methods a minimum loss of 20% of the phospholipid is obtained and with some procedures all of the lipid is removed (Cope and Williams, 1969a,b), although Mitchell (1969) reported retention of 95% of the cholesterol and 97% of the phospholipid of red blood cell stroma. Complete fixation of glycolipid and phospho-lipid with 30% loss of chlorophyll was noted with spinach chloroplasts (Ongun *et al.*, 1968). Robertson and Parsons (1970) found only a small loss of frog sciatic nerve cholesterol after fixation with glutaraldehyde and osmium tetroxide if the nerve was embedded directly in a resorcinol-formaldehyde resin, but about 50% of the cho-lesterol was removed by acetone dehydration prior to embedding with Epon. Shrinkage as a result of cholesterol loss was indicated by the finding that the major period lines seen by electron microscopy were separated by a distance of 160 Å when cholesterol loss was minimal and 130 Å when one-half of the cholesterol was removed.

Loss of neutral fat (mostly triglyceride) is commonly 100%, and 50% retention appears to be about the best that can be obtained (Casley-Smith, 1967; Cope and Williams, 1967). Improved retention of cholesterol was found when fixation was carried out in the presence of digitonin (Frühling and Penasse, 1969; Williamson, 1969; Scallen and Dietert, 1969). Subsequent work has generally been in agreement with the earlier observations of Korn and Weisman (1966). Both protein and lipid loss were determined by Dallam (1957) who found that losses from whole tissues, mitochondria, and microsomes with osmium tetroxide fixation were from 10 to 37% for protein and 5 to 30% for lipids. Although glu-taraldehyde fixation prior to treatment with osmium does not appear in general to change the extent of lipid loss greatly, it does appear to fix some phosphatidyl ethanolamine (and presumably also some phos-phatidyl serine) to protein (Gigg and Payne, 1969).

Treatment of myelin with various solvents was found to alter X-ray diffraction spacings (Rumsby and Finean, 1966a,b,c). Alteration of spacings observed with X-ray diffraction was also noted with osmium fixation and dehydration (Moretz *et al.*, 1969). The data demonstrate alterations of membrane structure by the methods commonly employed. The electron microscopic appearance of membranes does not appear to be correlated in any simple manner with the extent of lipid extraction (Cope and Williams, 1969b). It is apparent that many treatments alter lipid content and membrane structure, and it is thus difficult to draw precise conclusions from the spacings of lines on electron micrographs. Even when lipid is not removed, there is no assurance that it has retained its true *in vivo* relationship to other membrane components. Furthermore, findings and interpretations differ a great deal. Thus, Stempak and Laurencin (1970) failed to observe the typical unit membrane by high resolution electron microscopy of very thin sections. Rather, they observed a series of black dots and suggested that the unit membrane arises as a superimposition artifact of these dots when a section is too thick and the image not in proper focus. Reasons for erroneous interpretations of light and electron microscopic sections are discussed in detail by Elias (1971). Difficulties are also encountered in the interpretation of X-ray diffraction data because assumptions must be made and their choice may be influenced by the concept of membrane structure the investigator is inclined to favor. Thus, the results from the two methods thought for a long time to give excellent proof of the Davson-Danielli lipid-bilayer model of the cell membrane do not appear to be so definitive and clearly present major problems of interpretation.

Interpretation difficulties are also encountered with other physical methods (optical properties, nuclear magnetic resonance, infrared spectroscopy, and calorimetry). Despite the difficulties, data obtained by these methods are generally interpreted to indicate the existence of lipid bilayers with lipid-lipid and lipid-protein interaction by apolar bonds as well as by ionic interaction. The model proposed by Rouser (1971) and Rouser *et al.* (1971b) is in accord with these interpretations, although the lipid bilayers in the model are depicted as lying flat over the protein surface rather than perpendicular to it.

The usual presentation of the classic lipid bilayer is with molecules of the same general structure (glycerolphospholipids, sphingomyelin, and cerebroside). Other larger molecules also occur in membranes. Clearly, gangliosides, ceramide polyhexosides, and chlorophyll cannot be incorporated into membranes in the manner commonly shown for bilayers of smaller molecules. Also, some membranes contain lipids with polar groups on both ends (xanthophylls and sulfolipid of some algae).

Lipids of some mycobacteria are extremely large molecules consisting of fatty acids with about 100 carbon atoms each as well as polar groups. These lipids cannot be visualized as occurring in the classic bilayer. The problems of arrangement are, however, greatly simplified with the new model in which lipid lies over the protein which it can coat on both sides.

ACKNOWLEDGMENTS

The experimental work in the authors' laboratories was supported by Grants NS-01847, NS-06237, and NS-03743 from the Institute of Neurological Diseases and Stroke of the National Institutes of Health. Dr. Gerald Simon made important contributions in the work on brain lipids of different animal species, and Dr. Charles Altschuler provided many of the samples of normal human brain used in our studies. Dr. Nicholas Nicolaides and Dr. Richard Hammerschlag gave invaluable aid in preparation of the manuscript.

References

Acheson, N. H., and Tamm, I. (1967). *Virology* **32**, 128.

Adams, R. G. (1967). *J. Lipid Res.* **8**, 245.

Adams, R. G. (1969). *J. Lipid Res.* **10**, 473.

Adams, D. H., and Fox, E. (1969). *Brain Res.* **14**, 647.

Agrawal, H. C., Banik, N. L., Bone, A. H., Davison, A. N., Mitchell, R. F., and Spohn, M. (1970). *Biochem. J.* **120**, 635.

Akiyama, M., and Sakagami, T. (1969). *Biochim. Biophys. Acta* **187**, 105.

Anderson, R. E. (1970). *Exp. Eye Res.* **10**, 339.

Anderson, R. E., and Maude, M. B. (1970). *Biochemistry* **9**, 3624.

Anderson, R. E., Maude, M. B., and Feldman, G. L. (1969). *Biochim. Biophys. Acta* **187**, 345.

Anderson, R. E., Feldman, L. S., and Feldman, G. L. (1970). *Biochim. Biophys. Acta* **202**, 367.

Ansell, G. B. (1971). *In* "Chemistry and Brain Development," Proc. Advan. Study Inst. Chem. Brain Develop., Milan (R. Paoletti and A. N. Davison, eds.), Advan. Exp. Med. Biol., Vol. 13, pp. 63–74. Plenum, New York.

Ansell, G. B., and Spanner, S. (1971). *Biochem. J.* **122**, 741.

Anthony, J., and Moscarello, M. A. (1971). *FEBS (Fed. Eur. Biochem. Soc.), Lett.* **15**, 335.

Armstrong, M. L., Connor, W. E., and Warner, E. D. (1969). *Arch. Pathol.* **87**, 87.

Ashworth, L. A. E., and Green, C. (1964). *Biochim. Biophys. Acta* **84**, 182.

Avrova, N. F. (1971). *J. Neurochem.* **18**, 667.

Awasthi, Y. C., Chuang, T. F., Keenan, T. W., and Crane, F. L. (1971). *Biochim. Biophys. Acta* **226**, 42.

Bader, H. (1964). *Biophysik* **1**, 370.

Bahr, G. F. (1957). *Electron Microsc., Proc. Stockholm Conf., 1956* pp. 107–108.

Balakrishnan, S., Goodwin, H., and Cumings, J. N. (1961). *J. Neurochem.* **8**, 276.

Banik, N. L., and Davison, A. N. (1967). *J. Neurochem.* **14**, 594.

Banik, N. L., and Davison, A. N. (1969). *Biochem. J.* **115**, 1051.

Banik, N. L., and Davison, A. N. (1971). *Biochem. J.* **122**, 751.

Banik, N. L., Blunt, M. J., and Davison, A. N. (1968). *J. Neurochem.* 15, 471.

Basford, J. M., Glover, J., and Green, C. (1964). *Biochim. Biophys. Acta* 84, 764.

Bass, N. H. (1971). *Advan. Exp. Biol. Med.* 13, 412–424.

Baxter, C. F., Rouser, G., and Simon, G. (1969). *Lipids* 4, 243.

Beattie, D. S. (1969). *J. Membrane Biol.* 1, 383.

Ben Abdelkader, A. B., and Mazliak, P. (1970). *Eur. J. Biochem.* 15, 250.

Benton, J. W., Moser, H. W., Dodge, P. R., and Carr, S. (1966). *Pediatrics* 38, 801.

Bernhard, K., Lesch, P., and Neuhaus-Maier, S. (1969). *Helv. Chim. Acta* 52, 1815.

Berry, J. F., Fletcher, T. F., and Bovis, M. (1969). *Lipids* 4, 623.

Blok, M. C., Wirtz, K. W. A., and Scherphof, G. L. (1971). *Biochim. Biophys. Acta* 233, 61.

Blough, H. A., and Lawson, D. E. M. (1968). *Virology* 36, 289.

Blough, H. A., and Merlie, J. (1970). *Virology* 40, 685.

Blough, H. A., and Weinstein, D. B. (1967). *Virology* 33, 459.

Boon, J., Broekhuyse, R. M., van Munster, P., and Schretlen, E. (1969). *Clin. Chim. Acta* 23, 453.

Borggreven, J. M. P. M., Daemen, F. J. M., and Bonting, S. L. (1970). *Biochim. Biophys. Acta* 202, 374.

Bosmann, H. B., and Case, K. R. (1969). *Biochem. Biophys. Res. Commun.* 36, 830.

Brady, R. O. (1970). *Chem. Phys. Lipids* 5, 261.

Braun, P. E., and Radin, N. S. (1969). *Biochemistry* 8, 4310.

Broekhuyse, R. M. (1968). *Biochim. Biophys. Acta* 152, 307.

Broekhuyse, R. M. (1969). *Biochim. Biophys. Acta* 187, 354.

Broekhuyse, R. M. (1971). *Biochim. Biophys. Acta* 218, 546.

Broekhuyse, R. M., and Veerkamp, J. H. (1968). *Biochim. Biophys. Acta* 152, 316.

Bruckdorfer, K. R., and Green, G. (1967). *Biochem. J.* 104, 270.

Bruckdorfer, K. R., Graham, J. M., and Green, C. (1968). *Eur. J. Biochem.* 4, 512.

Bürger, M. (1956). *Medizinische* No. 1, 561.

Butschak, G. (1970). *Arch. Geschwulstforsch.* 35, 227.

Bygrave, F. L. (1969). *J. Biol. Chem.* 244, 4768.

Bygrave, F. L., and Bücher, T. (1968). *FEBS (Fed. Eur. Biochem. Soc.), Lett.* 1, 42.

Camejo, G., Villegas, G. M., Barnola, F. V., and Villegas, R. (1969). *Biochim. Biophys. Acta* 193, 247.

Carnegie, P. R. (1971). *Nature (London)* 229, 25.

Casley-Smith, J. R. (1967). *J. Roy. Microsc. Soc.* 87, 463.

Chevallier, F., and Giraud, F. (1966). *Bull. Soc. Chim. Biol.* 48, 787.

Chevallier, F., and Petit, L. (1966). *Exp. Neurol.* 16, 250.

Chevallier, F., D'Hollander, F., and Simonnet, F. (1968). *Biochim. Biophys. Acta* 164, 339.

Clausen, J. (1969). *Eur. J. Biochem.* 7, 575.

Clausen, J., and Berg Hansen, I. (1970). *Acta Neurol. Scand.* 46, 1.

Compans, R. W., Holmes, K. V., Dales, S., and Choppin, P. W. (1964). *Virology* 30, 411.

Conner, R. L., Mallory, F. B., Landrey, J. R., Ferguson, K. A., Kaneshiro, E. S., and Ray, E. (1971). *Biochem. Biophys. Res. Commun.* 44, 995.

Cooper, R. A. (1969). *J. Clin. Invest.* 48, 1820.

Cooper, R. A., and Jandl, J. H. (1969). *J. Clin. Invest.* 48, 906.

Cope, G. H., and Williams, M. A. (1967). *J. Roy. Microsc. Soc.* 88, 259.

Cope, G. H., and Williams, M. A. (1969a). *J. Microsc.* 90, 31.

Cope, G. H., and Williams, M. A. (1969b). *J. Microsc.* **90**, 47.
Cotman, C., Blank, M. L., Moehl, A., and Snyder, F. (1969). *Biochemistry* **8**, 4606.
Cotmore, J. M., Nichols, G., Jr., and Werthier, R. E. (1971). *Science* **172**, 1339.
Cremer, J. E., Johnston, P. V., Roots, B. I., and Trevor, A. J. (1968). *J. Neurochem.* **15**, 1361.
Cumings, J. N., Goodwin, H., Woodward, E. M., and Curzon, G. (1958). *J. Neurochem.* **2**, 289.
Cumings, J. N., Goodwin, H., and Curzon, G. (1959). *J. Neurochem.* **4**, 234.
Cumings, J. N., Thompson, E. J., and Goodwin, H. (1968). *J. Neurochem.* **15**, 243.
Cuzner, M. L., and Davison, A. N. (1968). *Biochem. J.* **106**, 29.
Cuzner, M. L., Davison, A. N., and Gregson, N. A. (1965a). *J. Neurochem.* **12**, 469.
Cuzner, M. L., Davison, A. N., and Gregson, N. A. (1965b). *Ann. N. Y. Acad. Sci.* **122**, 86.
Cuzner, M. L., Davison, A. N., and Gregson, N. A. (1966). *Biochem. J.* **101**, 618.
Dalal, K. B., and Einstein, E. R. (1969). *Brain Res.* **16**, 441.
Dallam, R. D. (1957). *J. Histochem. Cytochem.* **5**, 178.
Davidson, J. B., and Stanacev, N. Z. (1970). *Can. J. Biochem.* **48**, 633.
Davidson, J. B., and Stanacev, N. Z. (1971). *Biochem. Biophys. Res. Commun.* **42**, 1191.
Davison, A. N. (1969). *Sci. Basis Med.* pp. 220–235.
Davison, A. N. (1971). *In* "Chemistry and Brain Development," Proc. Advan. Study Inst. Chem. Brain Develop., Milan (R. Paoletti and A. N. Davison, eds.), Advan. Exp. Med. Biol., Vol. 13, pp. 375–380. Plenum, New York.
Davison, A. N., and Gregson, N. A. (1962). *Biochem. J.* **85**, 558.
Davison, A. N., and Wajda, M. (1959). *J. Neurochem.* **4**, 353.
Davison, A. N., Cuzner, M. L., Banik, N. L., and Oxberry, J. (1966). *Nature (London)* **212**, 1373.
Dawson, R. M. C. (1965). *Biochem. J.* **97**, 134.
Dekaban, A. S., Patton, V. M., and Cain, D. R. (1971). *J. Neurochem.* **18**, 2451.
De Konig, A. J. (1964). *Biochim. Biophys. Acta* **84**, 467.
De Rooij, R. E., and Hooghwinkel, G. J. M. (1967). *Acta Physiol. Pharmacol. Neer.* **14**, 410.
Derry, D. M., and Wolfe, L. S. (1967). *Science* **158**, 1450.
De Vries, G. H., Norton, W. T., and Raine, C. S. (1972). *Science* **175**, 1370.
Dickinson, J. P., Jones, K. M., Aparicio, S. R., and Lumsden, C. S. (1970). *Nature (London)* **227**, 1133.
Dietschy, J. M., and Wilson, J. D. (1970). *New Engl. J. Med.* **282**, 1128, 1179, 1241.
Dittmer, J. C., and Douglas, M. G. (1969). *Ann. N. Y. Acad. Sci.* **165**, 515.
Dobiašová, M., and Linhart, J. (1970). *Lipids* **5**, 445.
Dobiašová, M., and Radin, N. S. (1968). *Lipids* **3**, 439.
Dod, B. J., and Gray, G. M. (1968). *Biochim. Biophys. Acta* **150**, 397.
Dvorkin, V. Y., and Gasteva, S. V. (1969). *Biokhimiya* **34**, 144.
Easton, D. M. (1971). *Science* **172**, 952.
Eichberg, J. (1969). *Biochim. Biophys. Acta* **187**, 533.
Eichberg, J., and Dawson, R. M. C. (1965). *Biochem. J.* **96**, 644.
Eichberg, J., and Hess, H. H. (1967). *Experientia* **23**, 993.
Eichberg, J., Whittaker, V. P., and Dawson, R. M. C. (1964). *Biochem. J.* **92**, 91.
Eichberg, J., Hauser, G., and Karnovsky, M. (1969). *In* "The Structure and Function of Nervous Tissue" (G. H. Bourne, ed.), Vol. 3, pp. 185–288. Academic Press, New York.

Einstein, E. R., Dalal, K. B., and Csejtey, J. (1970). *Brain Res.* **18**, 35.

Eisenberg, S., Stein, Y., and Stein, O. (1969). *J. Lab. Clin. Invest.* **48**, 2320.

Elias, H. (1971). *Science* **174**, 993.

Eng, L. F., and Noble, E. P. (1968). *Lipids* **3**, 157.

Eng, L. F., and Smith, M. E. (1966). *Lipids* **1**, 296.

Eng, L. F., Chao, F. C., Gerstl, B., Pratt, D., and Tavaststjerna, M. G. (1968). *Biochemistry* **7**, 4455.

Erickson, N. E., and Lands, W. E. M. (1969). *Proc. Soc. Exp. Biol. Med.* **102**, 512.

Eto, Y., and Suzuki, K. (1971). *Biochim. Biophys. Acta* **239**, 293.

Eto, Y., Suzuki, K., and Suzuki, K. (1970). *J. Lipid Res.* **11**, 473.

Eto, Y., Suzuki, K., and Suzuki, K. (1971). *J. Lipid Res.* **12**, 570.

Eylar, E. H. (1970). *Proc. Nat. Acad. Sci. U. S.* **67**, 1425.

Fang, M., and Marinetti, G. V. (1970). *Biochim. Biophys. Acta* **202**, 91.

Feldman, G. L., Feldman, L. S., and Rouser, G. (1965). *J. Amer. Oil Chem. Soc.* **42**, 742.

Feldman, G. L., Feldman, L. S., and Rouser, G. (1966a). *Lipids* **1**, 161.

Feldman, G. L., Feldman, L. S., and Rouser, G. (1966b). *Lipids* **1**, 21.

Fewster, M. E., and Mead, J. F. (1968). *J. Neurochem.* **15**, 1041.

Fillerup, D. L., and Mead, J. F. (1967). *Lipids* **2**, 295.

Fineau, J. B. (1953). *Experientia* **9**, 17.

Fishman, M. A., Prensky, A. L., and Dodge, P. R. (1969). *Nature (London)* **221**, 552.

Fleischer, S., and Fleischer, B. (1967). *In* "Oxidation and Phosphorylation" (R. W. Estabrook and M. E. Pullman, eds.), Methods in Enzymology, Vol. 10, pp. 406–433. Academic Press, New York.

Fleischer, S., and Rouser, G. (1965). *J. Amer. Oil Chem. Soc.* **42**, 588.

Fleischer, S., Fleischer, B., and Stoeckenius, W. (1967a). *J. Cell Biol.* **32**, 193.

Fleischer, S., Rouser, G., Fleischer, B., Casu, A., and Kritchevsky, G. (1967b). *J. Lipid Res.* **8**, 170.

Folch-Pi, J. (1955). *In* "Biochemistry of the Developing Nervous System" (H. Waelsch, ed.), pp. 121–136. Academic Press, New York.

Folch, J., Lees, M. B., and Sloane-Stanley, G. H. (1957). *J. Biol. Chem.* **226**, 497.

Freysz, L., Nussbaum, J. L., Bieth, R., and Mandel, P. (1963). *Bull. Soc. Chim. Biol.* **45**, 1019.

Freysz, L., Bieth, R., and Mandel, P. (1966). *Bull. Soc. Chim. Biol.* **48**, 287.

Freysz, L., Bieth, R., Judes, C., Sensenbrenner, M., Jacob, M., and Mandel, P. (1968). *J. Neurochem.* **15**, 307.

Frühling, J., and Penasse, W. (1969). *J. Microsc. (Paris)* **8**, 957.

Fujino, Y., and Nokano, M. (1969). *Biochem. J.* **113**, 573.

Fumagalli, R., Niemiro, R., and Paoletti, R. (1965). *J. Amer. Oil Chem. Soc.* **42**, 1018.

Galli, C., and Cecconi, D. R. (1967). *Lipids* **2**, 76.

Galli, C., and Fumagalli, R. (1968). *J. Neurochem.* **15**, 35.

Galli, C., White, H. B., Jr., and Paoletti, R. (1970). *J. Neurochem.* **17**, 347.

Galli, C., White, H. B., Jr., and Paoletti, R. (1971a). *In* "Chemistry and Brain Development," Proc. Advan. Study Inst. Chem. Brain Develop., Milan (R. Paoletti and A. N. Davison, eds.), Advan. Exp. Med. Biol., Vol. 13, pp. 425–435. Plenum, New York.

Galli, C., White, H. B., Jr., and Paoletti, R. (1971b). *Lipids* **6**, 378.

Ganguly, M., Carnighan, R. H., and Westphal, U. (1967). *Biochemistry* **6**, 2803.

Gautheron, C., Petit, L., and Chevallier, F. (1969). *Exp. Neurol.* **25**, 18.

Gerstl, B., Eng, L. F., Hayman, R. B., Tavaststjerna, M. G., and Bond, P. R. (1967). *J. Neurochem.* **14**, 661.

Gerstl, B., Eng, L. F., Hayman, R. B., and Bond, P. (1969). *Lipids* **4**, 428.

Gigg, R., and Payne, S. (1969). *Chem. Phys. Lipids* **3**, 292.

Graham, J. M., and Green, C. (1969). *Biochem. Pharmacol.* **18**, 493.

Graham, J. M., and Green, C. (1970). *Eur. J. Biochem.* **12**, 58.

Habermann, E., Brandtlow, G., and Krusche, B. (1961). *Klin. Wochenschr.* **39**, 816.

Hajra, A. K., Seguin, E. B., and Agranoff, B. W. (1968). *J. Biol. Chem.* **243**, 1609.

Hallinan, T., Duffy, T., Waddington, S., and Munro, H. N. (1966). *Quart. J. Exp. Physiol. Cog. Med. Sci.* **51**, 142.

Hamberger, A., and Svennerholm, L. (1971). *J. Neurochem.* **18**, 1821.

Handa, S., and Burton, R. M. (1969). *Lipids* **4**, 205.

Hauser, G. (1968). *J. Neurochem.* **15**, 1237.

Hemminki, K. (1970). *FEBS (Fed. Eur. Biochem. Soc.), Lett.* **9**, 290.

Herschkowitz, N., McKhann, G. M., Saxena, S., and Shooter, E. M. (1968a). *J. Neurochem.* **15**, 1181.

Herschkowitz, N., McKhann, G. M., and Shooter, E. M. (1968b). *J. Neurochem.* **15**, 161.

Herschkowitz, N., McKhann, G. M., Saxena, S., Shooter, E. M., and Herndon, R. (1969). *J. Neurochem.* **16**, 1049.

Hildebrand, J., Stoffyn, P., and Houser, G. (1970). *J. Neurochem.* **17**, 403.

Holm, M. R. (1968). *J. Neurochem.* **15**, 821.

Holton, J. B., and Easton, D. M. (1971). *Biochim. Biophys. Acta* **239**, 61.

Honnegger, C. G., and Freyvogel, T. A. (1963). *Helv. Chim. Acta* **46**, 2265.

Horrocks, L. A. (1967). *J. Lipid Res.* **8**, 569.

Horrocks, L. A. (1968). *J. Neurochem.* **15**, 483.

Hrachovec, J. P., and Rockstein, M. (1959). *Gerontologia* **3**, 305.

Idler, D. R., and Wiseman, P. (1968). *Comp. Biochem. Physiol.* **26**, 1113.

Ishizuka, I., Kloppenburg, M., and Wiegandt, H. (1970). *Biochim. Biophys. Acta* **210**, 299.

Jacob, H. S. (1967). *J. Clin. Invest.* **46**, 2083.

Johnson, J. D., and Cornatzer, W. E. (1969). *Proc. Soc. Exp. Biol. Med.* **131**, 474.

Johnston, P. V., and Roots, B. I. (1970). *Int. Rev. Cytol.* **29**, 265.

Jones, J. P., Ramsey, R. B., and Nicholas, H. J. (1971). *Life Sci.* **10**, 997.

Jungalwala, F. B., and Dawson, R. M. C. (1970). *Biochem. J.* **117**, 481.

Kaiser, W. (1969). *Eur. J. Biochem.* **8**, 120.

Kaiser, W., and Bygrave, F. L. (1968). *Eur. J. Biochem.* **4**, 582.

Keenan, T. W., and Morré, D. J. (1969). *Biochemistry,* **9**, 19.

Kerr, S. E., Kfoury, G., and Djibelian, L. G. (1963). *Biochim. Biophys. Acta* **70**, 474.

Khan, A. A., and Folch-Pi, J. (1967). *J. Neurochem.* **14**, 1099.

Kishimoto, Y., and Radin, N. S. (1959). *J. Lipid Res.* **1**, 79.

Kishimoto, Y., Davies, W. E., and Radin, N. S. (1965). *J. Lipid Res.* **6**, 532.

Klein, F. (1968). *Bull. Soc. Chim. Biol.* **50**, 101.

Klein, F., and Mandel, P. (1968). *Bull. Soc. Chim. Biol.* **50**, 1967.

Klenk, H. D., and Choppin, P. W. (1969). *Virology* **38**, 255.

Klenk, H. D., and Choppin, P. W. (1970). *Virology* **40**, 939.

Koppikar, S. V., Fatterpaker, P., and Sreenivasan, A. (1971). *Biochem. J.* **121**, 643.

Korn, E. D., and Weisman, R. A. (1966). *Biochim. Biophys. Acta* **116**, 309.

Kreps, E. M., Manukyan, K. G., Smirnov, A. A., and Chirkovskaya, E. V. (1963). *Biokhimiya* **28**, 978.

Kreps, E. M., Manukyan, K. G., Patrikeeva, M. V., Smirnov, A. A., Chenkaeva, N. Y., and Chirkovskaya, E. V. (1966). *Fed. Proc. Fed. Amer. Soc. Exp. Biol.* **25**, T277. (Transl. Suppl.)

Kreps, E. M., Smirnov, A., Chirkovskaya, E., Patrikeeva, M., and Krasilnikova, V. (1968). *J. Neurochem.* **15**, 285.

Kritchevsky, D., Tepper, S. A., DiTullio, N. W., and Holmes, W. L. (1967). *J. Food Sci.* **32**, 64.

Kruger, S., and Mendler, M. (1970). *J. Neurochem.* **17**, 1313.

Lafranchi, E. (1938). *Arch. Sci. Biol. (Bologna)* **24**, 120.

Langley, G. R., and Axell, M. (1968). *Brit. J. Haematol.* **14**, 593.

Lapetina, E. G., Soto, E. F., and De Robertis, E. (1967). *Biochim. Biophys. Acta* **135**, 33.

Lapetina, E. G., Soto, E. F., and De Robertis, E. (1968). *J. Neurochem.* **15**, 437.

Larsen, W. J. (1970). *J. Cell Biol.* **47**, 373.

Lees, M. B. (1965). *Ann. N. Y. Acad. Sci.* **122**, 116.

Lees, M. B. (1966). *J. Neurochem.* **13**, 1407.

Lees, M. B. (1968). *J. Neurochem.* **15**, 153.

Lees, M. B. (1969). *J. Neurochem.* **16**, 1197.

Leitch, G. J., Horrocks, L. A., and Samorajski, T. (1969). *J. Neurochem.* **16**, 1347.

Lenaz, G., Sechi, A. M., and Borgatti, A. R. (1969). *Boll. Soc. Ital. Biol. Sper.* **44**, 2180.

Lesch, P. (1969). *Clin. Chim. Acta* **25**, 269.

Lesch, P., and Bernhard, K. (1967). *Helv. Chim. Acta* **50**, 1125.

Lowden, J. A., and Wolfe, L. S. (1964). *Can. J. Biochem.* **42**, 1703.

Luck, D. J. L. (1963). *J. Cell Biol.* **16**, 483.

Lunt, G. G., and Rowe, C. E. (1968). *Biochim. Biophys. Acta* **152**, 681.

MacBrinn, M. C., and O'Brien, J. S. (1969). *J. Neurochem.* **16**, 7.

McColl, J. D., and Rossiter, R. J. (1950). *J. Cell. Comp. Physiol.* **36**, 241.

McIlwain, H. (1959). "Biochemistry of the Central Nervous System." Little, Brown, Boston, Massachusetts.

MacMillan, V. H., and Wherrett, J. R. (1969). *J. Neurochem.* **16**, 1621.

McMurray, W. C., and Dawson, R. M. C. (1969). *Biochem. J.* **112**, 91.

McMurray, W. C., McColl, J. D., and Rossiter, R. J. (1964). *In* "Comparative Neurochemistry" (D. Richter, ed.), pp. 101–107. Pergamon, Oxford.

McSharry, J. U., and Wagner, R. R. (1971). *J. Virol.* **7**, 59.

Mandel, P., and Nussbaum, J. L. (1966). *J. Neurochem.* **13**, 629.

Medda, J., and Bose, A. (1967). *Wilhelm Roux' Arch. Entwicklungsmech. Organismen* **159**, 267.

Meissner, G., and Fleischer, S. (1972). *Biochim. Biophys. Acta* **255**, 19.

Meldolesi, J., Jamieson, J. D., and Palade, G. E. (1971). *J. Cell Biol.* **49**, 130.

Menkes, J. H., Philippart, M., and Concone, M. C. (1966). *J. Lipid Res.* **7**, 479.

Mesdijian, E., and Cornée, J. (1969). *C. R. Soc. Biol.* **163**, 2358.

Millington, P. F., and Critchley, D. R. (1968). *Life Sci.* **7**, 839.

Mitchell, C. D. (1969). *J. Cell Biol.* **40**, 869.

Moretz, R. C., Akers, C. K., and Parsons, D. F. (1969). *Biochim. Biophys. Acta* **193**, 1.

Morgan, C., Howe, C., and Rose, H. M. (1961). *J. Exp. Med.* **113**, 219.

Murphy, J. R. (1962). *J. Lab. Clin. Med.* **60**, 86.

Murphy, J. R. (1965). *J. Lab. Clin. Med.* **65,** 756.
Napier, E. A., Jr., and Olson, R. E. (1965). *J. Biol. Chem.* **240,** 4244.
Napolitano, L., LeBaron, F., and Scaletti, J. (1967). *J. Cell Biol.* **34,** 817.
Neerhout, R. C. (1968a). *J. Lab. Clin. Med.* **71,** 438.
Neerhout, R. C. (1968b). *J. Pediat.* **73,** 364.
Nelson, G. J. (1967). *Biochim. Biophys. Acta* **144,** 221.
Nielsen, N. C., Fleischer, S., and McConnell, D. G. (1970). *Biochim. Biophys. Acta* **211,** 10.
Norton, W. T. (1971). *In* "Chemistry and Brain Development," Proc. Advan. Study Inst. Chem. Brain Develop., Milan (R. Paoletti and A. N. Davison, eds.), Advan. Exp. Med. Biol., Vol. 13, pp. 327–337. Plenum, New York.
Norton, W. T., and Autilio, L. A. (1965). *Ann. N. Y. Acad. Sci.* **122,** 77.
Norton, W. T., and Poduslo, S. E. (1971). *J. Lipid Res.* **12,** 84.
Norton, W. T., and Turnbull, J. M. (1970). *Fed. Proc. Fed. Amer. Soc. Exp. Biol.* **29,** 472. Abstr.
Norum, K. R., and Gjone, E. (1968). *Scand. J. Clin. Lab. Invest.* **22,** 94.
Nussbaum, J. L., Bieth, R., and Mandel, P. (1963). *Nature (London)* **198,** 586.
Nye, W. H. R., and Marinetti, G. V. (1967). *Proc. Soc. Exp. Biol. Med.* **125,** 1220.
O'Brien, J. S., and Sampson, E. L. (1965a). *J. Lipid Res.* **6,** 537.
O'Brien, J. S., and Sampson, E. L. (1965b). *J. Lipid Res.* **6,** 545.
O'Brien, J. S., Fillerup, D. L., and Mead, J. F. (1964). *J. Lipid Res.* **5,** 109.
O'Brien, J. S., Sampson, E. L., and Stern, M. B. (1967). *J. Neurochem.* **14,** 357.
O'Brien, J. S., Okada, S., Ho, M. W., Fillerup, D. L., Veath, M. L., and Adams, K. (1971). *Fed. Proc. Fed. Amer. Soc. Exp. Biol.* **30,** 956.
Onajobi, F. D., and Boyd, G. S. (1970). *Eur. J. Biochem.* **13,** 203.
Ongun, A., Thomson, W. W., and Mudd, J. B. (1968). *J. Lipid Res.* **9,** 416.
Palmer, F. B., and Dawson, R. M. C. (1969). *Biochem. J.* **111,** 637.
Palmer, F. B., and Rossiter, R. J. (1965). *Can. J. Biochem.* **43,** 671.
Paoletti, E. G. (1971). *In* "Chemistry and Brain Development," Proc. Advan. Study Inst. Chem. Brain Develop., Milan (R. Paoletti and A. N. Davison, eds.), Advan. Exp. Med. Biol., Vol. 13, pp. 41–51. Plenum, New York.
Paoletti, R., and Davison, A. N., eds. (1971). "Chemistry and Brain Development," Proc. Advan. Study Inst. Chem. Brain Develop., Milan. Advan. Exp. Med. Biol., Vol. 13. Plenum, New York.
Paoletti, R., Fumagalli, R., and Grossi, E. (1965). *J. Amer. Oil Chem. Soc.* **42,** 400.
Parsons, P., and Basford, R. E. (1967). *J. Neurochem.* **14,** 823.
Patterson, D. S. P., Sweasy, D., and Hebert, C. N. (1971). *J. Neurochem.* **18,** 2027.
Patterson, E. K., Dumm, M. E., and Richards, A. G., Jr. (1945). *Arch. Biochem.* **7,** 201.
Penick, R. J., Meisler, M. H., and McCluer, R. H. (1966). *Biochim. Biophys. Acta* **116,** 279.
Pfleger, R. C., Anderson, N. G., and Snyder, F. (1968). *Biochemistry* **7,** 2826.
Pietruszko, R., and Gray, G. M. (1960). *Biochim. Biophys. Acta* **44,** 197.
Pilz, H. (1968). *Deut. Z. Nervenheilk.* **194,** 150.
Plazonnet, B., Tronche, P., Bastide, P., and Komor, J. (1969). *C. R. Soc. Biol.* **163,** 398.
Poduslo, S. E., and Norton, W. T. (1972). *J. Neurochem.* **19,** 727.
Poincelot, R. P., and Zull, J. E. (1969). *Vision Res.* **9,** 647.
Porcellati, G. (1963). *Riv. Biol.* **56,** 185.
Porter, K. R., and Bonneville, M. A. (1968). "Fine Structure of Cells and Tissues," p. 181. Lea & Febiger, Philadelphia, Pennsylvania.

Prensky, A. L. (1967). *J. Amer. Oil Chem. Soc.* **44**, 667.

Prensky, A. L., Moses, A., Fishman, M. A., Tumbleson, H. E., and Daftari, B. (1971). *Comp. Biochem. Physiol.* **39B**, 725.

Pritchard, E. T., and Cantin, P. L. (1962). *Nature (London)* **193**, 580.

Quarles, R., and Folch-Pi, J. (1965). *J. Neurochem.* **12**, 543.

Radin, N. S. (1970). *Chem. Phys. Lipids* **5**, 178.

Radin, N. S., Lavin, F. B., and Brown, J. R. (1955). *J. Biol. Chem.* **217**, 197.

Raine, C. S., Poduslo, S. E., and Norton, W. T. (1971). *Brain Res.* **27**, 11.

Rawlins, F. A., and Smith, M. E. (1971). *J. Neurochem.* **18**, 1861.

Rawlins, F. A., Hedley-Whyte, E. T., Villegas, G., and Uzman, B. G. (1970). *Lab. Invest.* **22**, 237.

Reed, C. F. (1968). *J. Clin. Invest.* **47**, 749.

Reed, C. F., and Swisher, S. N. (1966). *J. Clin. Invest.* **45**, 777.

Reinišová, J., and Michalec, .Č (1966). *Comp. Biochem. Physiol.* **19**, 581.

Reva, A. D., and Rudenko, L. P. (1969). *Byull. Eksp. Biol. Med.* **68**, 38.

Ritter, M. C., and Dempsey, M. E. (1970). *Biochem. Biophys. Res. Commun.* **38**, 921.

Robertson, J. G., and Parsons, D. F. (1970). *Biochim. Biophys. Acta* **219**, 379.

Roeske, W. R., and Clayton, R. B. (1968). *J. Lipid Res.* **9**, 276.

Roodyn, D. B., and Wilkie, D. (1968). "The Biogenesis of Mitochondria," Methuen, London.

Roots, B. I. (1968). *Comp. Biochem. Physiol.* **25**, 457.

Rothfield, L., and Romeo, D. (1971). *Bacteriol. Rev.* **35**, 14.

Roukema, P. A., van den Eijnden, D. H., Heijlman, J., and van der Berg, G. (1970). *FEBS (Fed. Eur. Biochem. Soc.), Lett.* **9**, 267.

Rouser, G. (1968). *In* "Biochemical Preparations" (W. E. M. Lands, ed.), Vol. 12, pp. 73–80. Wiley, New York.

Rouser, G. (1971). *In* "Chemistry and Brain Development," Proc. Advan. Study Inst. Chem. Brain Develop., Milan (R. Paoletti and A. N. Davison, eds.), Advan. Exp. Med. Biol., Vol. 13, pp. 311–326. Plenum, New York.

Rouser, G., and Fleischer, S. (1967). *In* "Oxidation and Phosphorylation" (R. W. Estabrook and M. E. Pullman, eds.), Methods in Enzymology, Vol. 10, pp. 385–406. Academic Press, New York.

Rouser, G., and Kritchevsky, G. (1972). *In* "Sphingolipids, Sphingolipidoses, and Allied Disorders" (B. Volk and S. Aronson, eds.), pp. 103–126. Plenum Press, New York.

Rouser, G., and Solomon, R. D. (1969). *Lipids* **4**, 232.

Rouser, G., and Yamamoto, A. (1968). *Lipids* **3**, 284.

Rouser, G., and Yamamoto, A. (1969). *In* "Handbook of Neurochemistry" (A. Lajtha, ed.), Vol. I, pp. 121–169. Plenum, New York.

Rouser, G., Bauman, A. J., and Kritchevsky, G. (1961a). *Amer. J. Clin. Nutr.* **9**, 112.

Rouser, G., O'Brien, J., and Heller, D. J. (1961b). *J. Amer. Oil Chem. Soc.* **38**, 14.

Rouser, G., Bauman, A. J., Kritchevsky, G., Heller, D., and O'Brien, J. (1961c). *J. Amer. Oil Chem. Soc.* **38**, 544.

Rouser, G., Bauman, A. J., Nicolaides, N., and Heller, D. (1961d). *J. Amer. Oil Chem. Soc.* **38**, 565.

Rouser, G., Kritchevsky, G., Heller, D., and Lieber, E. (1963). *J. Amer. Oil Chem. Soc.* **40**, 425.

Rouser, G., Galli, C., Lieber, E., Blank, M. L., and Privett, O. S. (1964). *J. Amer. Oil Chem. Soc.* **41**, 836.

Rouser, G., Kritchevsky, G., Galli, C., and Heller, D. (1965a). *J. Amer. Oil Chem. Soc.* **42**, 215.

Rouser, G., Galli, C., and Kritchevsky, G. (1965b). *J. Amer. Oil Chem. Soc.* **42**, 404.

Rouser, G., Siakotos, A. N., and Fleischer, S. (1966). *Lipids* **1**, 85.

Rouser, G., Kritchevsky, G., Simon, G., and Nelson, G. J. (1967a). *Lipids* **2**, 37.

Rouser, G., Kritchevsky, G., and Yamamoto, A. (1967b). *In* "Lipid Chromatographic Analysis" (G. V. Marinetti, ed.), Vol. 1, pp. 99–162. Dekker, New York.

Rouser, G., Kritchevsky, G., Galli, C., Yamamoto, A., and Knudson, A. G., Jr. (1967c). *In* "Inborn Disorders of Sphingolipid Metabolism" (S. M. Aronson and B. M. Volk, eds.), pp. 303–316. Pergamon, New York.

Rouser, G., Kritchevsky, G., Yamamoto, A., Knudson, A. G., Jr., and Simon, G. (1968a). *Lipids* **3**, 287.

Rouser, G., Nelson, G. J., Fleischer, S., and Simon, G. (1968b). *In* "Biological Membranes" (D. Chapman, ed.), pp. 5–69. Academic Press, New York.

Rouser, G., Simon, G., and Kritchevsky, G. (1969a). *Lipids* **4**, 599.

Rouser, G., Kritchevsky, G., Yamamoto, A., Simon, G., Galli, C., and Bauman, A. J. (1969b). *In* "Lipids" (J. M. Lowenstein, ed.), Methods in Enzymology, Vol. 14, pp. 272–317. Academic Press, New York.

Rouser, G., Fleischer, S., and Yamamoto, A. (1970a). *Lipids* **5**, 494.

Rouser, G., Kritchevsky, G., Siakotos, A. N., and Yamamoto, A. (1970b). *In* "Neuropathology: Methods and Diagnosis" (C. G. Tedeschi, ed.), pp. 691–753. Little, Brown, Boston, Massachusetts.

Rouser, G., Yamamoto, A., and Kritchevsky, G. (1971a). *In* "Chemistry and Brain Development," Proc. Advan. Study Inst. Chem. Brain Develop., Milan (R. Paoletti and A. N. Davison, eds.), Advan. Exp. Med. Biol., Vol. 13, pp. 91–109, Plenum, New York.

Rouser, G., Yamamoto, A., and Kritchevsky, G. (1971b). *Arch. Intern. Med.* **127**, 1105.

Rumsby, M. G., and Finean, J. B. (1966a). *J. Neurochem.* **13**, 1501.

Rumsby, M. G., and Finean, J. B. (1966b). *J. Neurochem.* **13**, 1509.

Rumsby, M. G., and Finean, J. B. (1966c). *J. Neurochem.* **13**, 1513.

Sakagami, T., Minari, O., and Orii, T. (1965a). *Biochim. Biophys. Acta* **98**, 111.

Sakagami, T., Minari, O., and Orii, T. (1965b). *Biochim. Biophys. Acta* **98**, 356.

Sarzala, M. G., van Golde, L. M. G., DeKruyff, B., and van Deenen, L. L. M. (1970). *Biochim. Biophys. Acta* **202**, 106.

Scallen, T. J., and Dietert, S. E. (1969). *J. Cell Biol.* **40**, 802.

Schengrund, C. L., and Rosenberg, A. (1971). *Biochemistry* **10**, 2424.

Seminario, L. M., Hren, N., and Gómez, C. J. (1964). *J. Neurochem.* **11**, 197.

Sheltawy, A., and Dawson, R. M. C. (1969). *Biochem. J.* **111**, 147.

Shephard, E. H., and Hübscher, G. (1969). *Biochem. J.* **113**, 429.

Sherman, G., and Folch-Pi, J. (1970). *J. Neurochem.* **17**, 597.

Siakotos, A. N., and Rouser, G. (1965). *J. Amer. Oil Chem. Soc.* **42**, 913.

Siakotos, A. N., Rouser, G., and Fleischer, S. (1969a). *Lipids* **4**, 234.

Siakotos, A. N., Rouser, G., and Fleischer, S. (1969b). *Lipids* **4**, 239.

Simon, G. (1966). *Lipids* **1**, 369.

Simon, G., and Rouser, G. (1969). *Lipids* **4**, 607.

Singh, H., Spritz, N., and Geyer, B. (1971). *J. Lipid Res.* **12**, 473.

Skipski, V. P., Barclay, M., Archibald, F. M., Terebus-Kekish, O., Reichman, E. S., and Good, J. J. (1965). *Life Sci.* **4**, 1673.

Smith, M. E. (1968). *Biochim. Biophys. Acta* **164**, 285.

Smith, M. E. (1969). *J. Neurochem.* **16**, 83.

Smith, M. E., and Eng, L. F. (1965). *J. Amer. Oil Chem. Soc.* **42**, 1013.

Smith, M. E., Fumagalli, R., and Paoletti, R. (1967). *Life Sci.* **6**, 1085.

Smith, M. E., Hasinoff, C. M., and Fumagalli, R. (1970). *Lipids* **5**, 665.

Soto, E. F., Seminario de Bohner, L., and Calviño, M. del C. (1966). *J. Neurochem.* **13**, 989.

Spence, M. W., and Wolfe, L. S. (1967a). *J. Neurochem.* **14**, 585.

Spence, M. W., and Wolfe, L. S. (1967b). *Can. J. Biochem.* **45**, 671.

Sribney, M. (1968). *Arch. Biochem. Biophys.* **126**, 954.

Stahl, W. L., and Trams, E. G. (1968). *Biochim. Biophys. Acta* **163**, 459.

Stahl, W. L., Sumi, S. M., and Swanson, P. D. (1971). *J. Neurochem.* **18**, 403.

Stanacev, N. Z., Stuhne-Sekalec, L., Brookes, K. B., and Davidson, J. B. (1969). *Biochim. Biophys. Acta* **176**, 650.

Stempak, J. G., and Laurencin, M. (1970). *J. Microsc. (Paris)* **9**, 465.

Stoffel, W., and Schiefer, H. G. (1968). *Hoppe-Seyler's Z. Physiol. Chem.* **349**, 1017.

Stuhne-Sekalec, L., and Stanacev, N. Z. (1970). *Can. J. Biochem.* **48**, 1214.

Sun, G. Y., and Samorajski, T. (1972). *J. Gerontol.* **27**, 10.

Suzuki, K. (1965). *J. Neurochem.* **12**, 629.

Suzuki, K. (1967). *In* "Inborn Disorders of Sphingolipid Metabolism" (S. M. Aronson and B. W. Volk, eds.), pp. 215–230. Pergamon, New York.

Suzuki, K. (1970). *J. Neurochem.* **17**, 209.

Suzuki, K., Poduslo, S. E., and Norton, W. T. (1967). *Biochim. Biophys. Acta* **144**, 375.

Svanberg, O. (1970). *Acta Physiol. Scand.* **80**, 45.

Svennerholm, L. (1968). *J. Lipid Res.* **9**, 570.

Svennerholm, L., and Ställberg-Stenhagen, S. (1968). *J. Lipid Res.* **9**, 215.

Tamai, Y., Matsukawa, S., and Satake, M. (1971a). *J. Biochem. (Tokyo)* **69**, 235.

Tamai, Y., Matsukawa, S., and Satake, M. (1971b). *Brain Res.* **26**, 145.

Tenenbaum, D., and Folch-Pi, J. (1966). *Biochim. Biophys. Acta* **115**, 141.

Tettamanti, G. (1971). *In* "Chemistry and Brain Development," Proc. Advan. Study Inst. Chem. Brain Develop., Milan (R. Paoletti and A. N. Davison, eds.), Advan. Exp. Med. Biol., Vol. 13, pp. 75–88. Plenum, New York.

Tombropoulos, E. G. (1971). *Arch. Intern. Med.* **127**, 408.

Tsuyuki, H., and Naruse, U. (1964). *Sci. Rep. Whales Res. Inst.* **18**, 173.

Turner, J. D., and Rouser, G. (1970). *Anal. Biochem.* **38**, 423.

Vanderkooi, G., and Green, D. E. (1970). *Proc. Nat. Acad. Sci. U. S.* **66**, 615.

Vanderkooi, G., and Green, D. E. (1971). *BioScience* **21**, 409.

Vanderkooi, G., and Sundaralingam, M. (1970). *Proc. Nat. Acad. Sci. U. S.* **67**, 233.

Vanier, M. T., Holm, N., Ohman, R., and Svennerholm, L. (1971). *J. Neurochem.* **18**, 581.

Vernadakis, A., Casper, R., and Timiras, P. S. (1968). *Experientia* **24**, 237.

Vorbeck, M. L., and Martin, A. P. (1970). *Biochem. Biophys. Res. Commun.* **40**, 901.

Webster, G. R., and Folch, J. (1961). *Biochim. Biophys. Acta* **49**, 399.

Weinstein, D. B., and Marsh, J. B. (1969). *J. Biol. Chem.* **244**, 4103.

Wells, M. A., and Dittmer, J. C. (1966). *Biochemistry* **5**, 3405.

Wells, M. A., and Dittmer, J. C. (1967). *Biochemistry* **6**, 3169.

Westerman, M. P., Balcerzak, S. P., and Heinle, E. W., Jr. (1968). *J. Lab. Clin. Med.* **72**, 663.

Westphal, U. (1961). *In* "Mechanisms of Action of Steroid Hormones" (C. A. Villee and L. L. Engel, eds.), p. 3. Pergamon, Oxford.

Wherrett, J. R., Lowden, J. A., and Wolfe, L. S. (1964). *Can. J. Biochem.* **42**, 1057.

White, H. B., Jr., Galli, C., and Paoletti, R. (1971). *J. Neurochem.* **18**, 869.

Wiegandt, H. (1967). *J. Neurochem.* **14**, 671.

Williamson, B., and Coniglio, J. G. (1971). *J. Neurochem.* **18**, 267.

Williamson, J. R. (1969). *J. Ultrastruct. Res.* **27**, 118.

Windeler, A. S., and Feldman, G. L. (1970). *Biochim. Biophys. Acta* **202**, 361.

Wirtz, K. W. A., and Zilversmit, D. B. (1968). *J. Biol. Chem.* **243**, 3596.

Wirtz, K. W. A., and Zilversmit, D. B. (1969). *Biochim. Biophys. Acta* **193**, 105.

Wirtz, K. W. A., and Zilversmit, D. B. (1970). *FEBS* (*Fed. Eur. Biochem. Soc.*), *Lett.* **7**, 44.

Wirtz, K. W. A., van Golde, L. M. G., and van Deenen, L. L. M. (1970). *Biochim. Biophys. Acta* **218**, 176.

Witting, L. A., Krishnan, R. S., Sakr, A. H., and Horwitt, M. K. (1968). *Anal. Biochem.* **22**, 295.

Wolfgram, F., and Katorii, K. (1968a). *J. Neurochem.* **15**, 1281.

Wolfgram, F., and Katorii, K. (1968b). *J. Neurochem.* **15**, 1291.

Wolman, M., Wiener, H., and Bubis, J. J. (1966). *Isr. J. Chem.* **4**, 53.

Wolstenholme, G. E. W., and O'Connor, M., eds. (1970). "Alzheimer's Disease and Related Disorders," 316 pp. Churchill, London.

Yakovlev, P. I., and Lecours, A. R. (1967). *In* "Regional Development of the Brain in Early Life" (A. Minkowski, ed.), pp. 3–70. Blackwell, Oxford.

Yamakawa, T., and Nishimura, S. (1966). *Jap. J. Exp. Med.* **36**, 101.

Yamamoto, A., and Rouser, G. (1970). *Lipids* **5**, 442.

Zborowski, J., and Wojtczak, L. (1969). *Biochim. Biophys. Acta* **187**, 73.

Author Index

Subject Index

A

Abetalipoproteinemia, 33–35, 310
N-Acetylneuraminic acid, 179
Acyl-coenzyme A desaturase, 106, 115, 124
Acyldihydroxyacetone phosphate, 242, 243
Acylglycerols, 235
S-Adenosylmethionine:Δ²⁴-sterol methyltransferase, 108–110
Age, lipids and, 261–350
Alkenylglycerols, 237
Alkylacylglycerols, 248, 249
Alkyldihydroxyacetone, 243
Alkyldihydroxyacetone phosphate, 243, 245, 248
Alkyl glycerolipids
    reactions used to identify, 239
    reduction of ketone group, 247, 248
Alkylglycerols, 235, 237
Alloxan diabetes, 151, 152
Apolipoproteins, 1
Arachidonic acid in brain, 149
Arthritis, rheumatoid, RE function in, 49

B

Bacillus subtilis, 120, 251
Batyl alcohol, 237
Blood-brain barrier, 147, 150, 172
Blood monocytes, 45
Brachydanio rerio, 149
Brain
    development of, 264, 265
        species differences, 265
    lipids in, *see* Brain lipids
    metabolic diseases of, 209–218
        gangliosides, 211–213
        glycolipids, 215–217
        neutral lipids, 213–215
        phospholipids, 217, 218
Brain lipids, 143–218, 261–350, *see also*
    specific substances
    analysis of, 263–266

biosynthesis of
    subcellular, 188
    young vs. adult, 187
    in cell-enriched fractions, 207–209
    chemistry and distribution, 185–187
    development and, 202–206
    effect of malnutrition on, 198–202, 265, 266
    enzymes and, 206
    fetal, 145
    human
        normal, 278, 279
        total, 276, 277
    polar, 278–288
    trace, 195, 196
Bromsulphalein, 60
n-Butyl palmitate, RES and, 63

C

Capillaries, lipids in, 312, 313
Carcinomas, plasma humoral recognition factor, 54–56
Cardiolipin, 154
4α-Carboxylic acid decarboxylase, 111
Central nervous system (CNS)
    lipids in, *see* Brain lipids
    microglia of, 45
Cephalin, RES and, 64
Ceramide(s) in brain, 166, 167, 170, 171, 264
Ceramide aminoethylphosphonate, 292
Ceramide dihexosides in brain, 264
Ceramide phosphorylethanolamine, 292
Cerebron, in brain, 173
Cerebroside(s), in brain, 264, 284, 291, 299, 314
    biosynthesis and degradation, 172
    fatty acids in, 146, 147, 149
    sphingolipids in, 172–174
Cerebroside esters in brain, 264
Cerebroside sulfate, 174
Cerebrotendinons xanthomatosis, 210, 213